Praise for
POWER UP

"I lost ten pounds in the first two weeks, and five more slowly over the next month. . . . I'm a terrible dieter—I usually give up by lunchtime on the first day—but *Power Up* was easy to follow because I didn't have to calculate grams of protein or calories. . . . I ate as much as I wanted as long as it wasn't tainted by the verboten foods. . . . In the stress log it became clear I was trying to do too much by myself, which resulted in anger and frustration. . . . Clearly I hadn't just lost my mojo—I'd lost my sense of humor. . . . [Dr. Merrell] recognizes that some alternative methods do work and that the mind plays a powerful role in our health, but he thinks antibiotics and immunization play a pretty important role, too. [Dr. Merrell's] book asks you to gut renovate six areas: your stress response, your diet, the toxins you use (everything from alcohol to carpet glue), your exercise regimen (or lack thereof) and our social and spiritual life (or lack thereof)."

—*Elle*

"One of the best-known proponents of integrative medicine . . . Merrell's advice is soundly based on established principles of healthy diet, regular exercise, and plenty of interpersonal relationships."

—*Library Journal*

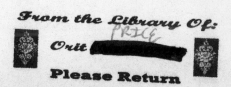

"Woody Merrell is the approachable, trustworthy, and compassionate physician we've always wanted—and he's here in these pages. Doctor Merrell draws on cutting-edge research to give us a comprehensive, sane, and fruitful path beyond health to vitality. Anyone can benefit from reading this book."

—Daniel Goleman, author of *Emotional Intelligence*

"*Power Up* is a must-read for anyone that wants to take their health and well-being to the next level. Dr. Merrell's focus on emotional fitness, dietary discipline, and exercise demonstrates that creating a balanced lifestyle isn't just about your health—it's about creating the foundation of a truly fulfilled and vital life."

—Anthony Robbins, author of *Awaken the Giant Within* and *Unlimited Power*

"My old friend, Dr. Woodson Merrell, has written this fine book sharing the important and skillful strategies he's learned and developed in his 15 years at the forefront of integrative medicine. He's been an enormous help to me and many of my friends, and I'm sure he will be helpful to many others. Give this book a try."

—Richard Gere

"Woody Merrell, M.D., is the doctor of the future. And *Power Up* is packed with exciting, health-enhancing secrets that you begin using immediately. Great stuff!"

—Christiane Northrup, M.D., author of *The Wisdom of Menopause*, and *Women's Bodies, Women's Wisdom*

"If you want to become healthier and also to transform your life, this book is for you. Dr. Woodson Merrell, one of America's leading pioneers in integrative medicine, is an utterly trustworthy guide. *Power Up* is a rich resource—good medicine, good science, and good sense."

—Larry Dossey, M.D., author of *Healing Words* and
Reinventing Medicine

"In today's world, there are countless doctors that are specialists, but Woody really treats the patient first; not only the disease. His unique ability to bring together Eastern and Western philosophy creates what I call a whole healing, which is for the mind, body, and spirit. This book will open the door to understanding that we all deserve optimum health and how to achieve it."

—Donna Karan

"I read this entire book in one sitting! I found I just didn't want to put it down. It really is a compelling read. Dr. Merrell's book reminds me why it's important to take care of our whole selves. The 21-Day Program is such a simple and empowering way to reconnect with your own source. I'm so thankful that Dr. Merrell put his wisdom into a book that I can refer to again and again."

—Cindy Crawford

"Well written and informative book. If you ever feel like you have no energy . . . by following the tips recommended in this book you will experience an increase in your energy levels. . . . Dr. Merrell's plan really does make a difference and I highly recommend this book!"

—RebeccaReads.com

*f*P

Woodson Merrell, M.D.

with Kathleen Merrell

POWER UP

Charge Up Your Health

Free Press
New York   London   Toronto   Sydney

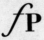

Free Press
A Division of Simon & Schuster, Inc.
1230 Avenue of the Americas
New York, NY 10020

First Free Press trade paperback edition September 2009

FREE PRESS and colophon are trademarks of Simon & Schuster, Inc.

For information about special discounts for bulk purchases,
please contact Simon & Schuster Special Sales at
1-866-506-1949 or business@simonandschuster.com

The Simon & Schuster Speakers Bureau can bring authors to your
live event. For more information or to book an event contact the
Simon & Schuster Speakers Bureau at 1-866-248-3049 or
visit our website at www.simonspeakers.com.

Designed by Katy Riegel

Manufactured in the United States of America

1   3   5   7   9   10   8   6   4   2

Library of Congress Cataloging-in-Publication Data

Merrell, Woodson C.
Power up : unleash your natural energy, revitalize your health,
and feel 10 years younger / Woodson Merrell, with Kathleen Merrell.
        p.   cm.
Includes index.
1. Fatigue.   2. Health.   3. Energy metabolism.   I. Merrell, Kathleen.   II. Title.
RB150.F37M47   2008
613—dc22   2008017455

ISBN 978-1-4165-6816-2
ISBN 978-1-4165-6817-9 (pbk)
ISBN 978-1-4165-7017-2 (ebook)

For Caitlin and Isabel,
our true sources of vital energy and boundless love.

Contents

A Note on Using Power Up   *xiii*
Introduction   1

PART I
Transforming Energy: Six Ways to Reclaim Your Vitality   17

   1. Power Mind, Boundless Energy   19

   2. Power Food, Your High Performance Fuel   55

   3. Power Detox, Remove Toxins, Increase Vitality 89

   4. Power Exercise, the Energy Factory   131

   5. Power Rest, How to Recharge Your Battery   159

   6. Power of Connection:
      Cultivate Spirit, Access Positive Energy   185

PART II
21 Days to Optimal Energy: Power Up, Cleanse, Maximize   207

PART III
Menus and Recipes   273

Recipe Index   365
Acknowledgments   367
Index   369

A Note on Using *Power Up*

THIS BOOK IS divided into three parts: The why, the how, and the food. The "why" of the book in Part I will provide powerful motivation for many of you who will be committed to taking on the 21 Day Plan after understanding the latest information on how your body makes energy and stays healthy. But for those of you who want to cut to the chase and skip the explanation of Part I, you may go straight to the "how"—the Plan in Part II on page 207. The Plan puts the six fundamentals of Part I into action, providing a daily guide for powering up your energy and retooling your health. But promise that as you work through the plan over the next three weeks you go will back to Part I and read the background and science underlying *Power Up*. Here you'll pick up on a wealth of useful information on how to increase your energy, and after reading the compelling evidence you will realize (as I have) that this is not a fad—this is the medicine of the future.

Introduction

JUNE CAME TO ME late on a Friday afternoon over twenty years ago at the beginning of my private medical practice. She brought with her a dossier with tests, scans, and results from procedures she'd undergone for four years in a quest to regain her wellness and youthful energy, on top of which she'd placed a cover sheet summarizing a chronology of her health events. Yet while she clearly wasn't well, the tests all showed that she wasn't ill, though she obviously felt awful and had no energy. At the bottom of her chronology page she had written, "My goal is to regain my energy, recover my health, and not to have to worry all the time about if I can or can't make plans or feel well enough to live my life fully." My heart went out to her.

June's problems were sporadic, but frequent enough to keep her from feeling well much of the time. She'd had a series of colds that deteriorated into chronic sinus congestion. After numerous visits to ear, nose and throat specialists, she'd had surgery for nasal polyps, which gave her some relief, but she continued to suffer from sinus infections every few months. She subsequently developed intermittent digestive problems with bloating and cramping, and trouble sleeping. For the past year she said she'd felt constantly fatigued. Too tired to exercise, June was overeating just to keep herself going.

Trying to make sense of all of the pieces of her puzzling fatigue, I looked for an overarching illness that could explain what had brought her to me with a sense of urgency over wanting better health, and especially more energy. But I, like the many physicians she had seen before me, couldn't find anything specifically wrong with her. I took almost every moment of that one-hour first visit to elicit the details of her medical history, but, looking back, I now see that one of the most important moments was when I asked her what had occurred in her life when the troubles began. Initially, she said everything was fine—successful marriage, two children, thriving real estate career—but it turned out she was not leading the charmed life she tried to present to the world. She became quite emotional as she related to me that she'd grown in a different direction from her husband, was relatively estranged from her mother who'd recently died from breast cancer, and harbored guilt over not spending enough time with her children.

As our time ran out I realized with frustration that I didn't have much to add in terms of conventional diagnoses. Wanting to say something positive I told her that over the weekend she needed to think about how to reduce the stress in her life. I asked her to return for a follow-up Monday to go over the few tests I could think of that had not been done—and I hoped I'd have a diagnostic brainstorm in the interim.

What happened when she came back three days later set my practice on a new course. And ultimately this new direction for treating patients evolved into the program at the heart of this book. On Monday, June walked into my office, dramatically more buoyant. She thanked me profusely for my time Friday, and said she had not felt this good in years. I tried not to let my jaw drop—by medical school standards I'd done virtually nothing. She said that being able to open up about the stressors in her life was the best medicine she had had in four years. She felt as if an energy switch had flipped on inside her. She had felt so much better after admitting that she had these stresses that on Sunday she'd even gone out for a light jog. Having named some of the energy-draining situations in her life, she was now determined to face them and take charge of her life again.

I worked with June to overhaul her diet, to help her stick with a regular exercise program, to reduce her stress, and to evaluate her home and office for potential environmental triggers of sinus infections. I also recommended that she use a few nutritional supplements. After two months, the sinus problems and bowel complaints disappeared, her sleep improved markedly, and June had more energy than ever before. Reflecting on the healing experience she'd been through, June told me that the most important part of her journey was that this new energy helped her feel connected again—to her family, to herself (with a better lifestyle) and to the world around her.

Since then, I have been constantly seeking ways to increase people's innate healing energy so that they can return to wellness. I have worked with thousands of people who, like June, came to me after visiting many other doctors, often finding little improvement. Many of them have had one medical problem lead to another until they find themselves with a host of chronic issues that drain their energy and keep them from living life to the fullest. Many people who come to me are not sick, but they're working on getting there, for example, with recurring colds or headaches, nagging fatigue, digestive problems, and unremitting stress that weaken them and make them susceptible to more serious illness. Many others are just pushing themselves way too hard, hoping not to get sick, but undermining their health in ways that will inevitably catch up to them. Sound familiar?

I did finally find the common thread that tied together all June's varied problems—and most other people's chronic complaints. That common link is energy. My patients were losing vital, health-giving energy in, at first, little, and then, increasingly, big ways. They weren't really sick, but they weren't well, either. They needed to stop leaking energy and shore up their bodies, minds, and spirits.

In order to develop a true healing program to treat this widespread energy deficiency, I needed methods that worked quickly as well as methods that kept working long-term. There was no single medicine or magic pill—and to this day there is no single medicine or magic pill—that could cure any deficiency of vital healing energy. So I looked into the latest medical and scientific studies on energy to find out more about what energy *is* and why my patients didn't have enough of it. If I could figure out where energy comes from—the source—if I could figure out how we make energy and how we lose it, maybe I could help my patients get and create more of it and increase their capacity to heal and achieve their optimum potential. I immersed myself in the sciences of metabolism (how the body extracts energy from food) and cellular respiration (how cells make energy) and psycho-neuro-immunology (how the body communicates its needs across systems, for example, from the nervous system to the immune system). I examined the growing research about the effects of our emotions and psychological states on our health, and also investigated the latest science on the effects of environmental toxins on various systems in the body.

I uncovered a lot of connections between physical energy and mental energy that had not been part of my Western medical school curriculum at Columbia University College of Physicians and Surgeons, or my internship and residency at New York City's Roosevelt Hospital. It became clear that people needed to urgently identify their underlying energy problems in order to improve their health. I also delved into other cultures' ancient methods for creating energy. I learned profound, beautiful ways that indigenous cultures view health—in all of which energy is at the core of their philosophy and practice. I sat at the feet of some great masters of Tibetan, Native American, Ayurvedic (Indian), and traditional Chinese medicine. Their systems see body, mind, and spirit as a whole, a single-energy system. Their treatments, including meditation, herbs, acupuncture, and tai chi, have simple physical components but deep overall effects—especially on energy. I have found them to be surprisingly compatible with a modern Western medical practice and daily lifestyle.

Besides these ancient traditions, I also trained in newer complementary approaches such as homeopathy, functional medicine (the nutrition science that studies food's effect on cell function and energy), and manipulative body work. And I kept going deeper into my study of energy until I arrived at the convergence of quantum physics and spirituality—two fields that actually share many views of the interconnected nature of energy and reality. Quantum physics has shown that matter at its most fundamental level operates as a web of interconnected energy fields in constant communication with each other.

Ultimately, I pulled everything I learned in my quest into a practical program for creating healing energy and for optimal health for my patients. For the last twenty years I have worked with many extraordinary people and helped them win back their health and regain a youthful, vital energy. Now, I want you to have that same experience—to feel as good as you can, and even better than you ever have. *Power Up* presents the long-lasting six-step program that I developed for my patients to increase their energy, as well as a complete *21-Day Plan* for revitalization.

My goal for every patient—and now for you as you embark on the healing journey of the *Power Up* program—is to help you transform from being an energy *consumer* to being an energy *producer*. You can live a fully sustainable life—without stimulants or cravings or prescription drugs or feelings of total burnout. I will show you how.

I've seen from my own practice—and from reading decades of other doctors' and researchers' concerns in the medical literature—that more people than ever before need the help that *Power Up* provides. There is an epidemic of fatigue in the United States. While fatigue is not classified as a disease, it is debilitating and makes you more vulnerable to developing a disease. No fewer than 75 million people admit to feeling "extreme fatigue" at work. Epidemiologists estimate that 38 percent of the workforce is fatigued, directly contributing to $100 billion in additional healthcare costs, accidents, and lost productivity for corporations. (Fatigue triples the chance that a worker will lose productivity.) Almost 1 million people have been diagnosed with the most severe form of fatigue, chronic fatigue syndrome, which is not well understood but is thought to be an immune system disorder—when the body doesn't have the energy to heal itself—with possible viral origins. The accepted practice of running on empty in our twenty-four hour consumer society is a major health and economic issue. Pundits have quipped that it's taboo to say you're tired, but I think it's time to alter the national dialogue and begin to solve this pervasive problem and bring back our greatest natural resource—human energy.

The most common solutions to the perplexing dilemma of energy loss are counterproductive self-treatments—240 million pounds of coffee beans were sold last year; Americans consumed $3 billion worth of caffeine-packed energy drinks like Red Bull; sleeping pill prescriptions were up 60 percent; and the new drug to increase alertness (Provigil) racked up $800 million in sales in its first year on the market. But these things don't address the sources of your energy drains and they don't rejuvenate your inner source of natural energy.

Loss of energy is one of the top five complaints to doctors, but that's only the tip of the iceberg. It's been estimated that 66 percent of people who visit their doctors while experiencing debilitating exhaustion never even mention the problem! This is primarily because of a widespread belief (mostly accurate) that doctors don't have a treatment for being tired. The truth is that only 3 percent of people with fatigue are found to have anything wrong with them when they are tested for the many things that can cause fatigue—a hypothyroid condition, anemia, heart disease, nutritional deficiencies, infectious diseases, immune deficiencies, or autoimmune diseases. Physicians are trained to stay within the precepts of Western medicine, using pharmaceuticals and surgery as their main tools. As a result, questions and recommendations about factors in their patients' lifestyles that should be a cornerstone of healthcare are often neglected. So many physicians have a difficult time helping their deeply tired patients—who often don't have an underlying medical disorder.

With *Power Up* I offer a fresh, unique perspective on the possibility of energy creation that unifies Western medical science with Eastern mind-body and energy practices. As a doctor of internal medicine with a busy private practice, as well as an educator and researcher at both Columbia University College of Physicians and Surgeons and Albert Einstein College of Medicine, I have helped lead the development of a new medical discipline, integrative medicine. This new approach to health and healing, which emphasizes a partnership between doctor and patient, utilizes the best of indigenous, complementary/alternative, and conventional approaches, which we individualize to each person's needs. Integrative doctors look at the whole patient, not just the disease, and we consider the emotional, spiritual, dietary, environmental, and lifestyle influences that can affect health and healing. I would never tell a patient just to cope with exhaustion because, to me, living each day with full vital energy is the essence of being well. I'm not a disease mechanic. My job description, and the goal of this book, is to promote your well-being. Energy is at the core of our quest for optimum health.

Many of the most common illnesses—such as hypertension, coronary disease, diabetes, and high cholesterol, as well as functional problems such as headaches, irritable bowel, and arthritis—originate in your lifestyle. Patients beginning to slip into diseases primarily created by lifestyle mismanagement often come to me after they've seen a conventional doctor who's addressed the developing problem with a pharmaceutical and, sometimes, general advice on how to lead a healthier life. My patients and I have usually been able to prevent or reverse these problems with exactly the program I put forth here in the *21-Day Plan*. The lifestyle changes you need to make are really quite simple: they focus on balancing and regenerating energy. I get such great satisfaction when a person who thought he was sentenced to a lifetime of disease-management medications (such as statins for high cholesterol or steroid inhalers for asthma) makes transformative lifestyle changes that allow him to taper off, and eventually stop, the medication merry-go-round.

Over the years I have found that many people have a difficult time believing in the connection between energy, health, and lifestyle—until they begin to understand that their mind, body, heart, and spirit are part of an interconnected web, rather than a collection of parts. Every thought, every emotion, every heart beat has the potential to resonate throughout the body due to the nearly instantaneous communication between cells that constantly takes place. Complex as these interconnections are, the process of making energy in the body has been very clearly demonstrated.

The Science of Personal Energy

From a strictly medical point of view, energy is a measurable biological commodity. Scientists working in biomolecular medicine have created a much clearer picture of how this common energy that powers life works and how the body creates energy. They have also made new discoveries into why the body begins to experience fatigue and slide into poor health. Last summer, I was amazed to read in the scientific journal *Genetics* that the dean of mitochondrial genetics at the University of California now equates the human energy generating system of the mitochondria to the concepts of chi and vital energy that have provided the basis of diagnostics in Traditional Chinese Medicine for 2000 years ("Mitochondria as Chi," *Genetics,* June 2008). Working independently in myriad disciplines from neuroscience to exercise physiology to nutrition and mind-body medicine, researchers have begun to delineate the sources of energy in your body and identify new ways to tap them. In *Power Up* I will show you how to apply the results of these findings to create more abundant energy and achieve more vibrant health.

Your body stays near 98.6 degrees throughout your life, which could be for the better part of a century, by making its own thermal energy day in and day out. Scientists have identified the carriers of the energy your body creates; they are present in every cell of the body—everywhere from your skeleton to your brain—as tiny rechargeable battery-like packets of available energy called adenosine triphosphate (ATP). The act of making these molecules of energy, also known as energy metabolism, depends on some very primitive DNA called mitochondrial DNA. Mitochondria are like tiny factories—thousands of them are within each and every cell (with DNA as the plant supervisor)—and they work ceaselessly to transfer the potential energy from food, air, and water into active human energy. With a complex cycle of chemical transformations that requires many essential vitamins and other nutrients, mitochondria are able to extract about 40% of the energy available in food and turn it into ATP, the universal currency of energy in your body that can be used anywhere to do any kind of work, from fueling your heartbeat, to providing the chemical energy to process thoughts, mustering the biological energy to attack a flu virus, or supplying the power to create a human life if you are pregnant.

The energy system in your body is highly dynamic, it constantly recycles energy, and it's exquisitely sensitive to change. Your activity level, your environment, the food you eat, the water you drink, your stress levels, your emotional state, the amount of sleep you've had, the type of body fat you have—are all factors that can affect your energy-generating system. What makes the body's energy supply so susceptible to shifts in the biological machine is the fact that the energy packets of ATP cannot be stored. ATP is constantly made on demand, used up, and quickly recycled, which makes the energy your body works so hard to manufacture quite fleeting—though almost infinitely replaceable if you properly care for and maintain your body.

The amount of energy your body is required to make every day is absolutely astonishing. At any given moment you've got about three ounces of energy (ATP) in your body—just enough to power ten seconds of intense exercise, or an all-out sprint to catch a train. And then your body starts all over again constantly remaking ATP thousands of times a minute. Even a sedentary person recycles an amount of ATP each day equal to about 75% of his total body weight (a 180-pound man would recycle almost 135 pounds of ATP just sitting on the couch with the flipper). A person running a marathon can recycle twice as much energy as a sedentary person—that would be a whopping 270 pounds of pure energy molecules processed by that same 180-pound guy while running a marathon. Considering the hefty energy requirements for keeping a body going, it is no wonder that people develop problems and inadequacies with their energy-generating system.

Energy metabolism—which is how biologists describe the body's energy-making activities—plays an important role in health and aging. The healthy functioning of mitochondria is a key component in longevity, according to a wide range of research—from a leading gerontologist in England to neuroscientists at UCLA. Weight loss researchers are even beginning to look at ways of manipulating the body's rate of energy expenditure as a way of losing weight. This is based on a recent finding that a specialized kind of body fat cell called brown adipose burns more calories than the more common white body fat (as little as 2 ounces of brown fat can burn up a full 20 percent of your daily calories). Using this latest research, and my decades of experience with patients, *Power Up* can improve your body's ability to extract and transform energy from your environment.

The message of energy philosophy behind *Power Up*—that your body is designed to be an energy *creator*, not an energy *consumer*—is easily translated to daily living by following the 21-Day Plan. Exhaustion does not have to be the inevitable by-product of coping with continual stressful demands. I will teach you how to build your energy through all your waking hours. Your mental acuity and creativity will increase day by day, as will your health. As you work with the 21-Day Plan—with its numerous methods for relaxation, exercise, eating for energy, emotional balance, sleep, spiritual development, and detoxification—you will find that all of your physical and mental systems function more efficiently and work together to support your energy needs.

Specifically, *Power Up* will show you:

- A new perspective on illness and health that stimulates and incorporates your inherent healing energy;
- The six essentials of energy creation: Power Mind (stress management), Power Food (diet), Power Exercise, Power Detox, Power Rest, and Power of Connection (spirituality);
- The latest scientific breakthroughs on how the body generates energy and ways you can maximize your body's energy-making mechanisms;
- How to think about, conserve, and create energy the way Eastern cultures do, with simple ways to practice energizing meditation and yogic breathing;
- Complementary/alternative approaches to curing fatigue and improving health, such as acupuncture, herbs, and body work;
- A 21-day, step-by-step plan—complete with recipes—for increasing energy.

The book is organized into three parts: Part One, "Transforming Energy, Six Ways to Reclaim Your Vitality"; Part Two, "21 Days to Optimal Energy"; and Part Three, "Menus and Recipes." Each part stands alone as a usable guide to energy creation. But taken together, all of the parts will magnify and deepen your understanding of how to increase energy and create a uniquely personal, healthy lifestyle.

Part One, "Transforming Energy, Six Ways to Reclaim Your Vitality," will help you identify your own energy issues with the Energy Quiz. It also recounts patients' stories of their energy epiphanies and reveals the latest scientific research. My goal is for you to come away from Part One with an appreciation of the miraculous web of emotional-physical-spiritual well-being that underlies vitality and health. And you will learn the relatively simple, straightforward things you can immediately do in your daily life to renew your energy.

CHAPTER ONE
Power Mind, Boundless Energy

This chapter explains recent discoveries about the link between thought patterns, stress, and energy production. It will give you a clear idea of the plan I've developed for using your mind to reduce stress as easily—and stresslessly!—as possible. It reveals how stress saps your energy and health because of its effects on myriad systems (hormonal, cardiac, nervous, digestive). *Power Mind* gives a clear prescription for managing and reducing stress—and for freeing up energy you can use to regain health.

CHAPTER TWO
Power Food, Your High Performance Fuel

Power Food reveals the latest information from the emerging science of functional medicine, a new nutrition science that emphasizes the molecular basis of how food produces energy. Food consists of molecules that provide substrates for rebuilding and creating energy. Food also sends specific signals to your DNA. Also in *Power Food* is cutting-edge science on the treatment of food allergies and sensitivities and the growing role of superfoods and supplements in achieving optimum health and energy— all of which are incorporated into the menus of the 21-Day Plan.

CHAPTER THREE
Power Detox, Increase Vitality by Removing Toxins

According to a study by the Centers for Disease Control, 148 different industrial chemicals circulate in the average American's bloodstream. Every individual varies in his or her capacity to process toxins—much of which depends on lifestyle factors. This program includes a one-day juice cleanse that has been shown to increase the efficiency of your energy-creating mechanisms. *Power Detox* drives home the critical importance of following the personal environmental clean-up protocol I've developed.

CHAPTER FOUR
Power Exercise

A fourth key to understanding energy is realizing that the human body is built to move. A sedentary lifestyle dramatically inhibits energy creation. Even moderate exercise (30 minutes three times a week of brisk walking), has been shown to increase the number and efficiency of mitochondria to produce energy. It also helps repair the nervous system by producing brain peptides that are critical for retaining a youthful mind. *Power Exercise* also gives easy, practical suggestions to act on right away and throughout the 21-Day Plan for moving and increasing energy.

CHAPTER FIVE
Power Rest, How to Recharge Your Battery

Recharging your battery is all about rest . . . whether this means resting between exercises sessions or sleeping properly every night. You probably don't get optimal sleep, which means your body doesn't have time to repair and renew, or to allow for proper energy creation. Lack of sleep is associated with some very common diseases, including heart disease, and weight gain! My program will show you how to overcome insomnia and sleep problems to significantly increase your energy and improve your health. Details on how to do this on a daily basis are in the 21-Day Plan.

CHAPTER SIX
Power of Connection: Cultivate Spirit and Gain Positive Energy

Though I'm a scientist I will not leave the unprovable out of my program or out of the energy equation. Energy does not exist in isolation; your energy goes beyond the boundaries of your body to interconnect with other energy sources—to the energy of others, to the energy of nature, to the energy of a higher power. Research has shown that cultivating connectedness leads to better health and increased longevity. The Power of Connection will explain current understanding of the role of spirit in the creation of energy and health. It also presents ways to jump-start connectedness and spiritual muscle in your own life.

Part Two, "21 Days to Optimal Energy," a practical, daily plan for implementing the changes that will turn your life from energy-starved to energy-rich. Each day will include advice from at least four and often all of the following categories: *Power Mind, Power Food, Power Exercise, Power Detox, Power Rest,* and *Power of Connection.* You can try some of the daily tips or try them all.

Part Three, "Menus and Recipes," contains your energy-packed eating plan for each day. You will find 69 recipes, the majority of which are vegetarian, but also include fish and poultry.

Decades of investigation into the art and science of energy creation have only confirmed my wholehearted belief that each and every person regardless of age or health status can boost and renew his or her energy and health. This is reinforced by the success over twenty years of seeing patients using energy creation as the path for optimizing health. In the past year I have been gratified to hear from so many readers that this plan has transformed their lives—improved their health, increased their energy, and helped them lose weight at the same time. I want this book to open new doors in your life. I feel certain that your personal healing journey will be enriched and energized as mine has been by learning to build and expand your energy, the source of true healing.

Now, please take the Power Up! Quiz in order to evaluate your overall energy profile.

The Power Up! Quiz

To determine your energy profile rate your honest answers on the following scale:

0 never
1 rarely
2 sometimes

3 most of the time
4 always

Circle Your Score

1. I wake up with good energy.   0 1 2 3 4

2. My energy is as good as it has ever been.   0 1 2 3 4

3. I look forward to each new day.   0 1 2 3 4

4. I have a feeling of joy in my life.   0 1 2 3 4

5. I am able to focus and finish tasks easily.   0 1 2 3 4

6. I have a good memory.   0 1 2 3 4

7. Exercise gives me energy.   0 1 2 3 4

8. My physical stamina is good.   0 1 2 3 4

9. I don't feel a need to rest during the day.   0 1 2 3 4

10. I drink less than 2 cups of coffee a day.   0 1 2 3 4

11. I drink a liter of water each day.   0 1 2 3 4

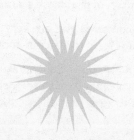

12. I do not need stimulants.	0 1 2 3 4
13. I get plenty of vitamins.	0 1 2 3 4
14. I feel alert after meals.	0 1 2 3 4
15. I'm not cranky.	0 1 2 3 4
16. I consciously manage my stress.	0 1 2 3 4
17. I am rarely ill.	0 1 2 3 4
18. My moods are stable.	0 1 2 3 4
19. My sex drive is good.	0 1 2 3 4
20. I feel younger than my age.	0 1 2 3 4
21. I am a vibrant member of my community.	0 1 2 3 4

TOTAL   _____

YOUR ENERGY PROFILE

Less than 30: **Neophyte**—You never have enough fuel. You need to make the commitment to learn how to manage and create energy.

30–40: **Novice**—Although you are aware of your deficiencies, you are an energy novice who wants and needs to develop new habits that both conserve and generate energy.

41–51: **Initiate**—You are an energy initiate. You respect your energy needs and use about as much fuel as you spend. Your energy levels are at risk of plummeting during times of stress.

52–62: **Adept**—Impressive! You are very good at balancing your energy, but must learn to generate more juice.

63 or more: **Grand Master**—Congratulations! You are ready to explore energy generation on an advanced level, and are already using energy to keep yourself healthy.

Check for Illness First

Before I place anyone on the 21-Day Plan I always screen for illnesses that could be causing fatigue. My most important job is to make sure every person I see is as healthy as possible—especially that he or she has no underlying, undiagnosed medical problems that could be causing fatigue. I expect you're picking up this book because you've already sought medical answers to your fatigue without success. But don't abandon your regular checkups. And as part of this general health care, you want to have regular periodic health evaluations and screening tests such as a colonoscopy by age fifty and a mammogram by age forty—or sooner depending on personal or family risk factors. There are numerous routine tests that just have to be done, even if you think you're perfectly healthy. Your General Practitioner knows about them and can help you schedule them. The 21-Day Plan presumes that you have been medically evaluated for existing conditions.

If you do have an existing medical condition, you can still embark on this plan along with your medical treatment, after clearing it with your own physician. Most everyone can follow this program, except that you cannot take the juice cleanse on day 10 if you have diabetes or are pregnant. People with heart disease and women who are pregnant should not take the saunas. And you should not take supplements without consulting your physician, especially if you have any serious medical conditions or are on medications. If you are experiencing ill health and fatigue, the following represent the most important categories of health concerns to have evaluated as part of a regular checkup.

Allergies	Hormonal imbalance
Anemia	Hypothyroid
Arthritis	Immune system
Asthma	dysfunction
Bowel dysfunction	Liver disease
Cardiac conditions	Medication side effects
Chronic infection	Nutrient deficiencies
Diabetes	Poor vision
Headaches	Tooth or gum disease

PART ONE

Transforming Energy

Six Ways to Reclaim Your Vitality

Chapter 1

Power Mind, Boundless Energy

JACK WAS IN HIS MID-FORTIES and had a family history of heart disease. A new patient, he arrived stressed and in a state of absolute depletion, complaining that he'd been forcing himself to get out of bed every day like a robot. This represented a dramatic downshift from his characteristic world-beating attitude, which had fostered his career as a top executive for a major corporation. He admitted to being deeply concerned about his health based on constant exhaustion, headaches, recurring colds, and the feeling of not wanting to get up in the morning. He said, "Maybe I've got a blocked artery, or a brain tumor! God knows what I've done to myself."

He was halfway through a multi-year contract that would make him eligible for a big payout, and he was planning to work right through that contract. Unfortunately for him, his company had developed catastrophic problems almost the day he'd arrived and he had been in a state of constant crisis management, working seven days a week.

I took all of the samples necessary for thorough testing and conducted a complete physical exam, which confirmed my initial impressions that Jack was basically healthy—by conventional physical standards. But in my opinion he was working on getting sick through a lifestyle that was completely out of balance with inordinate stress that he was managing poorly. He needed a break from the constant stress that was bathing his body in adrenaline, cortisone, and other stress hormones that damage cells over time.

My initial comments about relaxation got nowhere. Like many people I see, Jack felt he was not a person who could relax. He said he couldn't sit for ten minutes and do nothing—his downtime consisted of a high-intensity workout at 6:30 in the morning. He knew he was under high stress, but so was everyone else, and he simply had to turn the company around and not whine about it. Meditation was out of the question—it made him feel anxious and nervous and defeated.

I decided to introduce him to the powers of relaxation by giving him acupuncture. Acupuncture, used in China for thousands of years to promote relaxation, has been a mainstay of my stress management practice for decades: I had him lie down on an exam table with a pillow under his head, dimmed the lights, and gave him acupuncture on some primary stress points.

I returned to the room fifteen minutes later and removed the needles. He sat up with tears in his eyes. He said that he understood by the relaxation he felt during acupuncture how stressed he had been the last two years. He asked if he could use my phone, and called his office to tell his staff he'd be back in two weeks. He left that day for a truly life-saving vacation.

Three weeks later, Jack saw me again, ready to take control of his health and learn some relaxation exercises (he still won't call it meditation!). Then he got through the grueling last two years on his contract, for which he largely credits his morning relaxation exercise (focusing on his breathing for at least five minutes before getting out of bed) and breathing techniques that he uses throughout the day.

JACK'S CASE of stress-induced fatigue is extreme; not many people would attempt to work four years without a break! What is *not* unusual about Jack's situation, though, is that Jack (like so many people who come to see me) had no idea that stress—and his failure to address it—was causing his exhaustion and lethargy. The majority of people I see in my practice wildly underestimate both the amount of stress in their lives and the negative side effects of that stress. **Stress—and more important how**

you perceive it—is the single most pervasive factor that determines the state of your energy.

When you experience stress, the energy that your body needs increases, often significantly. For the short term, most of us have the capacity and reserve to meet these energy needs, but over time—with chronic exposure to stress—the body may not be able to keep up. Initially Jack was energized by the challenges of his new job; he was practically addicted to the adrenaline rush, but as happens with so many people, he couldn't sustain life on overdrive. He was depleted, felt exhausted, and, while he hadn't yet become sick, he was working on getting there.

Jack did not recognize that stress was the most pervasive detrimental influence on his health and energy. Nor did he know that managing it is possible and that the tools for managing it are very simple. Many people—including physicians—don't know this, either.

I spend the majority of my time as a physician pulling people back from the brink of illness, and most often the first step is to put into place a program of stress management that engages the power of the mind to reduce stress and the collateral damage caused by stress. By "mind" I do not mean a series of thought processes in an isolated region of the brain that orders the body to do something. By "mind" I mean your thoughts and emotions and your body working together as one entity. This was a novel concept thirty years ago, but has been established as a scientific fact—albeit an underappreciated one. Every cell in your body has a mindful intelligence that receives input, analyzes it, and sends out messenger molecules through the nervous system and the blood stream to communicate with the rest of the complex, weblike matrix of your body. **In this way, thoughts effect physical changes, and physical changes cause a reciprocal change in thought.** The intelligence of every cell in the body makes relaxation exercises such as meditation and breathwork so effective in combating stress. Using the power of your mind to stop the stress that undermines your health is essential to your well-being and to maintaining your energy.

Stress—or as I like to think of it, the mind that's running on overdrive—is now considered to be a leading factor in numerous illnesses: notably obesity, cardiovascular disease, gastrointestinal disorders, and chronic pain. By some estimates, up to 80 percent of all illnesses are stress induced. Research shows that for some heart patients, mental stress is as dangerous, as smoking cigarettes. Stress has been associated with slower, more complicated postoperative recovery; dysregulation of the immune system; and decreased blood flow to the heart muscle. **By shifting from being at the mercy of your stress to being in control of your stress you can affect a dramatic increase in energy, and as a result you will be less likely to get sick.**

Not all stress is bad—athletes and concert pianists will tell you that a touch of anxiety enhances their performance. The type of stress that causes damage manifests as a chronic sense of pressure that is beyond one's control. Energy-draining stress can arise from anything that disrupts your balance: Unrealistic deadlines at work, moving to a new home, marital disharmony or a new marriage, a change of job, financial difficulties—or all of the above. Your nagging concerns, your worries, your efforts to adapt to a new situation (whether welcome change or not) will take a toll on your energy.

We all try to compartmentalize our stress, but recent discoveries in neuroscience have shown that it is impossible to separate the workings of your mind and emotions from the mechanical functioning of your body. When you transform the pattern of your thoughts and emotions away from anxiety, fear, frustration, and anger toward tranquility, calm, and hopefully a greater sense of joy you also transform your energy. It is possible to harness the power of your mind—especially via the use of the mind-body techniques detailed in the second half of this chapter—to achieve just such a transformation.

If you're wondering why your general practitioner hasn't mentioned any of this, consider that most medical scientists still work under the old paradigm that drugs and antibiotics and other magic bullets are the best way to cure disease and kill bacterial and other "invaders" that make you sick. So scientists have for the most part used this radical new information about the body's global response to stress to search for more pharmaceuticals—antidepressants, antianxiety drugs, and sleeping pills. **Yet thousands of articles have proven that simple, nondrug, mind-body exercises can reduce stress, anxiety, and depression and improve sleep.** And after decades of experience, I have seen first hand that shock-and-awe medicines—while they can be useful in the short term and when dealing with advanced, severe problems—are often unnecessary. Simple, consistent, energy-promoting relaxation exercises and a realistic coping plan can counteract the deleterious effects of stress. You do not need the latest prescription medication advertised on television.

Stress is not the only cause of energy depletion; you'll learn about other lifestyle factors in every chapter of this book. While most people know that a diet of Twinkies is bad for you, few realize a constant emotional diet of stress is equally bad. You need to toss out the emotional Twinkies!

With this book, I am here to help you just as I help my patients. With the information in *Power Mind*—and more incrementally with the 21-Day Plan—you will be able to begin to transform the jagged stress in your life into a boundless stream of energy.

The Mind-Body Connection

I went to medical school in part because I wanted to understand the scientific reasons that meditation, yoga, and other Eastern philosophies and health practices—all of which have energy as their core concept—effect changes in the body. The essence of the healing process in Asian Medicine is tapping into vital energy or life force called Qi (Chi)—for which there is no correlation in Western Medicine. For example, in China acupuncture is understood to work by placing needles at specially designated points that access stagnant Qi (thought to cause illness or pain) and get it moving again. Such powerful practices had captured my imagination as a curious undergrad in the 1960s, but my Western mind craved a scientific explanation. When I entered the Columbia University College of Physicians and Surgeons in 1972, however, I quickly found there was little science available to explain them. Now, thirty years later, the story is much different. Scientists (spurred on by ever more powerful tools such as functional MRIs for watching molecules in action) have made tremendous headway in unraveling the mysteries of the mind-body connection. The massive volume of information has even spawned a scientific discipline called psycho-neuro-immunology (PNI), whose scientists try to understand the complex interplay between emotions and illness.

Mind-body research has brought about the equivalent of a Copernican revolution in physiology. The ideological wall that separates mind from body—constructed by scientific rationalists beginning in the seventeenth century with Descartes—has come crashing down. Whereas Copernicus figured out that the earth was not at the center of the universe, neuroscientists—working on the level of molecular activity much smaller than a single cell—have figured out that the brain is not running the show from your head. Rather, intelligent molecules distributed throughout your body are constantly sending and receiving information that directs nearly instantaneous changes in cells widely dispersed throughout our bodies. To be sure, much of the information comes from the brain via highly developed nervous system structures, but input from the brain is not the only information your body has to act on. **Your immune system, your heart, your gut, and your endocrine system all operate intelligently—independently and interdependently—through messenger molecules called neuropeptides. You think and feel with every inch of your body!**

You are what pioneering neuroscientist Candace Pert calls a "body-mind," a complex web of informational, electromagnetic, and chemical messengers constantly processing and responding to the environment, to thoughts, to emotions, and to physical processes. Pert dubbed these messengers "molecules of emotion," because so many neuropeptides (such as the feel-good hormones serotonin and endorphins) are associated with emotional states. These products of our intelligence operate on a global level throughout the body telling the DNA inside our cells what to do. For example, when you are stressed and start feeling depressed, not only is the serotonin in your brain reduced, but the intestinal cells, the cells lining your blood vessels, the platelets in your blood vessels are all reacting with their own serotonin production. On the other hand, laughter has been shown to help prevent blood-vessel complications in diabetes and improve the balance of immune antibodies throughout the body—especially for people with allergies and rheumatoid arthritis. In a wonderful study from Japan published in the United States, nursing mothers who laughed while watching the Charlie Chaplin movie, *Modern Times,* had higher levels of the beneficial hormone melatonin in their breast milk, which reduced their babies' previously diagnosed allergic skin reactions to latex and dust! The mind's intelligence (and sense of humor) is transmitted by a complex network of nerve fibers and chemical messengers that are located everywhere in your body—not just in the five pounds above your neck. When you have stressful thoughts, your entire body goes into stress response mode by initiating physiological processes that consume energy and can damage cells, leading to fatigue and, ultimately, to disease. When you have positive thoughts you stimulate positive changes in the brain that improve cell functioning throughout the body, including down-regulating inflammatory processes that cause chronic pain and that negatively effect the immune system.

The body's ability to adjust to its own milieu is nearly instantaneous. The very content of your thoughts, and the corresponding neuropeptide

The Proof Is in the Shoestring: Telomeres

For skeptics, here is hard scientific proof of the mind-body connection. The top science honor in the United States, the Lasker
Prize, was awarded a couple of years ago to Elizabeth H. Blackburn, a cell biologist at the University of California at San Francisco, for coming up with proof at the cellular DNA level that
psychological stress causes aging; ergo, the body truly is connected to the mind. Dr. Blackburn studies telomeres, protective
caps at the end of each chromosome (the carrier of DNA inside
the cell) that keep chromosomes from unraveling, very much
like the plastic tip on the end of a shoestring. Without telomeres
your chromosomes would be much more subject to damage,
and to unwanted combining with other chromosomes, creating
unhealthy mutations such as tumors. Scientists believe the length
of your telomeres determines your biological age—the longer
they are the younger you are. Unlike the tip of a shoestring,
which eventually falls off and allows the string to fray, telomeres
are programmed to repair themselves with an enzyme called
telomerase. Trouble crops up, however, when this enzyme-based
self-service system gets out of whack and allows the telomeres
to permanently shorten. Before Dr. Blackburns's research, genetics were the only explanation for differences in telomerase
ability to repair a telomere and keep a person young. But when
she studied mothers of chronically ill children, Dr. Blackburn
found the longer a mother had been caring for a chronically ill
child, the lower her level of telomerase and the shorter her
telomeres had become. This is considered the first evidence that
stress accelerates aging inside each chromosome. The inside
scoop is that Dr. Blackburn is a front-runner for the Nobel Prize.
Her current area of investigation? Telomeres and cancer.

activity generated by them, can change the rate at which your body uses
energy from moment to moment. In landmark studies of transcendental
meditators conducted at Harvard by Herbert Benson, M.D., a founding
father of the mind-body medicine movement, overall energy consump-

tion dropped by as much as 17 percent with the simple act of meditation. "They were burning less body fuel by thinking differently," says Benson. If you come away with nothing else from this chapter, I want you to remember that your thoughts are part and parcel of your body. If you are at all engaged in transforming your health and energy, you must also be engaged in transforming the content of your thoughts and emotions.

When my patients try to shrug off their stress as unavoidable, I try to make them see that stress is like a gateway drug to more serious stuff. Stress leads to other, more damaging states—such as depression and anxiety (it is estimated that 20 percent of the nation has undiagnosed anxiety). Unmanaged stress sets up a vicious cycle that becomes self-perpetuating—for example, people develop recurring headaches or irritable bowel syndrome from chronic stress; or they turn to unproductive emotional outlets—like heavy drinking or smoking—that displace the original stress but cause all sorts of other problems, not the least of which is significant loss of energy. Your mind has the power to make changes that will reduce stress, save energy, and avoid negative emotional states that sap even more energy once they are set into place. My patient Jack was about to reach this tipping point into the more serious stuff. His cellular batteries, the mitochondrial DNA inside each cell responsible for making energy, were beginning to get worn down from all the stress. **Research now even shows that stress can reduce the number of cells in a primary memory center of your brain and shrink a segment of your cells' DNA, called a telomere, a protective cap on the end of each chromosome that determines your biological age!** If it all boils down to shortening your life, will you begin to do some of the relaxation exercises that reduce stress? I hope so. First, let's go on a little tour of the body, so you can understand how the *Power Up!* stress reduction program works.

The Anatomy of Stress

Up to this point I've been describing your body's cells and how they respond to stress in a very general way. All cells have the same basic structure—a cell wall with receptors responsible for allowing information molecules to pass in and out; cytoplasm (the cells' soupy interior) containing nutrients, enzymes, and messenger molecules that relay information; and a nucleus that holds the cell's "brain"—the DNA, which directs cell function, repair, and regeneration on an ongoing basis—as well

as the mitochondria, special DNA inside each cell dedicated solely to generating energy day in and day out (see Chapter 2 for more on mitochondria). But as similar as cells are in basic structure, they are also highly
specialized. Each has its own shape and function—whether it's a nerve
cell, an immune cell, an intestinal cell, a heart muscle cell—each plays a
role within a larger system of the body. Some of these systems are more
immediately affected by stress than others. Indeed, the body has three
main mechanisms geared specifically for handling stress: the autonomic
nervous system (ANS); the hypothalamic-pituitary-adrenal (HPA) axis;
and the neuropeptide web. Familiarity with these systems will help you
understand the latest research that shows how relaxation exercises turn
down the volume on your stress response mechanisms.

The Marvelous Cell

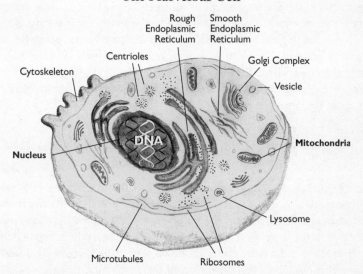

The millions and millions of cells that make up every part of your body have an intelligence of their own in the genomic DNA inside the nucleus; they make their own energy
supply from food and oxygen utilizing the DNA inside the mitochondria, and communicate with all the other cells through receptors and messengers that pass through the cell
wall and deliver crucial information to the genomic DNA.

Autonomic Nervous System (ANS):
Your fight-or-flight mode.

The body's massive nerve fiber network, the autonomic (automatic) nervous system is responsible for continual, subconscious functioning of all vital organ systems—heart, lungs, intestines, to name a few. Recognized as being responsive to stress as early as the nineteenth century, the ANS speeds up vital systems and provides a burst of energy in response to stress—preparing you to run from the proverbial saber-toothed tiger or modern mugger. It accomplishes this through two mirror-image operating modes: *sympathetic*, also known as the fight-or-flight mechanism, which releases adrenaline to speed up metabolic processes in response to a perceived threat; and *parasympathetic*, which releases the neurotransmitter acetylcholine (via the body's longest and largest nerve, the vagus) to slow down and reverse the frenetic activity caused by the *sympathetic* response. *Sympathetic* activation halts digestion (considered nonessential when preparing to fight or flee) and accelerates blood pressure, heart, and respiration rates, causing the body to expend considerably more energy during stress. Scientists now also believe the *sympathetic* system is involved in helping the body decide when to store food as fat, and when to use it for energy. The *parasympathetic* response (which can be deliberately activated with relaxation exercises such as a single yoga session) seeks to calm down the physiologic processes that have been put into hyperdrive by stress.

Hypothalamic-Pituitary-Adrenal Axis (HPA Axis):
Your Stress-Hormone Highway.

First identified as a stress response mechanism in the 1950s, the HPA axis is a network of glands that deliver information through hormones in the bloodstream, originating in the body's master gland, the hypothalamus (located in the lower part of the brain) and ending in the adrenals, two walnut-sized endocrine glands sitting on top of the kidneys. This basic survival mechanism, responsible even for shocking a newborn's body into drawing its first breath, causes the adrenals to bathe the body in adrenalin and cortisol, the principal regulatory hormones sent out in response to stress and in preparation for injury. Cortisol reduces inflammation, which is important because reducing inflammation is part of the initial healing process. However, repeated elevation of cortisol levels is

The Stress Hormone Superhighway

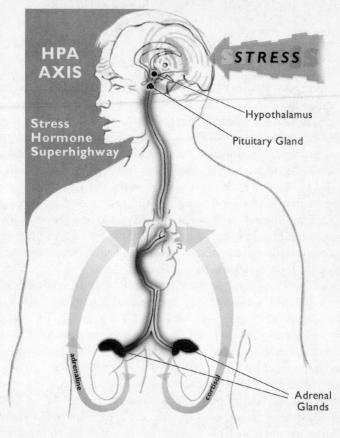

HPA AXIS

Stress Hormone Superhighway

STRESS

Hypothalamus

Pituitary Gland

adrenaline

cortisol

Adrenal Glands

Stress—both from external sources and from stressful thoughts—sets off a cascade of hormones including adrenaline and cortisol, which cause your heart to beat faster, your breathing rate to increase, your digestion to slow, and a number of other physiological responses that cause wear and tear on your body over time.

destructive: in its efforts to reduce inflammation cortisol also suppresses the immune system, and when chronically elevated cortisol raises blood pressure, increases blood sugar by blocking the effect of insulin, dampens memory, and causes the body to store visceral fat, the worst kind. All of these cortisol driven processes in response to stress require significant energy expenditure. Studies have shown that relaxation exercises result in lower cortisol and adrenalin production in response to stress.

Neuropeptide Web (NPW): Your Biochemical Internet.

First identified in the 1980s, this body-wide network of hormone-like chemical messengers, the neuropeptides, and their receptors gave a revolutionary new understanding of the mind-body connection, and helped explain how the body can respond so quickly to perceived stress. The neuropeptide web makes it possible for your psychological and physical states to have a back-and-forth exchange. Scientists were astounded to find that molecules that were associated with emotions (and thought to be limited to the brain)—such as endorphins, serotonin, and dopamine—could actually be manufactured and received in cells throughout the body. In fact, the cells lining the intestine produce more serotonin than the brain. The most celebrated neuropeptide, serotonin is responsible for maintaining mood, and provides the basis of action for the SSRI family of antidepressants such as Prozac. The cells lining the blood vessels also synthesize their own serotonin to help control blood pressure (a basis for the new triptan drugs for migraines). Likewise, substances previously only associated with the immune system (inflammation and immune response control molecules such as tumor necrosis factor and interleukins) are now known to be made in abundance in the emotional centers of the brain. And the immune cells (white blood cells) produce "brain" neuropeptides such as the pituitary's ACTH (which causes the release of cortisone), as well as endorphins, thyroid stimulating hormone, and growth hormones. Discovery of this neuropeptide web means that the stress response is far-reaching, with implications for every cell and organ system in the body. Through the neuropeptide web, the body responds to stress (both physical and psychological) with alterations in billions of cells' DNA leading to thousands of new chemical reactions in each cell that require tremendous energy production—all in the blink of an eye. By the same token, the body's response to a loving thought is equally dramatic, and infinitely more beneficial.

The effects of these three stress-response mechanisms have been subject to much research over the past decade, especially in mind-body science. The research so far has teased out the particularly dramatic effects that stress has on immunity, heart health, and the functioning of the digestive tract. By mapping the pathways of the autonomic nervous system, the HPA axis, and the neuropeptide web, scientists have begun to provide an explanation for the mechanism behind the link between stress and many different disease processes. Research has also established a firm connection between relaxation exercises and buffering of the three stress-response mechanisms.

Some of the most dramatic and compelling research on the control of stress has been done with the relaxation response, beginning with Herbert Benson's pioneering work beginning in the 1970s. Thousands of studies since then have shown that very simple techniques (meditation, guided imagery, biofeedback, and yoga among others) evoke a measurable decrease in the activity of the stress-response mechanisms, and improve health and energy. The relaxation response works throughout your body: It activates the calming parasympathetic nervous system of the autonomic nervous system, reduces output of stress hormones from the HPA axis and alters neuropeptide balance in the neuropeptide web—for example, increasing endorphins and serotonin.

A specific example of how stress effects your physical functioning is in work looking at Heart Rate Variability. Like the brain, the heart has its own measurable energy field. **I was amazed when I first learned that the heart's energy is five thousand times greater in strength than the energy produced by the next most electromagnetically active organ, the brain. The electromagnetic impulses of the heart can be measured up to ten feet away, and it's thought that others may sense your heart's energy by picking up on its energy field!** Researchers have been able to take advantage of the heart's formidable power output by recording changes in its rate, called heart rate variability (HRV). This measure of the duration between successive heart beats allows scientists to put together a detailed picture of the heart's response to stress.

One hallmark of an individual who handles stress well is greater heart rate variability—a sign of the heart's sensitivity to changing demands. Greater variability shows the heart is able to quickly return to a slower, resting state rather than constantly being in a fixed autonomic nervous system overstimulation-mode (through chronic exposure to adrenaline and other stress-induced hormones and neuropeptides). Unfortunately, millions of people are walking around with hearts that have been on too much stress—their heart rate variability is frequently out of whack, even in their sleep. This significantly increases the work of the heart—and such increased energy expenditure has been shown to result in heart disease as well as general fatigue.

The work on stress and heart rate variability over the last couple of decades parallels equally dramatic work on the effects of stress on many other organ systems. For example, researchers have found that stress (even something as purely cognitive as telling a lie) inhibits gastric activity after eating, which can cause indigestion. Scientists have proved that the sympathetic pathway of the autonomic nervous system acts as the inhibitor of digestion. By the same token, voluminous research shows that the relaxation response elicited by yoga, biofeedback, guided imagery, and meditation *reduces* the sympathetic activity of the autonomic nervous system, offering a no-risk method for improving digestion. In addition to relaxation exercises, certain supplements (herbs, vitamins, minerals, and others) that I will describe later in this chapter can also help tame stress. As someone who has exhaustively studied the literature and put it to practical use for decades, I can tell you with great certainty that the same pattern crops up over and over again: Stress activates mechanisms that, over time, cause low energy and poor health, and stress management is a simple way to reverse this damaging cycle.

We've all had the experience of stress making us sick. Now science has explained that this happens through the intelligence of our cells reacting to even just a stressful thought with biological changes all the way down to the smallest particles of DNA and the cell's energy generation mechanisms. Today we are only beginning to understand the subtleties of mind-body medicine, but you must accept the fact that the daily experience of life and its challenges directly affects your health and energy. Stress is a known risk factor for illness, and the greatest potential drain on energy. Actively working to transform your stress (the 21-Day Plan is a good jump start) is the single most powerful way to take back your vital energy and feel ten years younger.

Good Stress vs. Bad Stress

Several years ago a patient brought me a pillow embroidered with this bit of wordplay: "Stressed spelled backwards is desserts." I keep the pillow in my reception room in the hope that people will reflect on it as they wait to see me because it encapsulates one of the most important elements of stress management (not to eat more dessert!): **It is often your perception**

and handling of an event, and not the nature of the stressor, that determines its effect on you.

I mentioned earlier that for athletes and concert musicians, stress can lead to constructive outcomes—the adrenaline rush that releases a burst of energy before a game or performance can improve their playing. However, research has found that this is only true when a person has prepared thoroughly for a task. **The more control you perceive yourself to have over a stressful situation the less damaging the stress will be.** (For athletes and musicians control comes through practice and the resulting confidence.) In a fascinating study conducted at Yale University, adult men who were given no control over a laboratory-induced stress session for twenty minutes experienced a reduction in the activity of their natural killer cells (the first line of immune defense) that suppressed their immune systems for as long as seventy-two hours later. Those who were given control over the stress had no reduction in natural killer cell activity; their immune systems remained strong. In another study, painful stress after surgery was shown both to suppress immune function and to promote metastasis of cancer cells, but the proper use of pain medications to relieve the painful stress was shown to reduce those negative effects. The lesson is that health and immunity are not about stress per se, but about how you perceive and manage it.

Nowhere is the perception of stress better illustrated than in the latest research on the link between Type A personalities and heart attack risk. For many years scientists thought that all Type A personalities—hurried, high-achieving, risk-taking people—had a greater chance of developing heart disease than non-Type A personalities simply because Type As invite more stress into their lives. However, it turns out there are healthy Type As and unhealthy Type As—the difference is in their emotional coping style and how they perceive the stressors in their lives. A higher risk of heart attack exists only for Type A personalities in combination with a hostile coping style (characterized by anger and frustration in response to stress). Type A people with positive attitudes and optimistic coping styles live longer and have no greater risk of heart disease than the general population. The veil of emotions through which you perceive your stress to a large degree determines the toll it will take on health and energy.

Let's revisit Jack, whose case history introduced this chapter. He was definitely a Type A person, but he'd undergone a change in coping style, from feeling hopeful to feeling frustrated. This is a problem that people often develop when stress becomes chronic and fatigue sets in. Jack had in fact developed the two most damaging forms of stress: His was constant (remember he wouldn't take a vacation) and it had begun to feel beyond his control (he felt he was at the mercy of the misfortunes of the company he was running). In the medical world Psychologists have come up with rather intimidating terms for these problems: *allostatic load*—I call this the tipping point—which is the amount of stress you can take before it makes you sick; and *locus* (or perception) *of control*, which is the amount of control you perceive you have over a given stress versus perceiving the stress as imposed upon you. **Making sure you don't reach your tipping point, and gaining the perception of being in control are the keys to a good stress management plan.**

Two Ways to Turn Bad Stress Into Good Stress

- **Move Your Tipping Point:** The point beyond which cumulative exposure to stress causes fatigue and illness is a moving target. For each person, the tipping point is different and it can vary from day to day. There are many stories about people who survive catastrophic emotional or physical situations and tragedies and go on to lead healthy lives. On the flip side we all know people who collapse at seemingly trifling stress (the cable guy never showed up). The point is that you simply cannot allow stress to accumulate, no matter which kind of stress affects you. You've got to come up with ways to offload your stress. You probably can't take a vacation every other week, but you can constantly downshift your stress response with relaxation exercises. Over time, relaxation exercises can move your tipping point, increasing your limit of tolerance so that stressful situations don't bother you as much, and allow you to maintain your energy for other challenges.
- **Create the Perception of Control:** The thought (even if it seems initially like an illusion) that you can exercise personal choice in a stressful situation has been found to be the single greatest predictor of effective stress management— regardless of whether or not you actually have control! Taking conscious steps to control your stress, even if it's something as simple as taking calming breaths just before a major meeting, is an important part of the transformation toward a more energetic life.

Incredibly, I have found that it is in the most difficult periods of people's lives that they tend most often to underestimate the amount of stress they have, and therefore do nothing to cope with the additional burden. Jack's lack of self-awareness and absence of coping mechanisms put him on the brink of chronic fatigue and illness. At his first treatment with me, I was able to induce physical changes (slowing his metabolism with acupuncture by activating the parasympathetic nervous system, releasing mood-enhancing neuropeptides, such as endorphins and serotonin) that altered his physical awareness and his mental outlook and put some distance between Jack and his stress. Jack got a glimpse of what he could achieve by shifting his chemistry from stress-driven back to its natural balance, something he would later learn to do daily with relaxation exercises.

What's Your Coping Style?

Often the biggest obstacle to developing a stress management plan is your accustomed coping style. Taking an assessment of your coping style can begin to help you improve it. The first step is to think about how you typically cope. In my experience, people generally fall into one of five basic coping categories:

HELPLESSNESS—You are overwhelmed, incapable of reacting.
DENIAL—You don't recognize the presence of stress; eventually it catches up with you.
STOIC ACCEPTANCE—You may recognize stress, but repress it rather than attempt to deal with it
FIGHTING SPIRIT—You are not afraid to engage the stressors, often head-on, but sometimes this can lead to exhaustion.
RESILIENCE—You look for links between thoughts, feelings, and reactions, and come up with a reasonable coping strategy.

Regardless of your accustomed coping style, I want you to move toward resilience. The ability to detach from your stress, to place it in perspective, and come up with a plan for coping is the healthiest approach. When you are resilient you make the decisions, your emotions don't run the show. You are able to come up with a plan because you are not denying or repressing the need for one (in a recent study, suppressing emotions was associated with heart disease, especially for women). And for the most part you are able to let go of the stress. Daniel Goleman, psychologist and author of the bestselling book, *Emotional Intelligence*, has succinctly defined the desired attitude as self-awareness. "Self-awareness is not an attention that gets carried away by emotions, overreacting and amplifying what is perceived. Rather, it is a neutral mode that maintains self-reflectiveness even amidst turbulent emotions . . . It is the difference between, for example, being murderously enraged at someone and having the self-reflexive thought, 'This is anger I'm feeling.' " Many people might think this sort of detachment requires decades of psychotherapy, but, at the risk of sounding like a broken record, practicing relaxation exercises—like those detailed in the second half of this chapter—helps to cultivate just such a healthy perspective. For example, by practicing a brief breathing exercise in the 21-Day Plan, you can stop the cascade of stress responses triggered by an experience, and thereby provide a little distance for reflection.

Back in the 1950s my mother constantly reminded my brothers and me of the message of a popular New York minister and author, Dr. Norman Vincent Peale, who promoted the idea of the power of positive thinking. At the time we were too young (and certainly not introspective enough) to realize the importance of his message. He was even perhaps a bit ahead of his time (one of the first in a long line of self-help gurus), yet he was saying things that humankind has known for millennia: The key to a healthy life is in using the power of positive thinking. It is not what confronts you but rather the attitude you bring to a situation—and the tools you have for managing your attitude—that matters most. Now, as a physician, I have seen firsthand what my mother and Dr. Peale knew decades ago: Thoughts have the power to transform lives. **Your thoughts are the best medicine you have for dramatically improving your health. Your mind is the best tool you have for dramatically increasing your energy supply.**

A Guide to the Best Relaxation Exercises

Practicing just one of the recommended relaxation techniques—whether it's meditation, breath work, yoga, or tai chi—will bring positive energy into your life. Some of the techniques in this guide—such as breath breaks—simply trigger the relaxation response, while others like acupuncture have broader applications. It really doesn't matter which technique you choose, numerous published studies have shown that all relaxation techniques—which promote an altered state of relaxed concentration or focused reverie—have beneficial effects, including a decrease in energy consumption. The laboratories of Herbert Benson's Mind/Body Medical Institute at Harvard have demonstrated the healing influence that relaxation techniques can exert over numerous medical conditions such as high blood pressure, irregular heartbeat, chronic pain, insomnia, impotence, the side effects of cancer therapy, surgical recovery, and fatigue. Mind-body relaxation techniques are a means of releasing tension in the mind and halting the destructive march of the biochemical processes set into motion by that tension. The release of mental anxiety (which affects your entire physiology) in turn allows healing energy to flow.

The Relaxation Response

Opposite of the stress response, the Relaxation Response is a group of beneficial physiological changes that occur when a person achieves a state of psychological relaxation. It is most easily achieved by practicing any mind-body relaxation technique that focuses attention repeatedly on a sound, word, thought, phrase, visual image, or even a muscular activity that allows you to disregard other thoughts.

The top stress-management techniques described here—all elicit the relaxation response—have been used with great success by thousands of my patients. Many of these techniques were developed by other cultures over many years—in some cases thousands of years ago. Most of these techniques have been subject to rigorous testing by Western scientists over the past thirty years. There is something for everyone here, whether you dislike sitting still or can't stand to hear the word meditation. You can do this for yourself, and in fact you probably already know how. The best general description I've ever heard of the type of relaxation exercise that down-regulates the stress response comes from Belleruth Naparstek, a gifted psychotherapist and author of *Staying Well with Guided Imagery!*

Belleruth likens the altered state of relaxation achieved through these exercises to what you do when you get on a crowded elevator.

> When we are in a crowded elevator, and strangers are uncomfort-
> ably close to us, our defense is to stare straight ahead, concentrat-
> ing on an imaginary spot on the elevator door or on the lit floor
> indicator above the door, blocking out our perceptions of the
> people breathing down our necks.

This is a perfect example of turning down the volume on a stressful
situation. You don't have to be a monk sitting on a mountaintop to be
able to evoke an altered state, where all distractions cease. Many experts
have found ways to achieve the goal of relaxation, the point at which your
body's systems are operating with the least amount of effort. The best way
to find what works for you is through trial and error.

Have fun! Relaxation is a therapeutic intervention you can't overdo.

Establishing Breath Breaks

The supply of oxygen to your cells is a major determinant in how much
energy you make. By simply increasing the oxygen supply in your blood
with deep breathing exercises, you will be able to make more energy and
elicit the relaxation response, which simultaneously allows your body to
utilize less energy. Breathing involves chemical, mechanical, and cerebral
control mechanisms at many levels of the nervous system, all of which are
put into overdrive when you experience stress. Compared to other vital
functions such as heartbeat, breath rate is by far the easiest you can influence voluntarily. While breath work can be exceedingly powerful, especially when performed at an advanced level (such as kundalini yogic
breathing or Holotropic breath work), I consider it to be an entry-level
relaxation exercise—it can be easier for the novice than meditation. You
focus attention on your breath (the sound and sensation of the air moving in and out of your body) so you don't have to find a mantra or phrase
to repeat. The goal is to take deeper, slower breaths, which allows a general deceleration of the metabolism and stress-response systems, along
with a corresponding conservation of energy and improved alertness.

Patients have told me that this exercise transformed their lives by au-
tomatically reducing their stress. The key to this profound breathing

technique is to take abdominal breaths, which means that the abdomen, rather than the chest, expands as you inhale. (By involving the diaphragm, you draw oxygen deeper into the lung cells and recruit muscles and neurotransmitters that significantly enhance the effects.) It's best to sit up straight with shoulders back to expand your lung capacity. As you become more aware of your posture through these exercises, you'll notice that you spend much of the day with shoulders slumped forward taking shallow chest breaths that promote anxiety.

Your Power Up! Breath Break*

1. Inhale slowly to the count of four—with abdomen expanding, chest relaxed, listening to your breath.
2. Pause for one count.
3. Exhale slowly and completely to the count of six—with abdomen deflating, shoulders relaxed and engaged, listening to your breath.
4. Pause for one count.
5. Repeat four times.

* Sit up straight for this exercise, shoulders back.

You can take breath breaks any time—in the office, in the car, in a conference room, or on an airplane. By following these basic instructions you will unfailingly experience a softening of your upper body's usual tension, and a slower, more relaxed breathing pattern—even after you finish the exercise. Studies of this technique show that it results in slower pulse, lower blood pressure, relaxed intestinal muscles, lower cortisol and blood carbon dioxide levels. The nervous system alone utilizes about 20 percent of the oxygen you take in, so by reducing the nervous system activity you preserve energy. I recommend using this technique as often as you can—preferably every hour or two. Whenever you pass a mirror or window where you can see your reflection, check your posture and practice your breath work. **If you do only one thing to increase your energy, this breath break would be my choice.**

The M Word—Meditation

Many people are wary of meditation because of its association with sacred, esoteric, Buddhist, or Hindu religious practices. Some also worry that practicing meditation is somehow at odds with their own religious beliefs. But from my perspective meditation can be used with any religious practice. It is simply a tool for using the power of the mind, a very simple way to rest the mind—to let go of normal, everyday thought processes, especially the hundreds of worried, fearful, jealous, angry, or frustrated thoughts that tend to crowd into our consciousness, even when—sometimes especially when—we don't want them to. By allowing you to take a step back from the constant workings of the mind, meditation helps you gain greater insight into your thought processes and greater control of your emotions. It is the ultimate healing tool because it works subconsciously, on an energetic level where healing—and illness—take root. Practically speaking, meditation is a wonderful exercise for building a more resilient coping style, for cultivating self-awareness, and for quieting self-destructive tendencies—in short, it's just what the doctor ordered as part of an effective stress-management program.

Meditation at its most basic level, as it is used for stress management, is nothing more than slow breathing with a mantra—a neutral or positive word, phrase, or prayer repeated over and over again, such as Om, Peace, Now, or Calm. The rhythmic repetition of the mantra is an effective way to slow your breathing (by activating the calming parasympathetic nervous system) and to take your mind off anxious thoughts, thereby further dampening your stress response. There are a number of different meditation techniques, but the two most commonly practiced are single-pointed meditation—the aforementioned slow breathing, focusing on a mantra—and mindfulness meditation, which is basically slow breathing with the intention of keeping your mind in the present moment in an emotionally positive way. For example, when washing your hands, you consciously think of the beauty and usefulness of your hands and of the water running over them (not the dozens of thing you haven't gotten to yet today). Meditation is quite simply a change in thought patterns for the better. It is a direct way of replacing energy-draining negative thought patterns with energy-generating positive thought patterns.

Since the early 1970s when the Beatles introduced transcendental meditation to the public, researchers have been studying the mechanisms

Take Two "Oms" and Call Me in The Morning

Many beneficial physical changes occur with meditation. Numerous published studies have demonstrated the positive effects: Lower cortisol production in response to stress; less sympathetic (accelerating) and greater parasympathetic (calming) activity in the nervous system; improved heart rate responsiveness; reduced oxygen consumption; increased positive neurotransmitters, serotonin, and endorphins; increased (relaxing) alpha brain waves; increased immune responsiveness; and reduced pro-inflammatory molecules (cytokines). Meditation balances physiological processes—halting stress in its tracks, reducing energetic needs, and allowing energy to regenerate.

and effects of meditation. **One juicy research tidbit came recently from the University of California at Irvine where researchers were able to demonstrate a 50 percent reduction in lab-induced pain (as measured in the brain during an MRI) after people practiced meditation for five months.** At Jon Kabat-Zinn's Center for Mindfulness Medicine in the University of Massachusetts Department of Medicine, researchers showed that psoriasis patients who practiced a brief mindfulness meditation during light therapy (the standard treatment) had significantly faster healing than people who didn't meditate during treatment. One of the most astonishing recent studies came from the University of Calgary in Canada, where investigators were able to determine that meditation caused beneficial changes in the mix of T-cells (immune cells that fight cancer) in breast and prostate cancer patients. Every year new studies are published that attest to the power of meditation to effect beneficial changes throughout your body.

The nuts and bolts of how you meditate are relatively simple. It is best to sit with an erect spine in a comfortable position—if you lie down you might fall asleep. (It is not necessary to sit with legs crossed, though this is a good position for aligning your spinal cord from head to hips.) Choose a single point of focus: A neutral word such as the Sanskrit "om," peace, the sound of your breath—the exact mantra is less important than finding one that helps you let go of your thoughts. Especially in the beginning

it is best to meditate in a darkened room in order to reduce stimulation
and allow thoughts—and awareness of the outside environment—to re-
cede more easily. When you become aware that you are engaged in conscious thoughts, notice them, release them, and return to the single point
of focus. These are the basic instructions.

In the 21-Day Plan I ask you to do this for two minutes when you
wake up each morning, at a time when your stress hormones are nearly

---

A Happy Mantra

One of my favorite mantras comes from Thich Nhat Hanh, the
luminous Vietnamese monk who has published more than forty
books explaining Buddhism to the West. He offers a wonderful
point of focus for beginners with these two sentences: "Breathing in, I feel calm. Breathing out, I smile." You can simply say or
think "calm" when you inhale, and "smile" when you exhale.
Many people have told me this practice refreshes them even in
the midst of total stress.

---

doubling from their resting rate. This is a good practice for every morning, whether you're on the plan or not.

With practice, you will be ready to move on to the next level of meditation, allowing the focal point to dissolve and entering a deeply peaceful
state. This is the sweet spot of meditation. Once you are able to let go of
the mantra without conscious thoughts crowding in you've reached a
profoundly calm place—it's been described as nothingness or emptiness,
but I think of it as being completely in the present. The negative thoughts
of past and future worries that constantly swirl in your subconscious have
quieted. Rather than escaping from those thoughts, which is what happens when you watch television, for example, meditation allows you to
release negative thoughts. It's not just the effect of the 15 minutes you are
meditating—the nervous system is reset to a less reactive state for many
hours afterwards. With practice, meditation permanently cultivates a
more tranquil and positive mental attitude, which makes for a more effective coping style.

Mindfulness meditation differs from single-pointed meditation in
that it has an object: Your body, your feelings, your mind, the objects of

your mind. It may seem a little Kumbaya, but the idea is to radiate love toward the object. Mindfulness requires full attention. The idea is to keep your focus in the present moment, not letting in other distracting thoughts. It is the opposite of multitasking. Here is one example of mindfulness exercises from Thich Nhat Hanh, which can be easily practiced as you go about your day.

WASHING HANDS

"Water flows over these hands.
May I use them skillfully to preserve our precious planet."

From *The Energy of Prayer* by Thich Nhat Hanh

The beauty of a meditation exercise is you can repeat the same one over and over again, and receive ever-deepening benefits of enhanced tranquility and greater energy each time. The only limitation will be your own desire to get it right. There is no "right way." The process of meditation is what provides the benefits. There is no goal because the point is to be in the present moment. **Rather than spending your energy ruminating on the past or worrying about the future, you will find through meditation that your body has boundless energy for being in the here and now.**

Biofeedback

Biofeedback is what I call meditation for engineers. It is a decades-old, well-documented, stress-reduction method that employs an electronic device to guide you through a relaxation technique. Usually the device provides an audio or visual cue to slow the breathing to less than ten breaths per minute, a therapeutic zone shown in studies to reduce sympathetic activity, blood pressure, and stress. Biofeedback devices (from companies such as HeartMath, Stress Busters, and Resp-e-rate) employ sensors—most commonly attached to the fingertips—that record the biological markers of relaxation such as electrical skin resistance, and provide feedback (such as a change in tone of the audio cue heard through a headset) to signal the progress of your relaxation response. **Studies have** shown the ability to see how well you're doing significantly enhances any relaxation exercise's effectiveness, and the device itself provides a focus that keeps your mind from wandering to stressful thoughts.

Videogames have opened up a new realm of possibility for biofeedback. One of my favorite new products is a series of software programs from The Wild Divine Project (www.wilddivine.com), which uses phenomenal healers such as Deepak Chopra, M.D., Dean Ornish, M.D., and Andrew Weil, M.D. as interactive guides to the meditation session. The Wild Divine finger monitors plug into a USB port, and the software provides visually fanciful meditative imagery on the computer screen. In one segment you have to coax a rabbit out from behind a hedge simply through relaxation (my fourteen-year-old daughter is much better at this than I am!). The most extraordinary aspect of biofeedback is to be able to see how quickly you can improve your relaxation skills with a little practice.

Guided Imagery

Guided imagery is basically meditation with imagination. Many people find that it is easier to manage stressful thoughts with the distraction of specific imagery. The image can be preprogrammed and provided by audio recording, a book, computer software, or a therapist; or it can be a spontaneous image springing from your own imagination. The image has to be detailed enough so that it occupies sufficient cognitive space to stop you from reengaging with thoughts, worries, and concerns—so that it halts the cascade of stress responses. Often people start with a programmed image and then elaborate on that image with their imaginations.

Guided imagery can be extremely powerful, and has been found in recent studies to be especially effective in pain management and in helping insomniacs fall asleep faster by managing unwanted presleep worries. At the University of Washington Human Interface Technology Lab, cognitive psychologist Hunter Hoffman and his colleagues have been alleviating pain with a software program called Snow World. When a burn patient's bandages are changed it can feel like the experience of being burned all over again, so during wound care, patients wearing virtual reality goggles are immersed in an arctic landscape populated by smiling snowmen zipping about igloos and glaciers. Patients report a dramatic drop in pain, primarily, researchers believe, due to the complete shift of attention from the activity of wound care to the virtual world. It's also very likely that the snowy images help "put out the fire" in the viewer's minds.

For stress management, an image has to be relaxing, which varies tremendously from person to person. If someone had a terrible experience on the beach, then the ocean would not be a good image. For others, the ocean can be profoundly calming. First choose the general image then fill in the details. Here is one exercise that uses a mountain stream to create a relaxing world. The exercise will be more powerful if you evoke the place by listening to a recording of the sounds of the forest while you meditate.

MOUNTAIN STREAM MEDITATION

You are sitting on the bank of a clear, cold mountain stream;
You are surrounded by tall trees in an ancient forest;
You feel the gentle pressure of the soft forest floor underneath you;
You inhale deeply, taking in the crisp mountain air;
You become aware of the sound of birds in the trees above;
You watch beams of sunlight filter through the trees;
You see patches of deep-blue sky overhead;
You begin to focus on the site of the running water before you;
You watch the inches-deep water flow over rocks in the stream;
You notice pebbles moving along the streambed;
There is nothing else but you and the stream;
There is nothing else but you and the water;
You are one with this place;
You breathe in the rhythms of the stream;
You are the stream.

Stress Busting Body Work

Acupuncture

I have been using acupuncture in my practice for over twenty years, and consider it to be one of my most powerful tools for reversing the effects of chronic stress as well as for treating a multitude of stress-related conditions such as headaches, irritable bowel, asthma, and chronic back pain. In my experience, having acupuncture is a bit like having your car tuned up, everything just works better. The Chinese say that acupuncture raises and rebalances Qi (or vital energy). **Western medical research has demonstrated that it works through the nervous system, reducing inflammation, changing neurotransmitters, and turning down the stress responses of all the body's systems.** Many of my patients such as Jack report feeling energized and able to take further action to reduce their stress after just one session, which is about as close a definition to increasing vital energy as I can imagine.

Acupuncture is administered by inserting ultra-thin needles (six acupuncture needles can fit inside one hypodermic) at specific points depending on what the session is meant to address—the needles are so thin that most people don't notice them when they are going in. (General stress points are located in the shoulders, neck, hands and lower legs.) Treatments always require more than one needle placement because the idea is to provide balance—where one point is stimulated an equal and opposite point must also be stimulated.

As you receive the treatment, you usually either lie down or sit in a comfortable, supported position—usually in a darkened or softly lit room to enhance the relaxation. The needles' superfine points glide into the top layer of skin almost imperceptibly, creating a slight pinch. Many people report a sensation of invigoration—something like a shiver (what the Chinese call the De Qi sensation)—when the needles are inserted, followed by a sense of relaxation. A single session can last from 10 to 30 minutes. Dramatic effects can be achieved with one treatment, but a series of treatments produces more lasting results

Many people ask me how I know where to put the needles, and the answer to that question always leads back to China, where I first studied acupuncture in the late 1980s when the government was beginning to foster more scientific dialogue between East and West. The general position for all acupuncture points is in the muscular trigger point (the midpoint of a muscle, where nerve fibers and tension are most concentrated). The Chinese amassed a huge body of evidence through trial and error beginning two thousand years ago that established the acupuncture points most effective for eliciting global benefits. An experienced acupuncturist knows when he's hit the right spot by the feeling of De Qi. (Novices often learn to identify points with electronic sensors that measure changes in

How Does Acupuncture Work?

Hundreds of studies have been published since the late 1970s demonstrating that acupuncture buffers all three stress-response mechanisms. While acupuncture works by releasing tension at the point where the needles are inserted (locally it increases blood flow and decreases muscle strain), it also works at a distance from where the needles are inserted, generating beneficial changes in neurotransmitters. Similar to the relaxation response, but often more immediately powerful, acupuncture lowers sympathetic and raises parasympathetic activity in the autonomic nervous system and balances hormone levels in the hypothalamic-pituitary axis that governs the nervous systems' response to stress. Numerous studies have established that acupuncture can produce a dramatic shift in the neuropeptides governing mood, for example, sharply raising the level of feel-good endorphins. In short, acupuncture can significantly reduce stress, and its calming effects can last for days afterwards.

electrical resistance on the skin.) Historically, acupuncture in China has been used as part of a larger holistic system of traditional medicine that includes dietary changes, herbs, massage, and other techniques, but in the last century acupuncture has been recognized both in China and in the West as effective when used by itself.

I recommend that people receive treatment only from a licensed acupuncturist, but not necessarily a physician. In most states, it is illegal to administer acupuncture without a license, and states have regulations that govern education and licensing of acupuncturists—both physician and nonphysician. In some states, however, licensing guidelines are unclear and you should look for certification by the American Academy of Acupuncture and Oriental Medicine, a national certifying organization that issues the equivalent of board certification in acupuncture. (In Canada, the certifying body is the Acupuncture Foundation Institute of Canada.) In some cases when a person has complex medical problems it may be useful to see a physician acupuncturist, but for the majority of people with common ailments a nonmedical licensed acupuncturist is perfectly acceptable. Indeed, many of the most experienced acupuncturists are not physicians—they have spent a minimum of three years in full-time training just for acupuncture.

For the extreme needle-phobic there are other options for accessing acupuncture points. Laser acupuncture, magneto-acupuncture (employing magnets), and acupressure (using the hands to target points) are all alternatives to needling, in descending order of effectiveness. Laser and magnet therapy require a licensed acupuncturist. Acupressure (or shiatsu) is a massage technique that can be deeply affecting, and sometimes even difficult to endure as the tender trigger points are pressed and released.

Yoga

It is near impossible to go anywhere these days without seeing someone with a yoga mat in a bag over her shoulder, and considering the benefits its hard to argue against the craze. One of the world's oldest forms of exercise and mind-body techniques (continuously practiced in India for over three thousand years) yoga is the mind-body movement therapy most extensively studied by Western science—with numerous controlled studies comparing yoga to other restful nonyoga interventions, sham yoga, or no intervention. The many schools and styles of yoga include general stretching, breathing, and relaxation (hatha); strenuous energizing breath work (kundalini); deeply meditative and restorative (pranayama, Kripalu); therapeutic, oriented toward working with medical conditions (Iyengar); and intensely aerobic (power, urban, Ashtanga or Jivamukti yoga). Much of the benefit of yoga stems from moving and stretching the body in profound, often unaccustomed ways—often while doing yoga you will find yourself in a position you haven't assumed since childhood—and much benefit stems from the breath work and mental focus required. The challenging postures and deep breathing (known as prana) accomplished through yogic techniques developed over thousands of years and constantly updated by the many gifted yogis practicing in North America today offer a vast resource of healing potential.

In numerous clinical trials yoga appears to have widespread beneficial effects on fitness, stress reduction, and energy levels. **A single yoga session can involve the entire nervous system and thousands of muscles, many of which are accessory groups that haven't been activated in years.** The most powerful aspect of yoga is actually the breath work,

Six Gentle, Energy-Generating Yoga Postures

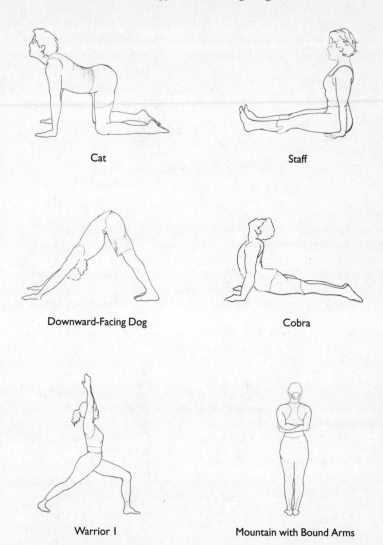

Cat

Staff

Downward-Facing Dog

Cobra

Warrior I

Mountain with Bound Arms

Here are some of my favorite energy-generating yoga postures. Getting into one of these postures requires specific steps. You should consult an instructor or an instruction video, and follow all of the preparatory steps required to complete the posture before attempting to try any of these.

which requires relaxed chest muscles and conscious control of the diaphragm in order to draw the air deeper. The overall effect is to energize corners of the body you forgot even exist, while calming the mind. By coordinating the rhythm of the breath with movement (for example, timing moments of exertion with exhalation) studies suggest the practice of yoga improves regulation of the autonomic nervous system. This vagal stimulation is thought to trigger a series of parasympathetic (calming) responses that buffer the effects of chronic stress. Amazingly, it doesn't take much yoga at all to achieve measurable results.

THE POWER OF YOGA

*Studies of yoga suggest the following beneficial effects**

After One 30-to-60-Minute Session	After Three to Eight Sessions	After Thirty Sessions
• Lowers heart rate	• Reduces cortisol (the master stress hormone)	• Reduces depression
• Lowers blood pressure		• Reduces anxiety
• Reduces fatigue	• Reduces blood pressure response to stress	• Accelerates cardiovascular recovery time from stress
• Reduces hostility		
• Induces digestion	• Activates antiinflammatory pathways	• Improves glucose tolerance
• Dilates arterioles	• Increases heart rate responsiveness	• Decreases visceral fat
	• Raises endorphin and serotonin levels (feel-good hormones)	• Reduces risk factors for arteriosclerosis, hypertension, and cardiovascular disease
	• Reduces the biochemical stress response	

* Compilation of numerous studies

The very real therapeutic effects of yoga perhaps explain its popularity. Numerous hospitals throughout the United States offer classes for therapy and rehabilitation, roughly 29 million Americans practice yoga and there are in the neighborhood of 70,000 yoga teachers. While I'm greatly in favor of this popularization, I am also concerned that it could lower the standards of yoga instruction. Recently, I heard about a combination wine tasting/yoga class, which sounds like fun, but is of dubious therapeutic value, to say the least. (For more on finding a good yoga instructor, see the 21-Day Plan, Day Eight.)

Once you learn the basic postures, you can practice yoga in a very small space in a relatively short time—at home, in the office, or on the road. If I had only one type of bodywork to recommend it would be yoga. It's a terrific way to reduce the perception of stress in your life, focus your attention on something that is good for you, and energize the forgotten recesses of your mind and body.

For more on yoga refer to Chapter 4.

Tai Chi

Tai chi is an ancient Chinese martial art that developed as an offshoot of qi gong, a major branch of traditional Chinese medicine. Tai chi combines controlled breathing with precise physical movements designed to build Qi (pronounced chee), or vital energy. Like yoga, there are multiple styles of tai chi (chen, yang, old wu, wu, and sun are just a few) all of which combine deep, diaphragmatic breathing with specific postures. Tai chi is a fluid practice; it entails performing a series of continuous movements that resemble a graceful slow-motion dance. Once restricted to highly secretive teaching within Taoist monasteries, tai chi classes are now more widely available. In my experience, patience is the only mandatory requirement for learning tai chi—not only because it is a slow-motion practice, but also because the postures are incredibly precise and require excellent muscle control.

Studies from several countries (of both healthy and chronically ill adults) suggest tai chi has similar effects on stress reduction as yoga—including lower blood pressure, reduced stress response, and enhanced heart function. **In a fascinating study from the Cousins Center for Psychoneuroimmunology of the University of California at Los Angeles Neuropsychiatric Institute, practicing tai chi for fifteen weeks improved older adults' immune response to a shingles vaccine.** Advanced practitioners claim to be able to manipulate energy (for example, releasing blocked energy) and nothing in my experience causes me to think this cannot be done. Several investigations offer evidence that tai chi reduces perceived stress and enhances stress-related coping, which is most likely a result of the focused attention required. In studies of elderly people, tai chi dramatically improved alertness, balance, and coordination. Quite simply, tai chi is a profound movement exercise that sharpens your mind, improves muscle tone and control, and is very likely to get your juices—and energy—flowing.

Supplements to Aid the Nervous System

If you are under a doctor's care for a medical condition, check with your doctor before taking any new supplements.

Nutriceuticals (nutritional supplements)

L-theanine: L-theanine is an amino acid, a natural nutrient comprising protein that is now sold in capsule form. L-theanine is one of my favorite calming aids: I liken it to a natural Valium, but without the drowsiness. It is found in green tea—and is the primary reason that the stimulants in green tea (theophylline, caffeine) provide a calming rather than a jagged lift. Studies have shown it reduces sympathetic nervous system activity—lowering heart rate and improving heart rate variability. It has also been shown to support the immune system. Much of L-theanine's calming and protective effect on the brain comes from its ability to block glutamate receptors—brain cell components that excite the nervous system and that need to be dampened for relaxation. Theanine has been shown to aid in raising beneficial brain neurotransmitters, including GABA, serotonin, and dopamine.

SAMe (S-adenosyl-methionine): SAMe is a very important nutrient for mood support. It is an active form of the amino acid methionine—the body converts the methionine in our food to SAMe. In this more active form, acting as methyl donor, SAMe has been shown to do three things, and do them well for many people: (1) help reduce arthritic symptoms (acting as an antiinflammatory), (2) help the liver detoxify, and (3) improve depression. SAMe provides the substrates the brain needs to make more mood-enhancing neurotransmitters, especially serotonin. (Precautions include needing medical guidance first if using SSRIs, and Parkinson's medications, and it can be overstimulating for some.)

5-HTP (5-hydroxy-tryptophan): 5HTP is another amino acid derivative. Its base, tryptophan, is also effective as a calming and antidepressant aid (serotonin is made from tryptophan)—but was removed from the market in the 1980s when a contaminated batch from Japan caused debilitating lung problems. Since then the more active form 5-HTP has safely been on the market, and used successfully to help induce a state of relaxation and improve mood. (Patients—especially those on SSRI antidepressants, antiseizure medications, and with Parkinson's and Down's syndrome—must consult their doctor before using.)

Magnesium: Magnesium is the second most common mineral in the body after calcium, and is extraordinarily important in many critical biological processes. It has been shown to help relax muscles, reduce vascular spasm in migraines and heart attacks, bronchial spasm in asthma, intestinal spasm in constipation, and blood vessel tension in hypertension. It also helps block the excitatory NMDA receptors in the brain, which is part of the explanation for its ability to calm some people. (Due to its huge range of physiological effects, and difficulty in measuring accurately in the blood, magnesium supplements should be used only with professional guidance.)

Botanicals (Herbs)

Chamomile (Chamomaelum nobile {Roman chamomile} or Matricaria recutita/chamomilla {German/English chamomile}): Certainly the best known of the relaxing herbs, chamomile has been used for centuries for its ability to calm the mind and body. It helps with stomach upset as well as emotional upset. Because of its pleasant taste, it is most commonly used as a tea or tincture. (Precautions pertain to its causing relaxation, with care in the daytime, and since it is in the ragweed family, people with these allergies should use with caution.)

Lemon balm (Melissa officinalis): This is another good-tasting herb that can be used as a relaxing tea. It has many active ingredients and, beside relaxation of the nervous system, has been shown to reduce stomach agitation (dyspepsia) and oral herpes. One interesting study showed reduced agitation in Alzheimer's patients. (Sedation is the main precaution.) *Other* calming herbs, such as valerian and passion flower, are better used as sleep inducters and are discussed in Chapter 5.

Lavender oil (Lavandula officinalis/angustifolia): Lavender oil has been used for centuries as a calming or sleep aid (depending on amount employed). Plus it smells beautiful. Lavender is administered by placing a couple of drops in an essential oil diffuser, or by diluting it with a neutral oil (such as almond oil) and rubbing into the skin—its active ingredients can be absorbed through the skin. (Don't take lavender oil internally, and be aware that its use can make you drowsy.)

Homeopathy: I was raised with homeopathy and use it daily in my practice for stress management, digestive disorders, upper respiratory allergic and asthmatic problems, and musculo-skeletal injuries to name a few. It is a medical discipline, first developed by a German physician in the nineteenth century, that utilizes dilute amounts of natural substances to stimulate the body's healing processes—in a manner likened to that of vaccines. A core concept in homeopathy is the restoration of a person's vital energy—leading to balance and amelioration of physical and psychological problems. Homeopathy is not intended to be primary treatment for serious or life-threatening diseases—it is too gentle for that. But for more limited physical problems, and for emotional issues it can be very beneficial. It is best used on the advice of a homeopathic practitioner who will take an extensive history. While reduction of stress and balancing of mood as both cause and effect in illness is a central part of homeopathic practice, there is no such thing as a homeopathic valium or valerian—each person's remedy is established by the totality of his or her unique characteristics.

Chapter 2

Power Food, Your High
Performance Fuel

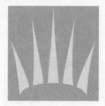

KATE, a working mom in her late thirties, came to me complaining of all-day fatigue, which despite her hectic life surprised her because she felt she had a healthy lifestyle and had recently lost ten pounds with a lower calorie diet. After quizzing her extensively on her new eating habits I discovered that she was consuming a diet high in wheat, and with too many refined carbohydrates. This resulted in late morning cravings for sugar, as well as for other foods that in susceptible people can drain rather than support energy. She also had been consuming caffeinated beverages that were contributing to a late afternoon crash.

The first step was to eliminate suspected food allergens—energy-draining foods. For the coming month she would have to avoid a number of the most common food sensitizers (wheat, eggs, nuts, red meat, dairy, caffeine, and alcohol), after which she would add them back one at a time every three days. This is the most accurate way to tell what foods your body reacts poorly to—better than any blood or skin test.

Right away Kate felt a difference when she eliminated wheat. She realized that she literally crashed after eating pasta! I recommended substituting nutritious "Old-World" whole grains such as spelt and kamut. We added nutrient-dense foods (such as morning energy shakes) and energy-enhancing noncaffeinated beverages throughout the day. Much to her surprise her energy zoomed back. Whenever she started back on wheat or caffeine, she felt a near-immediate decrease in energy.

FOOD MEANS DIFFERENT THINGS to different people: For foodies it's an art form to be celebrated and almost worshipped; for chronically overweight people it's a public enemy and sometimes secret lover; for the office-bound it's the hassle to get something, anything, delivered quickly; for many food represents the drudgery of daily preparation and for others it represents the sustenance of home. But for all people eating serves one vital purpose, and that is to provide fuel to support all of the body's processes. The most fundamental of these processes, necessary for any other cellular action to take place, is the creation of energy within the cell. Underlying life is energy: From energy all else flows. **With the 21-Day Plan, I'm going to reconnect you with the power of the energy in your food.**

Over the last half-century, as major food corporations have been liberating us from the labor of cooking from scratch, we've grown increasingly distant from the process of nourishing ourselves. We don't have to grow our food (an activity that imparts a tremendous appreciation for its energy and life force), we often don't have to cook it, and sometimes we don't even have to touch it with our hands, so clever is the packaging. It's no coincidence that, as food has become more convenient and is increasingly cultivated at greater distances from the majority of the population, we have as a people grown fatter and increasingly fatigued.

With this book I'm hoping you will see the wonder in the process that takes the potential chemical energy available in nature and transforms it into high-energy bio-molecules of life used to power every system in your body. Once a morsel hits your palate it begins the conversion into vital energy—this is one aspect of the food supply chain that hasn't changed a bit over the millions of years that people have been eating. But not all food holds the same potential to be transformed into energy. In the 21-Day Plan you will learn how to eat for more energy and health.

From a biochemical perspective your body is a massive nanotechnology manufacturing facility. Every day, food provides the raw materials your DNA uses to operate, maintain, repair, and, in many cases, replace parts. Most people think you only need DNA in order to inherit traits from your parents in the womb, but that couldn't be farther from the truth. DNA is the seat of intelligence in every cell that directs all processes within the cell on an ongoing basis—whether it's a pancreas cell producing insulin or a stomach cell aiding digestion. One of its critical functions is to make sure the cell survives by monitoring the cell's environment and regenerating itself. **As part of that process your DNA is programmed to replace almost every cell in your body every six months throughout your life. DNA provides the blueprint, but the integrity of the construction of this continually recycled-you depends largely on what you eat.** Energy, manufactured in each cell by special DNA located inside a tiny structure called mitochondria, drives this process of biofabrication, and the quality of your energy stems from the quality of your food. **When you eat whole plant foods, for example, your genes have the key to unlock the energy of the sun that is stored in leaves and stems, roots, seeds, and flowers.** When you eat processed foods full of synthetic preservatives, colorings, and flavorings, your body spends a great deal of energy separating out the artificial ingredients from whatever nutrients it can find.

The importance of eating whole plant foods has become increasingly clear with cutting-edge research from the field of functional medicine, a new scientific discipline founded by brilliant nutritional biochemist Jeffrey Bland, Ph.D., that explains at a molecular level how food—along with all aspects of lifestyle and environment—contributes to health and energy. Functional medicine offers a revolutionary new way of looking at food: The nutrients in food are molecular messengers that guide each cell's DNA. It turns out that whole plant foods carry incredibly sophisticated, health promoting signals for your genetic blueprint. **These messengers give food the potential to switch on beneficial aspects of your particular genome and switch off destructive aspects of your genome.** For example, the incorporation of fish or flax oil into your diet reduces the tendency for cell damage in chronic inflammatory conditions such as heart disease and arthritis. In this way food can be your best preventive medicine, helping you to avoid genetic predispositions to disease. By making food choices that deliver more pro-energy molecular messages and fewer energy-draining molecular signals you can reprogram your body to maximize energy—I will show you how.

Much of what I have learned treating patients over the years has to do with first eliminating foods that muck up the body's ability to heal itself and create energy. Like Kate, many people spend their days eating energy-draining foods. My role has been to rein in those impulses by teaching how and why some foods drain energy and others enhance energy. One way to remove energy drains is to detect food allergies and sensitivities that are symptoms of runaway inflammation set in motion by the immune system. Another way is to reduce or eliminate artificial stimulants. You should also avoid certain foods like burnt red meat, fried foods, and refined sugar that can lead to the creation of harmful chemical by-products called free radicals, which damage DNA and cause premature aging of cells. As you cull out foods with a negative effect on energy you will also begin to add foods with beneficial effects, which form the heart of the 21-Day Plan.

The medical establishment has been slow to leverage the importance of food to people's health and well-being, but there have been some very helpful advances in public policy. I am a great fan of food labels, which have become increasingly detailed as the chemistry of prepared foods has become more complex. It's crucial to know what you are eating, and to make choices that will promote energy and health rather than fatigue and accelerated aging. With this chapter you will have what it takes to understand what you are buying and eating, and to reclaim the energy that nature has to offer.

It's fashionable today to talk about food in terms of evolution and to note that our metabolism—which was fixed several hundred thousand years ago—and our instinct to eat when food is abundant haven't changed along with our lifestyle. Our ancestors were active hunter-gatherers, but we've become sedentary web surfers in a society overflowing with sugar-dense, fat-heavy, chemical-laden foods. Yet there are also many more clean and healthy foods available than at any time in recent history. Another aspect of evolution that I think is even more important is the increase in the average lifespan. **When there was a high probability of being killed by a saber-toothed tiger or smallpox or bubonic plague before age forty, it hardly mattered if you were suffering damage from free radicals or toxins that degrade health over the long term. But if you want to live to a ripe old age (average in the United States is now seventy-eight years) cumulative damage matters.** As you age (which is just another word for sustained damage to DNA), your cells get more and more depleted—think of wrinkles, but on the inside—and your body becomes less efficient at making energy, which is the basis for all functions. By consuming wholesome foods that cause minimal damage and promote maximum repair of cells, however, you can stave off the aging process, dramatically increase your energy, and begin to reverse many common health problems. With this book, you will learn how to eat for the new longevity.

Don't feel bad if you discover that your diet requires a great deal of revamping. You're in good company. Many senior medical school students don't know the first thing about food and nutrition, and I know many doctors who still don't understand it well. Advances in biochemistry and genetics are happening so quickly that it's an effort to keep up with learning about the role food plays in creating energy and health. The best advice I can give is to keep your diet simple and make changes thoughtfully so they will be lasting changes. Altering your diet is not something you can do overnight. **If I could I would turn back the clock on our collective dining lives—to an era when processed and packaged foods were not so readily available, and every patch of real estate wasn't replete with a coffee emporium selling scones and pound cake.** Since I can't, my goal is to help you embark on a thrilling journey back to nature—to connect you with the energy of the sun stored in plants, available to us as fruits and vegetables—and to bring life and vital energy to the daily process of nourishing your body.

Making Energy

All ... at are making energy every microsecond
... ular fires—food and oxygen delivered by
... **(derived from carbohydrates) is the**
... **ed with oxygen to make energy, there**
... **alled co-factors) essential for energy**
... **y has to acquire from what you eat.**
..., it breaks down every mouthful into glu-
... ozens of other nutrients (vitamins, minerals,
...s) that it absorbs and sends into the blood sup-
... process: The bloodstream delivers sugar, nutri-
... gen to each cell, and your cells' internal energy
... nondria) then use the nutrients to combine the sugar
... create energy. A heart attack caused by a clogged artery
... utdown in the fuel supply to the heart. Without the regu-
... nutrients and oxygen the heart can't make energy, and goes
into an... kly dying if the fuel line isn't restored.

The Energy "One-a-Days"

Here, some of the most important vitamins and minerals required for making energy: Vitamins B1 (thiamin), B2 (riboflavin), B3 (niacin) and B6 (pantothenic acid); biotin; iron; calcium; magnesium; vitamin C, zinc, and copper.

Every single one of the trillions of cells in your body can unlock the energy inherent in food and transform it into a sort of universal energetic currency called adenosine triphospate (ATP), available for any purpose. **A precise molecule of energy, ATP is made in the mitochondria of each cell. Even more amazing, each cell has the ability to determine how much energy it needs at any given moment.** At the core of the process of energy creation is a tiny structure within the cell called the mitochondrion—this is the body's energy factory. Each cell contains multiple mitochondria, depending on the cell's function. An energy-guzzling heart muscle cell can contain up to 100,000 mitochondria (comprising two-thirds of the heart's volume), whereas a short-lived sperm cell contains about ten mitochondria—with all due respect to the sperm, that's like the difference between a high-performance car battery and a triple-A. But the number of mitochondria (most cells contain about three thousand) is only one reason cells can make different amounts of energy.

The mitochondrion also has its own intelligence, that is, it contains its own DNA (inherited strictly from your mother) separate from the main DNA in the cell's nucleus. That mitochondrial DNA, when it's functioning properly, is immensely adaptive—capable of jump-starting its energy production rate on demand via a complex system of cell surface receptors, inner cell enzymes, and transport proteins—all of which regulate the amount of fuel entering the cell and the amount delivered to its energy factory. **This dance between regulatory mechanisms within the cell makes your body capable of incredibly intelligent energy creation.** For example, it allows your body to produce and consume much more energy when running a marathon than it will when you're sitting for a long car ride.

Once ATP has been made from sugar and oxygen in the cell's mitochondrial forge, it is released into the system as pure energy, leaving behind a sort of shadow molecule that goes back into the cell and waits to be once again transformed into ATP, like a microscopic recyclable battery. On average an ATP molecule of energy (of which your cells create billions every moment) gets recycled a thousand times per day. The process also generates heat, water, and toxic by-products called free radicals, but it results in the ultimate prize—that intangible animating substance we call energy. The ability to generate energy in each cell evolved over eons (molecular paleontologists have dated the origin of mitochondria back 1.6 billion years); our prowess for creating energy is what makes it possible to sustain the improbable complexity of the human body.

This miraculously complicated metabolic transformation from food and oxygen into energy is called the Krebs cycle. Trying to fully understand it has made medical students quake in their boots for generations. Most doctors have been content to memorize the Krebs for their exams and then forget it, but increasingly the Krebs cycle (and the nutrient spectrum required to complete it) has become the focus of nutritional science, and a rich area of research for preventive medicine. **The upshot of what scientists have learned about the Krebs over the past decade is that having a supply of nutrients sufficient for completing the cycle ceaselessly every day—and for keeping the mitochondria clear of damaging free radicals—is crucial to optimal health and energy.**

In an ideal world—where people eat a nutrient-dense, unpolluted diet and live stress-free, active lives—the mitochondria are efficient energy-generating machines capable of capturing 40 percent of the energy stored in food. Unfortunately, we don't live in an ideal world, and don't feed our systems the fuel needed to keep those millions of machines—performing the Krebs cycle over and over again—in good working order. **The Krebs requires basic elements worthy of a steel mill—iron, sulfur, copper, and zinc are all needed to make energy as well as at least a dozen other nutrients including the B complex vitamins and vitamin C.** All of those essential substances for making energy must enter the body by food—or supplements. I was shocked to find out a few years back that most people lack a full supply of the nutritional building blocks of energy when a definitive study from the Harvard School of Public Health determined that the majority of the adult population is deficient in vitamins and minerals. These deficiencies are considered to be subtle—**you may not have beri-beri, but your body is struggling to keep up with the nutritional demands of making energy.** Without sufficient nutrients, your cells have to beg borrow and steal from

Your Body's Energy Factory

CELL

GLUCOSE

Pyruvate

MITOCHONDRION

Actyl CoA

B Vitamins

CO_2

KREBS CYCLE

Minerals

O_2

B Vitamins

H

O_2

H_2O

ATP

ENERGY

KREBS CYCLE

Endoplasmic Reticulum

Nucleus

Ribisomes

Golgi Apparatus

Mitochondria

The multiple mitochondria within each cell of your body carry out a process called the Kreb's Cycle in order to manufacture energy from food and oxygen. Providing the nutrients necessary for the Kreb's Cycle is a key to maintaining healthy energy.

wherever they can (tissues, organs, neighboring cells), setting up a process of depletion that can lead to fatigue and ultimately disease.

In addition to often missing key nutrients for energy generation, your body's energy-making mechanisms are constantly under assault from environmental pollution (see Chapter 3) and three damaging internal processes—oxidation, inflammation, and glycation (see the "The Three Enemies of Energy," below). The mitochondria are routinely gummed-up, weakened, and sometimes even killed by these damaging processes, all of which are exacerbated (and some even created) by poor eating habits. The good news is you can eat foods that maximize your body's energy-generating capacity and minimize destructive processes in the cell discussed in detail later on. In the 21-Day Plan you learn how to do this by following the simple, delicious menus and recipes every day.

The Energy in Food

In conventional science the "energy" in food refers to the calories (the lion's share of which comes from sugars and fats). The traditional scientific worldview has come to realize that consuming too many calorie-dense foods is at the heart of many of our most common medical ailments— obesity, diabetes, heart disease, even cancer are significantly linked to overeating calorie-dense foods. **But the new science—based on our recently acquired understanding of the biological processes that take place inside a single cell—conceives of the energy in food as *all* of the constituents that contribute to the creation of energy: the calorie-carrying macronutrients (carbohydrates, proteins, and fats), along with the essential micronutrients including amino acids, vitamins, minerals, enzymes, and a host of other compounds that protect your DNA.**

Chronic overconsumption of macronutrient-dense sugars and meats, and chronic underconsumption of micronutrient-dense plants is a problem of epidemic proportion. I am always shocked by the fact that counting the potatoes in french fries and tomatoes in ketchup makes those two plants the most widely consumed vegetables in the United States. Since one of ketchup's main ingredients is sugar and french fries have more calories from the saturated fat in which they're cooked than in their potato base, this represents an extremely unhealthy state of affairs.

Empty, sugar-rich calories can give you a quick boost, but they ultimately do more harm than good. Your cells require a simple sugar molecule as the basic ingredient for making energy. **A sugar (or glucose) molecule's usefulness as an energy source, however, depends on several variables: how quickly that sugar gets absorbed, and whether or not it comes with a posse of nutrients that help convert the sugar into energy and clear the cell of free radicals created by the conversion process.** Eating sugar alone, say, in a doughnut, without essential nutrients forces the cell to use up some of its stores of micronutrients to convert the sugar into energy, and that sets off a process of depletion. **The best sugar source for energy comes from complex carbohydrates (whole grains,** brown rice, beans, lentils) that contain multiple energy-building and damage-controlling nutrients as well as fiber to slow the absorption of sugar to a steady stream.

Your cells also require protein to provide amino acids used for many critical cell functions like building muscle, hormones, and neurotransmitters as well as providing a back-up energy source. The problem is that the proteins most commonly consumed in the West come loaded with unhealthy fats. Red meat, while it does carry many energy co-factors like iron, zinc, folic acid, and the B vitamins, also delivers highly damaging saturated fats. The fats you need for optimum health are monounsaturated and omega-3 unsaturated fats (present in fatty fish, nuts, and olive oil, for example). These fats are key components in maintaining the integrity of your cells, and their constituent fatty acids can be used as fuel in an emergency. **A switch from refined to complex carbohydrates and from animal fats to fats from plants and fish will go a long way in improving your energy and endurance.**

Food pyramids foster the misperception that all foods fall into one of three distinct macronutrient categories—carbohydrates, proteins, or fats. This has led to the demonization of foods like carrots and eggs, which contain essential nutrients beyond the starches and fats that give them a bad rap. The reality is that foods cross boundaries; many foods contain a mix of macronutrients and micronutrients. I am a strong proponent of eating broadly within a spectrum that contains a balance of macronutrients (ideally 40 percent complex carbs, 30 percent lean protein, 30 percent healthy fats) packed with multiple micronutrients (see **"Power foods,"** page 80) including antioxidants, antiinflammatories, vitamins, minerals, and enzymes—all of which are essential for making and maintaining a vital energy supply.

At the risk of alienating dyed-in-the-wool devotees of "meat-sweet," which is what nutritional scientists disparagingly call the American diet, it's best to eat lean, plant-based foods. The typical meat-sweet diet is deficient in so many nutrients that it causes premature aging of nuclear and mitochondrial DNA (that means it makes you look and feel older and more tired than you should, and predisposes you to many debilitating health problems). Taking a multivitamin will help you extract more energy from food by providing energy's manufacturing co-factors, especially if your diet is heavy on meat and sugar, but if you really want to achieve optimal energy and feel ten years younger, you'll want to eat primarily nutrient-dense, unprocessed, plant-based foods. The 21-Day Plan

Calories Are Kindling

The calories in food provide the combustible material for creating energy. Different foods have different energy potential based on their calorie content. Nutritionists calculate calorie content based on the heat liberated when a specific food is entirely burned-up (in a device called a bomb calorimeter). Foods high in fat are the most calorie dense (over two times that of proteins and carbohydrates). A typical adult female who expends 2100 kCal of food energy each day would have to consume 420 celery stalks, 105 carrots, 26 eggs, yet only 1 1/4 cup of peanut butter to meet her daily energy needs. Filling up on vegetables and consuming moderate quantities of protein and carbohydrates along with small amounts of healthy fats is the best way to keep your fire burning all day long.

will take you through the baby steps you need to take to make this transition, and it will get you completely immersed in the nutrient-dense, energy-rich, plant-based diet. The 21 Day Plan involves interacting with produce (as I like to call it). Everyone who has done it reports a renewed sense of connection to the planet—and to the energy of the sun—by simply beginning to eat more glorious plants!

Talk to Your DNA

On a basic level, food is nothing more than a collection of genetic signaling molecules. When you eat a lot of sugar you signal your DNA to produce insulin. Tucking into a slab of Wagyu beef loaded with saturated fat can signal your DNA to create inflammatory molecules that among other mischief oxidize cholesterol, causing it to stick to the inside of your blood vessels. Eating fish signals your DNA to create antiinflammatory molecules that prevent harmful oxidation of fats. Every time you eat, you ingest substances that interact with your DNA, causing changes at the molecular level. If you want to tell your DNA to create more energy, you have to send the right signals.

So-called Energy

"Energy" seems to be the food industry's code word for drinks and snack bars packed with caffeine and sugar, which provide an immediate rush often followed by a crash. These so-called "energy" foods are actually energy substitutes: They mimic the effects of energy, but deplete your energy supply. If you use them as short-term fixes, make sure you also replenish essential nutrients, and get real rest. For making energy, catnaps beat caffeine, hands down.

Caffeine, probably the most widely used "energy" food, does not tell your DNA to make more energy, but rather tells your DNA to activate your nervous system. This may improve your sense of mental alertness, but the process of stimulating your nervous system actually *expends* energy. By contrast, aerobic exercise utilizes energy and burns calories, but it also causes the body to *create* more cellular energy factories. A jolt of caffeine consumes energy that in turn produces a rogue's gallery of damaging by-products. As a result, your DNA is told to clean up, which requires still more energy that could in fact be used for other purposes, like staying alert.

The way to coax your body into making more energy available for every task is to eat foods rich in the raw materials of energy manufacture, which signal your DNA to make energy. Sugar is the necessary foundation for creating an energy molecule (your body can make energy without sugar, but not at all efficiently), but the type of sugar you eat is absolutely critical. When you eat a complex carbohydrate, say a bowl of whole grain granola, you get starch that's converted into sugar, but you also get fiber to control the delivery of sugar and make you feel full, and the germ that contains hundreds of different phytochemicals—including the energy essentials zinc, copper, B complex vitamins, and vitamin E. Complex carbohydrates such as whole grains or beans allow the body to generate energy efficiently and mop up free radicals, sending pro-energy metabolic signals to your DNA. Better yet, eat your granola with almonds (that provide monounsaturated fats and amino acids, important energy co-factors) and a handful of blueberries (with antioxidants to sweep away toxic by-products.) That's the sort of snack that "tells" your DNA to manufacture clean energy.

Three Enemies of Energy—Inflammation, Oxidation, and Glycation

There are three processes within the cell that unnecessarily consume large amounts of energy, produce premature aging, and cause widespread damage: *oxidation, inflammation,* and *glycation*. All of these processes are affected by what you eat. Inflammation and oxidation are part of natural cell life, but when they happen in excess—from eating a typical Western diet, for example—they lead to cell damage and fatigue. The third cell-damaging process, glycation, is solely a result of sugar excess. Glycation is never a normal process, but it is becoming more prevalent in our society where highly concentrated sugar increasingly in the form of high fructose corn syrup is pervasive (you'll find it in bread, ketchup, salad dressing, and breakfast cereal to name a few sources). Minimizing these three processes is crucial to having high energy and good health.

I am asking you, as I do many of my patients, to eliminate the worst offenders that cause these processes. I realize it's asking a lot; many in-flammatory foods—such as sweets, meats, and cheese—taste delicious. (Keep in mind that everyone's vulnerabilities are different; part of this program is identifying which foods affect your body most.) But it's extremely important to protect cells from these three damaging processes, especially the cells in our most vital organs.

So here's the deal: I want you to read the case against these processes and decide for yourself. You be the jury, and send down a verdict on the offenders. The sentence I recommend: Banish the offending foods (see **Trouble Foods to Avoid,** below), and hold wild dinner parties with the many protective foods mentioned in this section and detailed in the **Power Foods** chart.

Inflammation

Inflammation is a powerful and wildly diverse immune response. Think of inflammation as your body's military defense network. It's a life-sustaining process by which the immune system identifies, attacks, and repairs damage from potentially injurious substances—without it we'd have no effective immunity. Like all defense systems, inflammation's use-fulness depends on its ability to recognize a substance as foreign, or not "self"—its target can be bacteria, a virus, a toxin, food, or even one's own tissue in the case of autoimmune disease. It can be seen in a broad range of anatomical events: from the redness, swelling, and heat that accompanies a sunburn to the bloating, pain, and diarrhea of inflammatory bowel disease; from the formation of plaque in your arteries to the hives, swelling, and trouble breathing initiated by a peanut allergy.

The retaliatory assault begins with a warning signal—that can be sent by just a single cell to far-flung locations in the body—carrying the message that defenses have been breached, and a potentially destructive process is underway. The immune system's first line of inflammatory defense, led by white blood cells, sends out multiple chemical messengers that mobilize the body's resources both locally and systemically to remove the bad guys. The most important of these immune messenger molecules are cytokines. Cytokines signal cells throughout the body to spring into action and send in reinforcements. In response, the immune system sends out a full defensive assault team: natural killer cells are the samurai warriors that engulf invaders; tumor necrosis factor is the flame thrower that disintegrates molecules; platelets are field docs ordered to stop bleeding; fibrin throws a sticky mesh over the area to hold it together. All the while neighboring cells release more cytokines to continue the inflammatory reaction. When the battle is won, to calm the warriors the body has a group of *anti*inflammatory substances—manufactured by cells and absorbed from foods—that turn the process off.

Chronic inflammation occurs when the inflammatory machinery doesn't get turned off. This is the abnormal process central to such common illnesses as coronary artery disease, diabetes, arthritis, Crohn's disease and ulcerative colitis, obesity, Alzheimer's, Parkinson's, and chronic fatigue. **Increasingly chronic inflammation is being suggested as the common link between *all* chronic illnesses.** For example, cancer researchers are only beginning to unravel the incredibly complex behaviors of the immune system's inflammatory molecules, which are thought to be able to either halt a tumor in its tracks or encourage its growth.

Lifestyle can magnify the inflammatory response—poor eating habits, high stress levels, and exposure to toxins (like tobacco smoke, air pollution, and heavy metals) can throw off the body's ability to maintain the balance between promoting and quelling inflammation, thereby creating a chronic state. **Food is a crucial factor in the inflammatory equation. Eating is the most constant and unremitting activity that can introduce proinflammatory "foreign" substances into the body, and can also introduce substances that calm inflammation.**

We now know that certain fats universally create inflammation and

How Fats Affect Inflammation

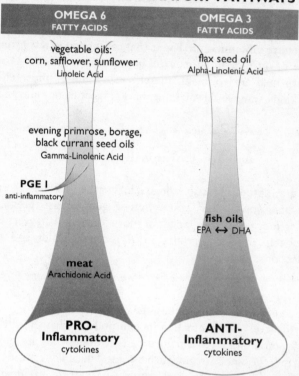

FATTY ACID INFLAMMATORY PATHWAYS

OMEGA 6 FATTY ACIDS	OMEGA 3 FATTY ACIDS

vegetable oils:
corn, safflower, sunflower
Linoleic Acid

flax seed oil
Alpha-Linolenic Acid

evening primrose, borage,
black currant seed oils
Gamma-Linolenic Acid

PGE I
anti-inflammatory

fish oils
EPA ↔ DHA

meat
Arachidonic Acid

PRO-Inflammatory
cytokines

ANTI-Inflammatory
cytokines

When digested, fats are transformed into substances that can either create or quell inflammation. On the *good* side of the divide (right) are foods that contain Omega-3 Fatty Acids that are transformed into *antiinflammatory* substances. On the *bad* side of the divide (left) are foods (for example red meat) that contain Omega 6 Fatty Acids, which are transformed into *proinflammatory* substances. Eating more Omega-3s can reduce damaging inflammation in your body.

others quell inflammation. There are two main classes of bad fats: The first includes saturated fat in meats, poultry, eggs, dairy, and some fish (shellfish, squid, and octopus all have cholesterol) and polyunsaturated fats in corn and safflower oil, all of which can be converted to arachidonic acid, a toxic substance the body uses to make proinflammatory cytokines. The other category of bad fats is man-made trans fats in margarine and baked goods, which directly cause inflammation. There are two categories of good fats as well: monosaturated (from olive and grapeseed oils); and omega-3 oils from flax, fish, nuts and seeds. These essential fatty acids (EFAs) are used by the body to make antiinflammatory cytokines. **Simply by switching from eating unhealthy fats to healthy fats you can dramatically reduce inflammation. Foods that contain good fats promote the creation of antiinflammatory cytokines and allow your DNA to operate in an optimal environment, thereby using energy more efficiently.** Which kind of fats would you rather have circulating in your system?

Are You Chronically Inflammed?

The symptoms: Muscle stiffness, joint aches, asthma, allergies, irritable bowel, slow wound healing, gum disease, premature aging, morning fatigue, longer or more frequent hangovers from moderate drinking, intense jetlag, recurring colds and sinus infections.

In addition to the mix of fats, the type of carbohydrate you eat also affects the level of inflammation in your body. Studies show that eating high glycemic index (GI), refined carbohydrates that are quickly absorbed into the blood stream (such as white wheat flour breads and pastas, potatoes, and white rice) causes an increase in inflammatory molecules. Conversely, when you eat low GI carbos (such as whole grains, beans, and legumes) there is a marked decrease in circulating inflammatory molecules.

Food allergies are another common source of inflammation. Most people are not surprised to learn that classic food allergies (which cause an immediate, acute reaction) produce inflammation. But most people don't know about the prevalence of more subtle delayed food allergies and sensitivities, which operate along slightly different inflammatory and immune pathways than immediate allergies. (For more on allergies see "Hidden Allergies," page 76.)

While I want you to eat fewer foods that cause inflammation, I also want you to eat more foods that calm it. As scientists have been elucidating the complex immune process of inflammation they have also

Power Foods that fight inflammation

Salmon, trout, almonds, walnuts, legumes, cruciferous vegetables, dark leafy greens, tea, grape skin, citrus, olive oil, turmeric, ginger, garlic, and rosemary.

learned a lot about what stops it. Cruciferous vegetables, legumes, nuts and seeds, olive oil, herbs and spices, and fatty fish all contain dozens of antiinflammatory compounds—including bioflavonoids, polyphenols, catechins, and anthocyanins. These compounds, which the human body cannot make, were developed by plants and fish to fight off their own inflammation and diseases, but can be used by our bodies to switch off the destructive activities of inflammatory molecules without weakening the immune response. Many of these compounds—for example, the flavanoids in turmeric—directly reduce the activity of the cell's internal DNA messenger NF-kB (nuclear factor-kappa beta) that can force the cell into inflammation hyperdrive. Food changes the messages getting to your DNA. **By eating foods that fight inflammation you free up your body's energy supply to be used for more productive pursuits and reduce the risk of developing one of the many diseases—including cancer, heart disease, and diabetes—that are now associated with inflammation.**

Knowledge of the importance of dampening systemic inflammation is leading to a frenzied search for new antiinflammatory pharmaceuticals such as NF-kB inhibitors (one of turmeric's specialties). In reality, the body has sophisticated mechanisms for managing the inflammatory process with a proper, antiinflammatory diet and healthy lifestyle—especially in the early stages of inflammation. Your daily sustenance should be low in inflammatory foods and high in foods that provide antiinflammatory substances along with the substrates (primarily essentially fatty acids) for manufacturing the body's own internal antiinflammatory brigade. Hence the adage: Food is your best medicine.

Oxidation

This particular enemy arises from the love-hate relationship most life-forms have with oxygen. Your ability to create energy efficiently—and support life—depends on oxygen. But while oxygen gives life to your cells, it also can be corrosive, with the ability to damage or oxidize cells (think of rust and tarnish). **The very act of energy creation invites oxygen into the inner, most vulnerable part of the cell—the nucleus and mitochondria—creating a number of highly destructive substances called free radicals as a natural by-product of energy creation (think of it as your mitochondrial smokestack).** You are constantly ingesting, absorbing, and creating free radicals, not only from your own metabolism, but also from certain toxic foods, air and water pollution, and sun exposure—they're everywhere!

Naked Genes

Compared to your cell's main, genomic DNA (which has a fairly sophisticated system of defense against free radicals) the energy-generating mitochondrial (mt) DNA is relatively naked—it's a small and simple structure, without the twisting spiral configuration, and is easily damaged by free radicals. When the mtDNA suffers damage the cell's ability to produce energy slows, like reducing the voltage on your battery.

These free radicals (most of which are known by the rather Jurassic title of reactive oxygen species) can easily damage your all-important mitochondrial and nuclear DNA and harm other delicate cell structures, including membranes that hold the cell together and enzymes that constantly break down debris. The body has a number of compounds designed to very efficiently eliminate free radicals, these are home-grown antioxidants continually produced by the cells (for those of you who work the *Scientific American* crossword puzzle, the big three natural antioxidants are glutathione reductase, superoxide dismutase, and catalase). **Problems arise, however, when the free radical bad guys outnumber your internal antioxidant good guys. This is when your body looks to nature to send in reinforcements in the form of foods that provide addi-**

tional antioxidants. Vitamins E, C, and the carotenes are prime examples, but there are hundreds of other compounds found in abundance in fruits (especially berries and citrus), vegetables (especially leafy greens and cruciferi like broccoli and cauliflower), and green tea.

My mantra for dealing with oxidation is: reduce exposure; increase protection. It's critically important to reduce the cumulative burden of free radicals.

First, if you smoke, please stop—free radicals are only the tip of the toxic iceberg that is a cigarette. Second, avoid free radical-promoting foods (charred meats, refined sugar, trans-fats, fried foods). Another good fix is to exercise more and moderately (overly intense aerobic activity generates free radicals); and work out as far away as you possibly can from car exhaust and other pollution. Avoid overimbibing alcohol to the point of getting a hangover, which is basically an overdose of toxins and free radicals. Drink adequate amounts of water (minimum six glasses a day), which will support your body's ability to excrete the neutralized free radicals and other toxins. By practicing relaxation exercises you can reduce the nervous system's enormous energy needs, and thereby reduce the free radicals that result from constant energy manufacture. But reducing free radicals is not as easy as it sounds. In addition to being in the environment, they are also ubiquitous, natural—albeit harmful—by-products of metabolism.

You can, however, make a dramatic impact on your body's ability to protect cells from free radical damage by simply eating more foods with antioxidants. You may have had it up to here with food and drink labels that scream the latest miracle antioxidant story. So let me make this easy. The best antioxidant foods are those that carry hundreds of multiple beneficial compounds, which can only be said of fresh fruits and vegetables. **I don't care how good food scientists are at their job, it is not possible to design a processed food with the complex antioxidant capabilities of a plant**—especially one that has been grown organically in nutrient-dense, pollution-free soil. You will find a more complete listing of antioxidant foods in the Power Foods chart, but **here is my short list of antioxidant foods to start eating now: blueberries, cranberries, green tea, broccoli, dark chocolate, carrots, spinach, kale, cantaloupe, yams, tomatoes, and citrus.** Color is of the utmost importance because plant pigments such as chlorophyll, carotenes, flavonoids, and anthocyanodins are antioxidants—in fact color may very well be part of a plant's own defense mechanism.

By eating a diet full of colorful plants (a so-called "rainbow diet") you will reduce oxidative stress and are very likely to reduce your chance of getting cancer and many other diseases. In their wonderful book *Healing Foods*, naturopaths Michael Murray and Joseph Pizzorno write, "Some experts have said—and we agree—that cancer is a result of a 'maladaptation' over time to a reduced level of intake of fruits and vegetables." While this may be an oversimplification I believe there's a great deal of truth in it. At the very least, when you become a devotée of produce you will protect your mitochondria from oxidation, and as a result you will protect your energy supply.

Glycation

OK, here we go with the sugar bashing. You've heard it before, but it's an important part of the energy story. When the body has too much circulating sugar—which is almost always a result of eating too many rapidly absorbed sugars from overly refined carbohydrates—the resulting excess glucose molecules will eventually start sticking to proteins, in a process called glycation. Glycation transforms the molecular structure of cells, damaging their function and making them die an early death. I call this sugar aging; it happens every time your blood sugar spikes.

Low *Glycemic Load** Carbs You Can Eat

Pumpernickel bread, plain steel-cut oatmeal, wholemeal rye bread, spelt multigrain bread, All-Bran cereal, muesli cereal, Kashi, Rye Crisp bread, lentils, beans, apples, cherries, grapefruit, kiwi, oranges, tomato juice.

* Note: *Glycemic Load* is below 10.

People often have a "that's-not-me" attitude toward the concept of sugar aging. This is partly due to a common misconception about how the body receives sugar. A food does not have to be made with table sugar (called sucrose) in order to deliver sugar to the cells. For example, white rice is rapidly converted into sugar even though it doesn't contain sucrose. Nutritional scientists have given us two ways to determine whether or not a food will cause a spike in blood sugar—glycemic index and glycemic load. Glycemic index (GI) is a measure of how quickly sugar is absorbed from a food; glycemic load (GL) is a measure of the amount of sugar a food actually delivers to the cells. Glycemic *load* is the more relevant number. Eating low glycemic *load* foods is the most critically important way to reduce glycation.

One hidden trove of sugars is the veritable mountain of new low-fat foods, which are routinely given extra sugar to make up for the loss in flavor from fat. This sets up a situation in which two scoops of full-fat ice cream carry a lower glycemic load (registering 6.1) than a typical cup of low-fat yogurt (registering 8.5 on the GL scale). (The ice cream has a lower GL because fat slows absorption of sugar, although this doesn't make ice cream a health food.) Mind you, both a serving of ice cream and of yogurt have a fraction of the glycemic load of a plain bagel (which racks up a whopping 25 points on the GL scale). Indeed, Americans get a full 42 percent of their sugar from baked goods. It's no wonder, since high fructose corn syrup (a highly concentrated manufactured sugar) is the second ingredient on most bread labels, even though this is a completely unnecessary ingredient for making delicious bread. The other hidden sources of sugar are all manner of nutrition drinks and bars, some of which deliver a mother lode of sugar. The spike in blood sugar created by these ubiquitous foods not only creates sugar aging, it also raises your body fat composition—as all sugars not immediately used for energy are stored as fat. And a spike in blood sugar inevitably takes a bite out of your energy supply.

When you eat a high glycemic load food, for example, a doughnut, you quickly produce (and just as quickly lose) a lot of energy—and you generate a lot of internal pollution in the process. Not a reasonable fuel, a doughnut will overtax the cell's ability to handle the excess rush of sugar without providing the co-factors necessary to make energy efficiently or to clean up the toxic by-products of your natural combustion. A complex carbohydrate (such as lentils or brown rice) generates a slow-burning flame that cleans up what little smoke it creates, whereas a refined carbohydrate (such as a plain bagel) produces a flash-fire that dies down quickly and throws off all sorts of damaging by-products that cannot be removed without depleting your cells of nutrients they need for other processes.

The Skinny on Bars and Shakes

Judging from the almost $4 billion that will be spent this year on meal replacement bars and shakes, people are willing to sacrifice taste for convenience. While I always prefer whole foods (a handful of trail mix is perfect in a pinch) some meal replacement choices are better than others. My primary concern is sugar. Many of the bestselling meal replacement drinks contain a lot of sugar and other carbohydrates (like sugar alcohols that don't raise insulin but do contribute to calories). Slimfast Meal-On-the-Go and Ensure Complete Balanced Nutrition contain 25 and 40 grams of carbohydrates, respectively, which is too much to process at one sitting. Making matters worse, the drinks do not contain fiber to slow down sugar absorption. If you must have a liquid meal, go for one of the higher protein formulas, which tend to have less sugar. For my money, the bars are a better bet because they contain complex carbohydrates with fiber. Even so, keep an eye on the sugar content, and beware of saturated fats, which are mixed into bars to give better mouth feel. Look for bars made with all natural plant ingredients with less than 12 grams of sugar, at least 6 grams of protein, and less than 6 grams of fat (with maximum 2 grams saturated fat). The best bars are made from whole foods; look on the ingredient label for nuts and seeds, whole grain fiber, and natural sweeteners like honey and fruit juice—some bars even have dehydrated fruits and vegetables, which I consider to be a bonus.

Hidden Allergies

There are three problems with foods in terms of reactivity and sensitivity. *Immediate* food allergies are often swift and severe as with peanuts and shrimp, and most people are acutely aware of these inflammatory triggers. *Delayed* food allergies are difficult to recognize because their symptoms can appear up to three days after exposure, in the form of rash, headache, and joint soreness among others. They can often be the source of constant fatigue. A third category is food chemical *sensitivities*. These are not true allergies, but are inflammatory reactions to chemical compounds in foods such as lactose intolerance and insensitivity to caffeine or fermented foods.

Classic food allergies (like an anaphylactic allergic reaction to peanuts or shrimp) and subtle food allergies (such as irritable bowel or eczema stemming from a subtle wheat or egg allergy) are both based on an immune system malfunction. White blood cells produce antibodies (IgE and IgG) that attack the food, often creating energy-draining and symptom-producing, inflammation and oxidation in the process. The difference is in the type of immune antibody involved: A classic allergy is the result of an immediate IgE antibody reaction; a subtle allergy is the result of a delayed IgG antibody reaction. Classic and subtle allergies have very different symptoms. The IgE response occurs quickly, resulting from an instant release of histamine and other chemicals and inflammatory cells that cause redness, itching, swelling, hives, or shortness of breath. The IgG response is slower to develop and harder to recognize, involving antibodies that can appear 2–3 days after exposure, causing myriad symptoms that often seem mysterious to people because they take so long to appear.

It's important to diagnose subtle allergies and sensitivities because they cause such an array of problems that often go unrecognized. While tests can be helpful for identifying delayed allergies, the gold standard for diagnosing hidden food reactivity (both allergic and sensitivity) is the elimination diet: For one month you stop eating the most common allergens such as wheat, dairy, peanuts, corn, shellfish, soy, citrus, nuts/seeds, chocolate, coffee, and fermented foods (yeast, alcohol, soy sauce, pickles, and cheese). I also cut out foods that people say they crave or eat a lot of because those often turn out to be offenders. After the month you add back the foods one at a time, for two to three days eating enough of each (usually twice per day) to challenge the system to cause symptoms if that food is a problem. (When an allergy produces a delayed reaction, eating a small amount of the trigger may not cause noticeable symptoms.) With a strictly enforced elimination protocol (the 21-Day Plan can be a starting point for this) you can pinpoint the cause of even subtle allergies (as well as other food reactions) with considerable accuracy.

Bottom Line: Trouble Foods to Avoid

Let me finish up this guide to energy drains with the list of what *not* to eat. Your goal is to avoid the three damaging inflammatory processes and to stop your body from wasting energy on repairing and cleaning up from foods that harm your cells. Here is what to eliminate along with a quick look at healthier substitutes. The 21-Day Plan offers practical, complete menus and recipes for avoiding these trouble makers.

Red Meat: With apologies to your local butcher, for the next twenty-one days I'd like you to take a break from eating red meat (beef, pork, lamb, and veal). It causes inflammation by promoting formation of unhealthy fatty acids, oxidation by introducing free radicals, and (if nonorganic) possible exposure to toxins from antibiotics, growth hormone and pesticide residues. Replace red meat with healthier protein options. After your twenty-one-day abstention, eat meat only sparingly if you must.

Trans Fats: Primarily found in packaged baked goods and margarine (fortunately, home-baked goods do not contain trans-fats), these cause premature aging of the circulatory system, accumulation of fat in the midsection, and damage to the DNA. Use a smidgen of butter and olive oil, and avoid trans fats for life.

Refined Carbohydrates: White flour, white rice, potatoes, sweets are too quickly converted to sugar—draining energy, promoting inflammation and glycation, and producing free radicals. Refined carbs are also easily converted to midsection fat. Swap with whole grains and unrefined sweeteners like honey

Wheat: So many people have become sensitized to the "New World" wheat that pervades our food supply. It's can be a major source of inflammation and refined carbohydrates. Swap this form of wheat for "Old World" wheat (spelt and kamut). For 5 percent of the population who are gluten intolerant, none of these grains is acceptable.

Cow's Milk: Another common allergen and sensitizer, cow's milk also contains saturated fat, which causes inflammation and is a potential source of antibiotics and growth hormone, which your body has to work to remove. For 21 days eliminate cow's milk (opt for soy or rice milk). For many people nonfat yogurt from cows is OK, but for those with true milk allergies there are other forms of yogurt from sheep, goat or soy that are better choices.

Coffee: Overstimulates your nervous system and sets you up for a crash. Wean yourself from coffee. Eliminate coffee for 21 days or at the very least drink half your current dose, substituting with more calming green tea or at least decaf coffee is even better.

Alcohol: By taking a break from alcohol you allow your detox mechanisms, especially in your liver, to work less hard and free up energy for repair.

Power Foods

Finally, here's what I want you *to eat* with gusto. Power foods will create the new, vital you. They'll provide all of the good stuff: sustained release of sugar with complex carbohydrates balanced by fiber and lean protein; a high level of nutrients to create energy and repair damage; substances that promote detoxification; and defensive superstars that fight inflammation and oxidation. When you eat these foods daily, you will absolutely renew your cells, increase your life force, and feel younger and more energized. Follow the recipes in the 21-Day Plan. The foods in the plan are by no means confined to the superstars in the Power Foods chart on the following page. All vegetables, whole grains, legumes, fish, nuts, and seeds can and should be welcomed into your world and prepared with a generous helping of TLC.

Naturally, if you're accustomed to eating a meat-sweet diet, these foods may not appeal to you at first glance, but I suggest you try our recipes because it's very likely you've had one or more of these items improperly prepared. Most people overcook food, leaving the greens wilted and sour; the garlic and oil burned and bitter; the beans and lentils soggy and heavy on the stomach or causing too much gas. Instead of boiling broccoli, I brown it in the oven with fresh olive oil and garlic. To rid fish of its fishy smell it's always washed first with lemon and salt then rinsed under water before cooking. Poultry is always cooked with aromatic

POWER FOODS

	Complex Carb	Lean Protein	Soluble Fiber	Good Fats	+Energy Nutrients	Fights Radicals	Antiinflammatory	Promotes Detox
Salmon, Trout		****		****	**		****	
Halibut/flounder/sole		****		**	**		**	
Eggs (poach or boil)		****			****			
Soy	***	***	***	**	**	**	**	**
Yogurt (plain is best)	*	***			***	**	****	
Whey protein powder		****	**		**		***	****
Almonds/alm. butter	*	**	**	***	**	**	***	
Walnuts	*	**		***	**		***	
Lentils	****	***	***	*	*		*	
Beans (red, black)	****	**	***	*	**	**	*	*
Wheat germ	**		**	**	****	***	**	**
Quinoa/spelt/kamut	****	*	****		**	**	**	**
Flax seeds	***			****	**	**	****	*
Olive oil				****	**	**	****	
Grapeseed oil				****	**	**	****	**
Spinach/kale	**		***		***			
Swiss chard	**		***		***	***		**
Broccoli/Brussels Sprouts	**		***		***	***	**	****
Watercress, arugula	*		**		**	**		****
Avocado				****	**	**	***	
Sea vegetables			*	*	****	***	**	***
Shitake/reishi			**		***	***	***	**
Fresh veggie juice	*		*/***		***	***	***	***
Onions					**	***	**	****
Garlic				*	***	***	***	****
Blueberries	*		**		**	****	**	***
Kiwi	*		**		****	****	**	**
Papaya	*		**		***	***	***	**
Grapefruit	*		**		**	**	**	**
Apples	**		**		***	**	**	**
Red grapes	**		*		**	***	*	*
Turmeric					***	***	****	***
Cinnamon/ginger					***	***	***	***
Green tea						****	***	**
Vinegar							**	**
Unfiltered honey						***	*	
Dark chocolate (70%)						****	*	
Red wine (moderate)						***	***	

spices to impart flavor. The 21-Day Plan offers many recipes to energize your kitchen.

Keep in mind my ideal balance: 40 percent complex carbohydrates; 30 percent lean protein; 30 percent healthy fats. In my experience most people eat either too much protein, too many saturated fats, or too many carbohydrates. Get accustomed to loading your plate with vegetables (have a vegetable and salad with dinner). Taking a small peach-sized portion of carbohydrates, and consume less protein than you're used to. **In our former agrarian society, when people had to catch their own fish or raise their own animals, protein was eaten sparingly and with great appreciation—I recommend that we all reconnect with that perspective.**

If you want to lose weight, watch your intake of fats and carbohydrates, and eat more steamed fish and veggies. While the fats in my plan are healthy, they do add calories. When you're trying to slim down, the trick is to eat foods that contain a lot of water and fiber with minimal calories such as greens, kale, collards, celery, lettuces, and fish. If you, like most people, are accustomed to carbohydrate-dense snacks, you will lose weight simply by following the 21-day meal plan. If you are the kind of person who operates on coffee and anything you can gobble as you run out the door you'll find that eating this new way will calm your nervous system and give you tremendous endurance. If you tend to panic when you feel hungry you'll also do just fine, because these foods have ample fiber and a reasonable amount of healthy fats, both of which are satiating. You simply have nothing to lose by eating the Power Foods way.

On convenience: By no means should you give up and have a cheeseburger if you can't get salmon and Swiss chard for dinner. Most towns now have food stores and restaurants that both prepare healthy meals and deliver. The goal is to eat lean protein, complex carbohydrates, and vegetables, preferably fresh, but frozen is certainly acceptable too (freezing actually preserves the nutrients in food that can be lost while it travels across country, sits in a warehouse and then on the grocery store shelf). A can of wild caught salmon prepared with lemon or a touch of low-fat mayo and a salad is a perfectly acceptable lunch. I am a big fan of frozen organic fruits and vegetables in a pinch and also recommend keeping fully cooked, organic frozen meals in the freezer, and stocking your pantry with organic (low-salt) canned lentil and bean soups.

When you're in a hurry, good intentions tend to go out the window. But this sets up a cycle of energy depletion just when you need it most. **When you think you don't have time to eat well, take a deep breath and realize that supportive nourishment may very well be the one thing that actually pulls you through a big challenge.** Whether you take an hour preparing a meal or five minutes, make sure that what you eat sends an energetic message to every cell in your body.

Supplements: When Good Food Is Not Enough

Many people come to me with bags full of supplements from the health food store—they've got megavitamins, antioxidants, high doses of obscure nutrients, herbs from remote corners of the planet, "natural" hormones from their latest nutrition guru, and all manner of proprietary formulas for everything from energy to sexual potency. They come looking for guidance, and sometimes even for more pills, and I almost always disappoint by telling them to throw most of it away. So often health food store clerks and "alternative" newsletters and websites take a one-size-fits-all approach to supplements, causing people to purchase and consume pills they don't need. **I am not a big fan of taking a lot of supplements regularly. I believe that most people can and should get the nutrients they need from food.** If after significant changes to lifestyle and diet there are still deficiencies, or if there is a disease process that requires a supplement, I will recommend one, but my goal is to use supplements only to jump-start a treatment and recovery protocol. I aim to avoid daily use of all but the most absolutely necessary supplements, which for many people is simply a quality multiple vitamin.

One compelling reason for my reluctance to supplement is that, because nutritional science is fairly new, researchers have only begun to unlock the compounds (most of them found in plants) that are beneficial to your health. Plus, there are inherent risks in using too much of any one extract or supplement. Ten years ago, most doctors and scientists didn't appreciate there is more than one type of vitamin E; now we know there are at least six types (tocopherols and tocotrienols); and some of them are more powerful at fighting free radicals, and even tumors, than others. The same can be said of subclasses of carotenes (the vitamin A family). When the entire carotene family is used together as it is found naturally in foods it strengthens the immune system and reduces the risk of cancers, but when a single member of the family, beta-carotene, is used alone it can actually cause lung cancer to spread more rapidly. Folic acid can help prevent heart disease and some cancers and birth defects, but may increase the risk of colon cancer. Selenium can protect the prostate from cancer and the heart from arteriosclerosis, but it can increase the risk of developing skin cancer. This is just a fraction of the cross-reactions and side effects of vitamins and minerals.

Understanding one vitamin or mineral, though, is child's play compared to analyzing any one herb, which entails discovering which of the hundreds of compounds found in a plant benefits health without producing side effects. When you look at what's on the shelves for just one herb, say echinacea, you don't know if the capsule contains the powerful leaf and root components, or relatively worthless stem parts. **Quality control is up to the honesty of the manufacturer who knows he is at little risk of his products being assayed for accuracy (consumer organizations such as consumerlabs.com and Consumer Reports are increasingly giving us important quality information).** Look for a label that says GMP, which means the manufacturer is complying with good manufacturing principles—making his products at near-pharmaceutical standards. Also look for an assay of the active ingredient in the product, indicating some due diligence at producing a high quality supplement. But despite these general guidelines, misinformation is rife, and without the help of a well-versed health care partner who can apply the latest research—and product knowledge—to your specific problem, it's very difficult to sort out on your own.

My recommendation is to complete the first fourteen days of the 21-Day Plan, following the balanced, nutrient-dense menus and recipes. In the third week of the plan if you want to try a supplement specifically to increase energy, I've listed some here that I have found often useful for jump-starting energy. The key is to try only one new supplement at a time so that you can determine its effects, if any. I usually give a supplement for at least a week before evaluating its impact on a patient's health and sense of energy (some take up to six weeks to have a notable effect). Naturally, if a supplement makes you feel poorly or even just a little strange, stop taking it immediately. Everyone's metabolism and nutritional profile are different, so it's impossible to predict how any one nutrient or formula of nutrients will affect you. My mantra with supplements is to err on the side of caution, and see your doctor before taking new supplements if you are being treated for a medical condition.

Co-enzyme Q10 (Ubiquinone): CoQ10 is an essential critically important nutrient, occurring naturally in the human body, required for the mitochondria to make ATP (your energy currency) and also as a necessary antioxidant for neutralizing the large number of free radicals generated as a by-product of creating ATP. Occasionally your body cannot supply enough CoQ10 for optimum energy. For example, the statin drugs, Lipitor and Zocor may deplete CoQ10; if you take a statin you might consider supplementing with CoQ10, especially during periods when there are heavy demands on your energy. This nutrient also has been shown to improve cardiac function in people with cardiac disease. CoQ10 goes right to the mitochondria to make the machinery more efficient. It's safe to use long-term, for example if you're taking statins, but not everyone needs it. If you're not deficient, taking CoQ10 won't give you more energy. (Rarely, a side-effect can be cognitive changes—feeling "foggy": if this happens, stop CoQ10 and the symptoms should clear quickly.)

L-carnitine: Carnitine is an amino acid that has many beneficial uses in the body. One of these is to facilitate the uptake into the mitochondria of fatty acids. Fatty acids not only help stabilize the mitochondrial membrane and provide some antiinflammatory protection, but are sometimes used as a back-up fuel source in the mitochondria—bypassing the usual glucose mechanism. This could be useful when one's glucose stores are low—during endurance athletic activities—and for people with chronic debilitating illnesses (including current ongoing research studies on fatigue in cancer). (Side effects are unlikely—as with many supplements, occasional stomach upset may occur if too much is taken on an empty stomach.)

Krebs Cycle Nutrient Co-Factors: Many people have insufficient stores of the critical vitamin and mineral co-factors needed for the mitochondria to produce energy. Inadequate diets, stress, toxic loads, and chronic health conditions can all deplete the body of essential nutrients. Taking a targeted multivitamin/mineral supplement can help put you back on the road to being able to produce more energy. The most important nutrients to look for are B complex, copper, zinc, and magnesium. Iron can be tricky, while it's an important nutrient co-factor, there are contraindications (for example, some men have high-normal hemoglobin counts and should not take iron supplements). (Note: while higher doses of water soluble B vitamins are quite safe, minerals and other vitamins have a greater potential for harm, so make sure to check with your health care provider before using these nutrients.)

Resveratrol: Resveratrol is a natural polyphenol found in grape skins and wine that is thought to be one explanation for the "French Paradox." It has been the subject of intense research with numerous studies, thus far mainly in animals, showing resveratrol's ability to reduce the risk of cardiovascular disease, obesity-related illness and insulin resistance as well as help prevent cancer. Convincing studies suggest resveratrol can increase the production of mitochondrial energy factories and prolong life. While wine contains some resveratrol, the amount needed to produce the health benefits demonstrated in studies can only be obtained by taking concentrated supplements. Studies suggest a 100 mg tablet per day is the optimum dose.

It Ain't Easy Being Green

The market for products promising that elusive fountain of youth of abundant vital energy is flooded with "green" drinks (also in powder form). These are nutrient-dense powders made from plant—primarily seaweed—compounds such as chlorella, spirulina, blue-green algae, and wheat grass, and mixed with other whole food ingredients. If you don't like to eat your veggies (optimally eight or nine servings a day), these drinks are not a bad idea because they deliver a bounty of vitamins, minerals, antioxidants, and other nutrients in a whole food form. These concentrated powders may even have benefits beyond the typical land vegetable in helping remove heavy metals from the gut.

Adaptogens

Adaptogens are an important group of herbs that can help the body to maintain energy. Studies show that adaptogens can strengthen the immune system, act as antioxidants, support the adrenal glands' ability to regulate cortisol, and help the body maintain muscle mass. Adaptogens do not simply increase energy, they also help maintain the balance between the body's energy-producing and -consuming mechanisms. Which herb works best is very idiosyncratic; it's like feeling a difference between aspirin and ibuprofen. People who have serious medical conditions or take medications should check with their doctor before taking any herb or supplement.

Cordyceps (cordyceps sinensis): One of my favorite herbs, cordyceps, is a mushroom that particularly excels at supporting the adrenal gland. It was originally used in China, where it remains popular, but is manufactured to pharmaceutical standards today in the United States. Studies show that it makes cells more efficient at using cortisol, so the adrenal gland can produce less cortisol and not work as hard. Cordyceps has been shown to be an excellent antioxidant, to increase cellular lifespan, to strengthen the immune system, improve the ability of the cell to metabolize sugar, help the liver detoxify more effectively, and increase sexual function and energy.

Ayurvedic Ashwaganda (Withania somnifera): This is a powerful balancing tonic, another of my favorites. Its use as an energy herb originated in India. While its mechanisms of action are quite different from cordyceps and ginseng its end result is similar: Ashwaganda improves the utilization of cortisone and metabolism of sugar, strengthens the immune system, and is both antiinflammatory and antioxidant. Ashwaganda has the added benefit of reducing the effects of stress—while stimulating the processes that enhance energy production, it also has a calming effect on the nervous system.

Russian Arctic Root (Rhodiola rosea): Russian Rhodiola has been used for decades by Russian cosmonauts and athletes to increase energy, and especially to increase stamina for endurance activities. Extensive research in Russia (and some good research in the United States) has shown that Rhodiola can improve cognitive function (particularly under stress) and increases mood by facilitating production of serotonin. It is thought to reduce stress by helping the body use cortisone more efficiently and dampening the autonomic nervous system's production of excess adrenaline. It is both an antioxidant and antiinflammatory agent. Unlike ashwaganda and cordyceps, Rhodiola can be overly excitatory. I recommend starting with a low dose of 100 mg in the morning. If you take it at night it might keep you awake.

Ginseng: Similar to cordyceps, ginseng has been used for thousands of years in China as a universal remedy for balancing energy, stress, mood, and immunity. In studies it's been shown to improve exercise performance and stamina and reduce fatigue. Like cordyceps, ginseng reduces the need for the adrenals to produce cortisol, and also allows the body to utilize sugar more effectively, and is an antioxidant. You will typically find two non-Siberian forms of ginseng in health food stores: panax (Asian) and panax quinquefolium (American). These two varieties can affect individuals differently. I have had patients who only get results from Asian ginseng and others who say only American works for them. Like Rhodiola it can be excitatory, so start at a low dose.

Siberian ginseng (Eleutherococcus): Not related at all to the true ginseng family (other than bearing a passing physical resemblance), eleutherococcus is one of the most widely used adaptogens. Research has shown it can increase stamina and energy without overstimulating the nervous system. As a balancing herb, Siberian ginseng is excellent for helping adapt to environmental, physical, or emotional changes.

Shizandra (Shizandra Chinensis): This Chinese herb is much less known in the West, but has been highly respected in Asia for millennia as a powerful adaptogen. It has been shown to improve energy, stamina, athletic performance, and recovery, as well as enhancing cognitive performance, particularly under stressful conditions. Historically it was used as one ingredient in multi-ingredient traditional Asian formulas, but more recently its powerful effect as a single herb has been recognized. As with many other adaptogens it helps support the liver's ability to detoxify.

Licorice root: In my four years of medical school, licorice was one of the few herbs ever mentioned—and we were warned *not* to use it because of its known ability to raise blood pressure. While bad for hypertensives, this makes licorice root particularly well suited for people with low energy and *low* blood pressure. While technically not classified a true adaptogen, licorice can be very effective in supporting the adrenal gland's functions. Most people who think they have eaten licorice have actually had a commercial preparation of anise-flavored sugar gel, with no (or minimal) flavoring from licorice. Licorice root comes in both chewable and capsule form.

Chapter 3

Power Detox, Remove Toxins, Increase Vitality

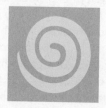

SAM, AGE THIRTY-TWO, came to me as a last resort. A lifelong asthmatic and allergy sufferer, he had been on maximal medications for years (nasal and lung steroid inhalers, bronchodilator inhalers, antihistamines, antiinflammatories, expectorants, with frequent rounds of antibiotics and oral steroids) but didn't feel that he was ever healing. "It's like I'm walking on eggshells, always afraid of a flare-up. My energy is constantly low because of worry and the medications."

His fears had come true one day a month prior to his first visit with me. He arrived at his office on a Monday morning where new carpet had been laid the previous Friday evening, and began having difficulty breathing. Within twenty-four hours he was on a respirator in the ICU with life-threatening asthma. Since then he had been placed on a number of different prescription medications for asthma. With no end to the drug regimen in sight the approach felt to him like a Band-Aid, not a cure.

As with most sufferers, his asthma was highly susceptible to all sorts of environmental triggers, such as dust, mold, and pollen, and the bout in the ICU had shown that he was also highly chemically sensitive (especially to volatile organic compounds such as carpet adhesive and solvents). I immediately began a twofold approach to reducing his immune system's tendency to overreact: First we worked together to remove triggers, and then I developed a treatment plan to build up his body's ability to process any unavoidable exposure to internal and environmental triggers. I ordered further tests to determine whether he had vitamin or mineral deficiencies, subtle food allergies, an overabundance of the immune system's inflammatory messengers, or possible organ (especially digestive) dysfunction—all of which could disrupt his body's ability to process environmental toxins. He tested abnormal in all of the above areas, which meant that taking a comprehensive approach to improving his overall health—rather than just treating his symptoms—would do his asthma a world of good.

We worked on rigorously cleaning his environment, with advanced HEPA filters at home and work, removal of caustic chemical cleaners, plastic shower curtains, dust mites, mold, and carpet adhesives—the list was extensive, but he was highly motivated after his bout at the ICU. I took him off many foods he was allergic to and put him on a more plant-based diet, removing animal products that cause inflammation. He began to take a number of supplements (including omega-3 fatty acids, magnesium, the spice turmeric, medicinal mushrooms, and probiotics for intestinal flora) to reduce inflammation, strengthen his ability to remove toxins, and support his immune system. I gave him acupuncture, initially twice weekly, then weekly to reduce inflammation and stress hormones. We included relaxation and imagery exercises combined with biofeedback breath training because anxiety can make asthma worse.

Within the first week he felt stronger, and after a month we began to slowly taper some of his medications. Now, two years later, he has remained symptom-free, using only occasional bronchial inhalers and seasonal allergy pills. He has maintained his healthier lifestyle, and says that he feels more energetic and "alive" than ever. He told me that he had thought before coming to me that he'd never heal, and that his healing journey had truly started when he realized there was a lot he could do to alter his frail condition.

YOU HAVE AN EXTRAORDINARY ABILITY to neutralize toxins. Unlike frogs and bees and many other endangered creatures, you have elaborate mechanisms throughout your body, headquartered in the liver, for removing stuff that doesn't belong inside you and that can harm you in many different ways. This is the system that you're depending on when you're waiting for a hangover to go away or recovering from a bout of food poisoning.

But not all detox systems are equal. The strength of your internal detox abilities depends on many variables. The amount of toxins you're exposed to; your vitamin, mineral, and nutrient levels; how much alcohol you drink; the amount of fiber you eat; how much exercise you get; your hydration levels, and even how much you sweat can affect your ability to isolate and excrete chemical compounds that don't belong—whether they are natural by-products of your own metabolism like free radicals; natural chemicals you've intentionally ingested like alcohol or caffeine; or one of the many industrial chemicals you are exposed to every day from air, water, and food. **While most everyone is built to clean up after their own metabolism, people today have a storehouse of industrial chemicals that have accumulated over a lifetime of exposure, which makes bolstering your internal detox a high priority.** In my experience, strengthening your detox mechanisms, releasing chemicals stored in your body, and reducing the continual onslaught of chemicals makes a huge difference in health and energy—as it did for Sam.

Even before there was such a thing as a lab, humans evolved a sophisticated detox system. This was meant to handle the by-products of normal metabolism such as the free radicals generated by energy production that damage cells. Your cells basically have a built-in combustion engine that needs constant pollution control. The detox mechanism also evolved to remove potentially harmful, naturally occurring chemicals in plant and animal foods. With industrialization we have significantly added to the list of substances the body must neutralize.

There are many unknowns about the long-term effects of having multiple industrial chemicals stored in your organs, fat tissues, and bloodstream. **At last count the Centers for Disease Control found 148 man-made chemicals in the average American blood sample, including alarmingly high levels of mercury.** The many negative ways in which the 75,000 commercial chemicals approved for use in the United States interact with your genes and interfere with how DNA directs cellular operations and maintains health are exceedingly difficult—almost impossible—for scientists to demonstrate. Unfortunately, there are so many chemicals in our environment with the potential to affect our health in so many different ways that it's difficult to determine which ones should be removed from use. Even so, I am optimistic that you can make changes to better cope with what is known as the body-burden of industrial chemicals.

A growing body of solid scientific evidence (much of it gleaned from studying how pharmaceuticals are metabolized) shows that we do process and excrete environmental toxins, and that we can make our detox system more efficient. **Diet, lifestyle, allergies, the health of your digestive tract, genetics, and medical history all play a role in determining how well your body handles your extensive exposure to man-made chemicals that is a defining characteristic of modern life.** This is the sweet spot of my interest in environmental medicine, and it is one of the new frontiers of medicine.

Global warming is only half the picture of what's become of all the industrial chemicals introduced since the nineteenth century; the accumulation of toxic chemicals in our food and water supply and the consequent increase in the body burden of toxins is the other half. **For many years I have researched methods to help my patients clean up their internal toxic load—it's a sort of Kyoto protocol for your body.** With the 21-Day Plan I will teach you how to use the latest research to improve your ability to detoxify, freeing up your resources to create energy rather than clearing out debris.

The Problem: Chemicals and Your Environment

First, let's take a look at what we're up against. The Environmental Protection Agency (EPA) in the United States estimates that over 5 billion pounds of toxic chemicals are released by industry into the nation's environment each year, including 75 million pounds of recognized carcinogens. In addition to this massive release of toxins into the air, water, and soil from industrial sites, chemicals enter your body directly from chemically treated and enhanced food and the dizzying array of man-made substances you come in contact with on a daily basis. Everything from car exhaust and plastic by-products to lawn fertilizers to pesticides on produce, drug residues in meats and milk, volatile organic compounds in paints and adhesives, cosmetics that penetrate the skin, and even pharmaceuticals and the capsules they're in randomly leave behind residues—

modern chemical footprints in the human body. The fact that we've survived our collective pillaging and disruption of the environment is a testament to the resilience of the human body. No one has studied the effects of this sort of low-level exposure to multiple chemicals over time, but it has been established that combinations of toxins have additive, or synergistic, effects, meaning that the presence of one toxin can magnify the effect of another. For example, it's been demonstrated that low doses of lead and mercury—low enough to be harmless to lab animals—can become fatal when the two are administered together. Linking chemical exposures to a specific disease [in a research study] is extremely difficult, partly because the exposures are vast and uncontrolled—they occur to millions of people over millions of square miles—and partly because the human detox enzyme system is so complex and individualized—your system may be different from your mother's, sister's, or daughter's. Of course, there's also precious little research funding (from government or industry) available to analyze the problem.

One thing is certain: When toxins are present in your body they cause excess energy expenditure that can lead to fatigue and disease. All toxins can damage DNA, both directly and via free radical generation: shortening the telomeres (tiny caps at the tips DNA-carrying chromosomes that protect against damage), and altering the structure of DNA to make it function less efficiently. **Mitochondrial DNA, which is inside the cell and is responsible for creating energy, is even more vulnerable to damage from exposure to toxins than your nuclear genomic DNA (see Chapter 2).** As cells cope with contaminants, they require additional energy (known as ATP) in order to package off and remove the toxins presented. On top of that, they also need energy to fix any cellular sabotage that occurred as a result of the exposure. The liver's role as master detox mechanism also requires additional energy for each additional toxin it's presented with. All of this explains why my program, which improves the efficiency of the detox system and reduces exposure to toxins, also helps your own energy.

Humans clearly can and do co-exist with enormous quantities of industrial chemicals (many people contain toxins in their bodies for decades without apparent harm), but in spite of the many obstacles to research, scientists have begun to make associations between pollution and many diseases—including various cancers, diabetes, obesity, asthma, reproductive disorders, cardiovascular and autoimmune diseases, and neurological development syndromes. In a review of research by the Silent Spring Institute, researchers identified 216 chemicals that were linked (in at least one animal study) just to breast cancer. These included pesticides, dyes, pharmaceuticals, and hormones. Twenty-nine of these chemicals are produced in the United States at greater than one million pounds per year, 35 are air pollutants, and 73 have been found in consumer products or as food contaminants. The ubiquitous presence of such chemicals should be reason enough for you to make an effort in shoring up your own natural detox mechanisms.

Perhaps even more disturbing was a study conducted on the umbilical cords of newborn babies. In a small study conducted by the non-profit Environmental Working Group, researchers analyzed umbilical cord blood collected at birth from a random selection of infants in the United States and found that it was laced with an average of two hundred industrial chemicals that entered the umbilical cord from the mother's body. Some of these substances were in concentrations that were six times those found in the mother. After birth the problem for many continues; breast milk is one method the body uses to expel fat-based toxins that it stores in the breast tissue. There's increasing evidence that women in the United States produce breast milk that contains residues of industrial chemicals. I actively encourage women to breastfeed—it's nature's healthiest food— but women of child-bearing years need to be particularly careful about avoiding toxins and following the program in the second half of this chapter for removing toxins before they get pregnant. Nobody can say for sure how these industrial chemicals—known carcinogens and nervous system toxins among them—affect your baby's earliest stages of development. No regulatory action can be taken without proof of cause and effect. But in the meantime research is beginning to hint at irreparable damage to nervous and reproductive systems.

You don't need to wait for the proverbial smoking gun to take steps to lower your body burden of toxins. In my practice, which is focused particularly on preventing illness, reducing exposure to chemicals, and making sure people are neutralizing them efficiently is a universal goal—it reduces the likelihood that you will develop a disease and it frees up energy otherwise occupied in keeping your body's detox mechanisms operating on overdrive.

Your Natural Detox System: How It Works

As indelicate as this may sound, here is one of the keys to survival in the twenty-first century: Your body has the ability to identify toxins and remove them by way of your urine, your breath, your bowel movements, and even through the pores of your skin. You have a large roster of enzymes and antioxidants that can defuse toxins and flush them out before they cause damage. These systems are present in every cell; but your gut and liver are specially high-powered detox machines. **The gut and liver regularly identify and package toxins to ship them out of your body on the scale of the post office at tax time.** If you eat conventional, nonorganic produce your urine contains a steady stream of pesticide metabolites (or residues). If you apply sunscreen, some of the chemicals in the sunscreen will be absorbed through your skin and found in your urine days later. Industrial chemicals can be detected in people's sweat. All of this is due to your natural detox system working to remove the toxins. Unfortunately, the body is not a perfect detox machine; some of the chemicals are left behind in your bloodstream and get stored, particularly in your fat cells.

My goal for every patient is to improve the body's natural detox system. At the end of this chapter, and in the 21-Day Plan, you will find my step-by-step program for boosting your body's detox mechanisms. But first, a quick primer on how your body does it, which will help you understand how the detox plan works and why it is so crucial to health and energy.

Your Gut's Instinct

Your body processes more than 25 tons of food over a lifetime, placing your gut on the frontlines of pollution control. Your intestinal tract can both absorb beneficial nutrients from food and drink and prevent absorption of harmful substances from food and drink. Unfortunately, the gut too often allows absorption of industrial chemicals and other harmful substances (like natural toxins in foods) on a regular basis, either because it does not recognize them as harmful or is simply too overwhelmed or damaged to reject them all. The twenty-foot expanse of mucous, cells, connective tissue, and muscle that constitutes your gut ejects toxins in four ways. First, fiber in your gut can absorb toxins and carry them away. Second, substances excreted into the inside of the gut by the cells lining it can try to neutralize toxins. Third, the intestinal cells forming the wall of your gut try to reject and neutralize the toxins attempting to be absorbed through them. And finally, the cells try to stick closely together using adhesive molecules between cells—forming a Maginot line if you will—to prevent offenders from sneaking in between the cells out of the intestines and into the surrounding tissues and blood stream. And if all the above systems within the gut fail—either because the gut is damaged or "leaky" or the cells don't even recognize the toxins as a threat and allow them to waltz on through—there's yet another line of defense just beyond the intestinal wall: the immune system composed of your lymphatic system with its white blood cells and drainage channels. Even with all the above defensive systems, however, toxins still escape through the gut into the rest of your body on a regular basis.

Sadly, the modern world hasn't been very good to your gut: medication piled upon medication; ever more powerful germs; damaging levels of stress with no relief; and the abysmal contemporary diet loaded with unnatural chemicals have all breached, and in some cases even shattered, the gut's defenses. **In a sense, evolution hasn't caught up to pollution, and the gut simply isn't equipped to keep up with all the toxins we dump into it now.** It has a limited ability to recognize and neutralize mercury, for example. After toxins like mercury or PCBs or organophosphate pesticides have made it past the gut, the next stop is your liver, where once again you're left with what evolution has given you, which in the case of the liver is a pretty sophisticated, but often overwhelmed detox system.

Your Liver: Gatekeeper and Detox Machine

While the liver's function includes making cholesterol and processing fats, proteins, and carbohydrates, much of its energy is expended detoxifying your body. All food absorbed by the intestines is shunted first to the liver before the body will allow it into the general circulation. Likewise, inhaled and topical agents can wind up in the liver for detox. Once the liver receives any chemical it must decide whether or not a substance gets a green light (beneficial nutrients pass through untouched); a yellow light (equivocal substances like triglycerides get tagged for reprocessing); or a red light (toxic substances from industrial chemicals to cigarette smoke get red-flagged for detox and elimination).

The liver's job goes way beyond identifying toxins, it is also able to transform the vast array of harmful molecules your body encounters (including alcohol, pollution, food additives, pharmaceuticals, or even flu viruses) into harmless molecules that can be easily sent out of the body as waste. (In its spare time it also produces 80 percent of the body's cholesterol needs, stores glucose in the form of glycogen, processes extra calories into triglycerides and other fats, and has an internal immune system.)

Fortunately with this huge list of critical responsibilities, the liver is constantly renewing itself—it is one of the body's fastest regenerating organs.

The liver accomplishes its remarkably precise clean-up in two phases that even the Maytag repairman could admire. First, it employs a large family of enzymes, called *cytochromes*, to turn specific toxins into general free radicals—this is known as **Phase I liver detox**. Secondly, the resulting free radicals (called toxic intermediaries) are then neutralized by the liver's highly sophisticated army of free radical fighting *conjugators*—this is known as **Phase II liver detox**. If you think of your liver as your internal washing machine, the liver enzymes of Phase I are the laundry pretreatment—they are a kind of "Shout!" for your bloodstream. Once the enzymes have removed the "stains," the Phase II conjugators step in as a sort of all-purpose Tide for your bloodstream. Working together, the two phases of detox are able to remove toxins from your body.

There are lots of molecular players in both phases of liver detox. During Phase I detox at least 120 members of the enzyme family known as cytochrome P450s pretreat the hundreds of thousands of toxins that your body encounters every day. Exactly which member of the liver enzyme family is involved in taming a particular toxin depends on the substance that's being neutralized. For example, caffeine, certain pesticides, some of the carcinogens found in cigarettes, and the polyaromatic amines found in charbroiled beef are all detoxified by the activity of one cytochrome known as CYP1A2. Certain antibiotics like erythromycin require a different cytochrome, CYP3A4, to be metabolized. The abilities of a particular cytochrome to properly detox a range of molecules can vary significantly from individual to individual, and this is often what accounts for different people's threshold of tolerance to different chemicals.

Idiosyncrasies in the cleaning power of a particular enzyme can be largely genetic, which is a white-hot area of scientific research at the moment. For example, when it comes to digesting caffeine, which is metabolized through your Phase I detox pathway, there are two types of people in the world—rapid caffeine metabolizers and slow caffeine metabolizers. The difference is due to a slight variation in the gene code for CYP1A2 (called a genetic polymorphism). About half of all Caucasians have the slow variant of the gene code, which means caffeine hangs around in their systems longer, versus only 14% of Asians. **In one fascinating study of 2,014 men and women published in *The Journal of the American Medical Association* (*JAMA*) in 2006, being a slow caffeine metabolizer was associated with a dramatically increased risk of heart attack for sub-**

Taming Toxins

LIVER DETOXIFICATION PATHWAYS

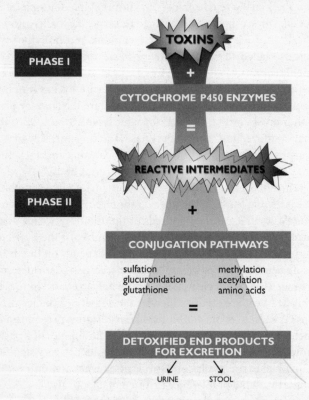

Your liver captures toxins (from food, chemicals, and your own metabolism) and transforms them into harmless substances to be eliminated. This process involves two steps. In Phase I the cytochrome P450 enzyme family targets a toxin and breaks it down into an intermediary substance (this is like putting Shout! on a stain). In Phase II, conjugators transform the intermediary substance into a harmless molecule to be excreted (this is like washing it out with Tide). Keeping these two phases well supplied with nutrients is a key to having a powerful internal detox system.

jects who drank more than four cups of coffee per day, whereas fast caffeine metabolizers drinking more than four cups per day had a reduced risk of heart attack compared to the control group. (Drinking one cup a day had no effect, regardless of genetic makeup.) That's a significant difference in heart attack risk for heavy coffee drinkers based solely on how your liver is genetically programmed to detoxify caffeine!

To say the least, this study suggests that if caffeine easily gives you the jitters, drinking more than one cup a day could be deleterious to your health. But it also demonstrates how the activity of your liver's Phase I enzyme detox system can have a profound effect not only on how you feel, but also on your overall health and energy. As the science of genomic medicine advances, researchers are continually discovering more about the body's various detox enzyme systems. For example, a European study published in the *Journal of the U.S. National Institute of Environmental Health* established that for men, an individual's gene code for Phase I detox of the industrial pollutant PCBs (found commonly in fatty fish) determined whether or not the presence of PCBs in the bloodstream caused a decrease in sperm count. Your liver's ability to detoxify can even affect your sperm count! One exciting result of the latest research is that simple blood tests are becoming available that allow your physician to measure many of these cytochrome detox capabilities, and doctors can use this information to better individualize dosages for drug therapies.

Beyond genetics, the other variable that affects how well your liver's Phase I cytochromes work is how busy they are: The more substances they have to face, the less chance there is that they will be able to fully detoxify all the substances they are responsible for. This is why, for example, grapefruit juice can affect drug dosages. Compounds in grapefruit juice, such as the coumarin paradisin (a plant oil that provides disease resistance), inhibit the ability of specific members of the cytochrome P450 family of enzymes to metabolize certain drugs. This allows the drugs to build up in the body, a process that can be very harmful, yet has also been used therapeutically. For instance, certain drugs (such as the potentially heart-toxic chemotherapy drug adriamycin) can be given in one-half to one-third the normal dosage when the patient drinks one glass of grapefruit juice a day. By monopolizing a Phase I detox system, grapefruit juice causes the drugs to hang around longer in the bloodstream.

This can be the case with any Phase I detox enzyme system: Any substance, for example a specific chemical in cigarette smoke, can monopolize a Phase I cytochrome and cause another substance, such as a specific pesticide, to hang around longer in your bloodstream, leaving the body no choice but to store it in your fat cells. In this way, overloading your detox enzyme system can cause chemicals to build up in your body as they wait their turn to be detoxified. This toxin gridlock can have deleterious effects on your health including disrupting your hormone balance, your nervous system, your immune system, and even your reproductive system. Because your Phase I detox system has this limited capacity, it's critically important to reduce your exposure to toxins.

Sometimes the opposite problem can arise: your Phase I detox system is going like gangbusters and your Phase II system cannot keep up the pace—usually due to a dearth of raw materials (nutrients) from food needed to get the job done. **Think of using a lot of Shout! on a stain and then not washing the shirt. You're left with a gross shirt.** Well, it's the same with your internal washing machine; if your Phase I system is working away and Phase II is inadequate, then you're going to feel gross—generally you'll have a hung-over feeling that won't go away.

As I pointed out at the beginning of this section, Phase II relies on an army of free radical-fighting antioxidants called conjugators. Conjugators are amino acids that specifically target free radical compounds from Phase I; they efficiently neutralize the compounds and allow them to be eliminated. These conjugators are continually made by your body, and they all can come from key nutrients that you must eat. Problems arise when either your Phase II conjugators are depleted or your Phase I system is on overdrive. When this happens you get a buildup of free radicals—you're oxidized or rusty! And you need more free-radical fighters fast. For tips on how to improve Phase II see the program at the end of this chapter.

The importance of maintaining balance between the two phases of the liver's detoxification processes is a critical open secret, but many doctors are clueless about it. Too many toxins/drugs/chemicals can overwhelm Phase I and lead to toxin buildup in the body, with resultant low energy and ill health. The flip side of this is that it is not uncommon for people to have normally functioning Phase I systems, but poorly functioning Phase II systems, thus setting up a situation of *oxidative stress*—with a buildup of large quantities of unquenched free radicals from Phase I that can also lead to illness and low energy. I often suspect that the liver's detox phases are out of whack when people tell me they feel like they've got a constant hangover—or, like Sam, when they're waking up fatigued and feeling like they never have quite enough energy. **In such cases, a detox program that reduces the toxic load presented to Phase I and is rich in food substances that increase Phase II detox can bring back**

vital energy. You will learn how to build a better detox system in the last section of this chapter, "Boost Your Detox System."

The Solutions: Zap Toxins and Build a Better Detox System

Reduce Your Exposure

At the risk of sounding like Dr. Strangelove, I have to emphasize toxins do have a remarkable talent for getting into your body, and the first step in any good detox program is to slow the flow. Consider the ways in which toxins can make their way into your cells:

- Chemicals can drift in through your nose and mouth as volatile organic compounds (VOCs) like paints and solvents, or simply as fine particles like most air pollution from car exhaust and industrial smokestacks.
- Toxins can be absorbed through your skin, as is the case with thousands of chemicals used in cosmetics (some of which are known carcinogens). Chemicals used in sunscreens (on average 4 percent of what's applied to the skin) have been found in people's urine up to five days after application—to get there they had to pass through multiple skin layers and into the bloodstream, potentially depositing some molecules for storage in fat cells, before being shuffled off to the liver for detox and excretion. For this reason, researchers recommend that infants (whose detox systems are not fully developed) be protected with nontoxic sunscreens specially formulated for them.
- Contaminants can enter with the water you drink—municipal water treatment plants are not designed to remove most industrial chemicals including pharmaceuticals. In a recent study by the nonprofit Environmental Working Group (www .ewg.org) 141 unregulated contaminants were found in public water supplies in forty-two states between 1998 and 2003 (52 were linked to cancer, 41 to reproductive toxicity, 36 to developmental toxicity, and 16 to immune system damage). One example, rocket fuel (perchlorate) is now found in the water supplies of over 20 million Americans. Perchlorate blocks the uptake of iodide, an essential nutrient added to salt

in the form of iodine to benefit public health. Perchlorate's tendency to shut iodide out of cells (especially in the breast and thyroid) is a problem because it is essential for fetal brain development and for regulating energy metabolism in adults. But the EPA has yet to set a drinking water standard for perchlorate or mandate that its presence in drinking water be reported to consumers. Translation: it's not illegal to have rocket fuel in your water and no one has to tell you it's there!

- North America's food supply—despite the existence of the FDA and the Canadian Food Inspection Agency—is laced with chemicals: Some, like PCBs and DDT, have been banned for years, but never leave the environment and are ubiquitously present at low levels—even in whole organic milk. Other toxins are still in use: Just last year Teflon was identified as a "probable human carcinogen" and Du Pont has agreed to stop using it (though not until 2015). Hundreds of new chemicals are introduced every year for use in farming and food manufacture.

Unlike the movie *Dr. Strangelove*, this chemical horror story is not a product of anyone's imagination—it's public information (much of it from the National Institute of Environmental Health Sciences and its excellent publication *Environmental Health Perspectives*). Between your respiratory system, your skin, and your digestive tract, your body is an open door to every conceivable toxin. With this cumulative load of chemicals in so many aspects of your life, it is essential to make a concerted effort to reduce exposure in any possible way. Here's how I would prioritize the project to zap toxins.

Eat Organics

Let's begin in a realm that has the greatest impact on toxic load and lends itself to maximum control: the food you eat. Food can deliver a toxic punch to your system in a number of ways. Almost any food can carry bacteria such as salmonella or E. coli; *conventional produce*—grown using agricultural chemicals such as pesticides and herbicides—can carry toxic residues; and any processed food—packaged in jars, cans, bottles, cartons, and plastic containers and made at an industrial facility by a food producer—can contain additives, preservatives, colorings, thickeners, dough conditioners, flavorings, or any one of the thousands of chemicals approved for use in commercial food preparation. More than 12,000 ingredients end up in the nation's food supply as a result of processing and curing according to Ruth Winters, M.S., in her marvelously detailed book, *A Consumer's Dictionary of Food Additives*. To give you more perspective on the chemical load in your food, manufacturers spend $1.4 billion annually just on flavorings and flavor enhancers, which represent a fraction of all additives. It's not only the ingredients in processed food, but also packaging that can leach substances into the food. The food industry has a lot of technical data to convince you these chemicals are safe to eat for a lifetime. But I'd rather you fill your stomach with the marvelous vitamins, minerals, fiber, phytochemicals, and beneficial oils that plants have to offer, especially because scientists are constantly discovering new important functions these wonderful natural food constituents perform. **Eating organics—food grown with old-fashioned methods such as soil composting and nontoxic pest management—is the best way I know of imbibing nature's bounty with minimal interference from synthetic chemicals.**

Beware Pesticide Loads

Buy organic versions of these fruits and veggies, whose conventionally grown versions were found by the USDA to have the highest pesticide loads:

Peaches	Cherries
Apples	Lettuce
Bell peppers	Grapes
Celery	Pears
Nectarines	Spinach
Strawberries	Potatoes

That said, it would be nearly impossible to buy only organic foods and, depending on where you live, this could also be an expensive proposition. But you can prioritize your organic food choices.

Produce: The United States Department of Agriculture—well aware of the dangers of consuming foods that contain pesticides and other agricultural chemicals—routinely tracks the quantity of man-made chemicals on produce. In the most recent ranking of produce according to chemical load (measured after washing and peeling), the USDA found peaches, apples, sweet bell peppers, celery, nectarines, and strawberries to have the heaviest toxic loads—one conventional apple can carry as many as 14 different pesticides! On the previous page is a list of the dozen most polluted fruits and vegetables; I recommend that you bring this list to the grocery store and commit to buying organics for these items. You get a break on onions and avocados, which have been shown to carry the least amount of chemicals. A good general rule of thumb is, the thicker the skin (for example, bananas, citrus, and avocados) the lower the amount of chemicals that have been absorbed into the flesh that you eat. Careful washing (especially with a safe citrus-based produce wash) is still in order, however, to prevent chemical residues on the produce skin from contaminating what's inside.

At this point most people ask me, "Well, what's so bad about pesticides?" Let's start with how most pesticides work—they are mostly neurotoxins built to fatally damage a pest's nervous system. In animal studies, many pesticides appear to target the dopamine-producing neurons in the brain involved in coordinating movement. **At the very least, it's advisable not to ingest even minute amounts of known neurotoxins on a regular basis. On another level, many pesticides have been shown to disrupt the body's hormone signaling mechanisms—altering levels of thyroid and estrogen among other deleterious effects.** In fact, scientists now place the majority of pesticides in a class of environmental pollutants known as hormone disruptors. (In high doses pesticides kill by being neurotoxins, but in relatively small doses with long-term exposure they can produce adverse reactions such as hormone disruption.) Such chemicals are implicated in epidemiological trends toward reproductive disorders (such as infertility) and hormone-based cancers like prostate and breast cancer. Finally, many pesticides are carcinogenic and others are tumor promoters. There are only a limited number of studies that evaluate the cancer risk for individual pesticides, though, and much more work is required before detailed assessments can be made.

I'm not willing to wait. I recommend avoiding foods grown with pesticides whenever possible. **It's never too late to change: Just five days of an organic food diet was enough to dramatically decrease the levels of**

pesticides measured in the urine of children in a convincing study con-ducted in 2006 at the Rollins School of Public Health, Emory University in Atlanta. In their conclusions, the study's authors wrote, "We were able to demonstrate that an organic diet provides a dramatic and immediate protective effect against exposures to organophosphorus pesticides." And for my money, that's reason enough to switch to organics.

Processed Foods: Any food that's prepared and packaged for you is "processed"—the Department of Commerce refers to the "process" as the transformation of livestock and agricultural products for final consumption. Just about everything in a package—salad dressing, hot dogs, cookies, milk, bread, cereal—is processed. Getting those products to the supermarket where they can sit on a shelf and look pretty requires food engineering, which for the most part involves industrial chemicals.

From the point of view of convenience, processed foods give people what they are often looking for—quick, cheap calories with a flavor punch. Processed foods also give the major food companies what they are looking for—revenue. At $511 billion in sales last year, the processed food industry is one of the largest manufacturing sectors in the United States.

Meat and dairy account for the largest portions of the processed foods on the market, but bakeries and tortilla manufacturing make up a surprising 10 percent of processed foods, while sugar and confectionaries account for another 5 percent. Classic soft drinks represent the absolute epitome of processed foods; they contain plenty of calories (in the form of high fructose corn syrup from a highly governmentally subsidized crop, corn) with usually no nutritional value.

The problem is that, when you eat a processed food, for the most part you don't know what you're eating! The inclusion of potentially carcinogenic nitrates in processed meats is one example. Another is the widespread use in processed foods of ingredients made from genetically modified (GMO) crops. **I was shocked to learn that 70 to 80 percent of processed foods contain GMO ingredients (on the other hand, no produce sold in markets contains GMOs thanks to consumer activism).** Processed foods routinely include corn syrup and corn oil made from GMO crops. The long-term health effects of eating foods that contain GMOs are unknown, but I have some concerns. For example, GMO corn is engineered specifically to tolerate more Roundup weed-killer. The result has been an increase with GMOs in the use of Roundup. Other GMOs have the ability to produce their own pesticides built into the

Of Lunch Meat, Bacon, and Hot Dogs

Studies demonstrate a connection between consumption of processed meats and stomach cancer, colon cancer, and bladder cancer. Processed meats (including sausage, bacon, hot dogs, and bologna) often contain nitrite or nitrate and N-nitroso compounds, which are potent carcinogens that can induce tumors in animal species. Processed meats also usually contain high amounts of salt, which can irritate the stomach lining and enhance the carcinogenic effects of compounds. Recent studies detailing these connections with more than 100,000 subjects are considered preliminary. Until there's further direct evidence of deleterious effects, food companies can continue to sell meats processed with nitrates and salt. But you don't have to eat them!

plant's DNA. None of this has been studied for long-term health effects. By avoiding processed foods you also avoid eating GMOs—which from my perspective is a very good idea.

Genetically mutated plants are only one of the unsavory ingredients you might encounter in a processed food. A bottle of America's top selling Italian salad dressing contains thirteen ingredients (not including water). **There is absolutely no healthy reason that a dish you can make at home with two ingredients—oil and vinegar (maybe a pinch of salt and a squeeze of lemon juice or teaspoon of mustard)—should contain 13 ingredients, including high fructose corn syrup, xanthan gum, calcium disodium EDTA, and food coloring.** You don't need that junk, especially on top of your beautiful organic vegetable salad!

I want you to buy your food one ingredient at a time—fish, broccoli, onions, garlic, olive oil, lettuce, apples, walnuts—you get the picture. I realize how difficult it is to avoid those miles of processed food aisles in the typical supermarket, but it's crucial that you do. My nutrition superhero, Marion Nestle, renowned nutritionist and professor of nutrition, food studies, and public health at New York University, puts it succinctly: "My rule of thumb is to never buy foods that have more than five ingredients. The more processed a food is, the more ingredients it is likely to have and the lower the nutritional quality." And I would add that the more synthetic ingredients in a food, the higher the chance that you are eating something bad for you that requires more energy to metabolize. Stick to the periphery of supermarkets where the fresh food is displayed—avoid the center aisles which are almost exclusively processed foods.

Milk and Red Meat: The value of buying organic milk is a subject of heated debate, though when you look at the facts it's pretty clear that buying organic milk is a no-brainer. The crux of the matter is in how farmers get cows to produce more milk. In her book, *What To Eat,* Marion Nestle points out that in an attempt to cut costs and meet demand over the past thirty years the dairy industry has doubled the amount of milk obtained from each cow in the United States, mostly by injecting the animals with hormones. The most widely used growth hormone is a genetically engineered version made by Monsanto officially known as recombinant bovine somatotropin (rbST). The dairy industry claims that milk from cows treated with rbST is indistinguishable from milk from cows not treated with rbST. Because most of the research about the effects of drinking milk produced by cows on hormones has been conducted by the dairy industry itself, judging the safety of such practices is difficult, but I'm not comfortable with the widespread use of genetically engineered hormones in a nutritional staple.

The milk story illustrates how the use of one man-made chemical solution often leads to the need for another—whether in animal husbandry, farming, or commercial food production. The practice of stimulating milk production with rbST increases the need for antibiotics—the broken skin at the site of the twice-weekly hormone injection is vulnerable to infection and the increased milk production also makes udders more vulnerable to infection. Choosing USDA organic milk—a standard that is monitored by the government—is the only way you have of guaranteeing that it won't come from cows treated with antibiotics or rbST, which is not allowed to be used in cows that produce milk labeled as certified organic. It is heartening that the number of organically raised cows in the United States has increased twenty-five-fold in the last twenty years. To put that in public health perspective, though, organic production still only represents 1 percent of U.S. dairy output.

Even more disheartening is the situation in the beef industry, where herds are subject to similar chemical exposures and there's much less reliable organic supply. The current surge of resistant E. coli infections in meat is partly the result of using suboptimal doses of antibiotics that select out for highly resistant bacteria. In the 21-Day Plan I recommend reducing your dairy intake and eliminating red meat altogether because I want you to avoid saturated fat as well as potential toxins.

Chicken: A lot of my patients, when asked to switch from red meat, start eating more chicken. Chicken is a pretty decent meat alternative: lower in saturated fat and associated arachadonic acid, especially if cooked with the skin off, which is where most of the saturated fat resides in chickens. But conventional American chickens can be polluted. Extensive use of antibiotics in conventional poultry farming has resulted in an increase in antibiotic resistant bacteria, especially Salmonella. Conventional chicken meat can also contain arsenic residues—a surprise to most people. Arsenic—a known carcinogen and poison (at higher doses than used in animal feed) is an animal feed supplement approved for use in conventionally raised chickens that many farmers use to control intestinal parasites. In recent research from the National Institute of Environmental Health consumption of conventional chickens was identified as contributing to significant amounts of arsenic exposure in the U.S. population. The only public health recommendation that came out of this disturbing revelation was to reduce the amount of arsenic allowed in the water supply (which no governing body even bothered to do). I recommend buying organic chicken. Birds sold under organic labels cannot legally be given arsenic or antibiotics. And because their feed is higher quality, they usually taste better.

Buying Chicken: When Being Label-Conscious Is a Good Thing: A chicken can only be as healthy as its upbringing, and the only way to determine that is to look behind the claims being made on the label. Problem is, it's hard to separate the hype from reality. The chart opposite explains what the labels mean in the U.S. marketplace, and which are worth paying for.

You will note in this chart a relatively new designation: "Certified Humane Raised and Handled." This signifies that the product meets standards set by the Humane Farm Animal Care Program, a nonprofit organization that partners with the ASPCA and other groups. The rigorous certification program requires producers to provide a nutritious diet, without antibiotics or hormones, and to raise animals with shelter, resting areas, sufficient space, and the ability to engage in natural behaviors. The "Certified Humane Raised and Handled" label is increasingly found on a variety of products including chicken, turkey, beef, lamb,

Chicken Label Claim	Standard/ Meaning*	Independently Verified*	Is It Worth the $?
"Certified Organic"	Set by USDA: No antibiotics, no growth hormones, no genetically engineered substances, no animal by-products in feed, no arsenic, minimal pesticides, access to outdoors (can be minimal).	Yes	**Definitely**
"Natural"	Set by USDA: No artificial flavor, no color, no chemical preservatives or synthetic ingredients.	No	**If other verified labels are not available**
"Free Range/ Roaming"	Set by USDA: Coop door open for at least 5 minutes per day, chickens may stay inside.	No	**No**
"Antibiotic Free"	Claim not allowed by USDA.	NA	**No**
"No Antibiotics Administered"	Set by USDA: No antibiotics used, preventively or therapeutically, during animal's life.	Only when specified on label.	**Yes**
"Hormone Free"	USDA does not allow hormones to be used in any poultry, so the label's meaningless.	NA	**No**
"Fresh"	Set by USDA: Chicken has never been frozen, processed or preserved.	No	**No**

(continued)

Chicken Label Claim	Standard/ Meaning*	Independently Verified*	Is It Worth the $?
"Certified Humane Raised and Handled"	Set by American Meat Institute: No growth hormones, no antibiotics, healthy living conditions.	Yes	**Yes**

* Source: www.greenerchoices.org

and eggs. Hopefully one day this will be the standard for all animal food we eat.

Fish: Fish provides the marvelous omega-3 fatty acids that we can't get enough of, yet paradoxically the fat that is so healthy for us is also the main repository in fish for storing environmental toxins—primarily mercury and PCBs, but also dioxin and pesticides (especially in farmed varieties). What's the problem with this stuff?

- Mercury is a non-biodegradable (it lasts forever) heavy metal, released into the air primarily from industrial sources (especially from coal-burning plants), that falls in rain and snow into the planet's water supplies. Industries have also disposed of it by dumping into the ocean, into migratory paths of fish. According to the EPA, mercury concentrations in fish can be 1 to 10 million times its concentration in water due to "bio-magnification" (when small fish with low mercury levels get eaten by bigger fish—like swordfish and tuna—the predator's mercury increases exponentially). When people eat mercury it targets the nervous system and the kidneys. The developing brain and nervous system of a fetus are most vulnerable, but adults are also at risk. In my practice, 80 percent of people eating fish (which is often tuna) frequently have mercury levels above limits deemed acceptable by federal regulatory bodies (which allow concentrations of mercury in food up to 1 part per million, which is more mercury than I'm comfortable with eating on a regular basis). Symptoms include numbness, fatigue, irritability, and loss of memory. Fortunately most of us can clear lower levels of mercury from our bodies within a

month of two if we discontinue eating foods contaminated
with it.

- PCBs (polychlorinated biphenyls) are industrial pollutants
used in a number of different ways including as engine
coolants, flame retardants, and in carbonless copy paper. PCBs
were banned from use in America in the 1970s, but, like DDT,
still persist in the environment and accumulate in fatty foods,
especially fish. PCB exposure regularly affects the brain, the
nervous and hormone systems. It can damage the immune
and reproductive systems, and has been linked to cancer as
well as increased rates of allergies.

- Dioxins persist in the environment as a result of industrial
processes, such as the production of certain herbicides and
disinfectants, waste incineration, and chlorine bleaching of
pulp at paper mills (small amounts of dioxins are also produced naturally during forest fires and volcanic eruptions).
Dioxin has a destructive effect on the immune system that
caused regulatory agencies in the United States and Canada
to classify it as a "probable human carcinogen." It also affects
the reproductive, endocrine, circulatory, and nervous systems.

Fish are not the only sources of exposure for these contaminants, but
they are the source of heaviest exposure. In addition to environmental
exposure, the fishing industry does not have tough standards for pesticide use in farming. While some farm-raised fish are relatively toxin free
(notably shrimp and tilapia), farm-raised fish can be treated with a combination of parasiticides and antibiotics, and in the case of farm-raised
salmon, even food coloring to make its flesh look pinker. What's more,
they can be fed corn or other grain, which reduces the amount of beneficial omega-3 fatty acids that come from the typical wild algae-based
diet. And the overcrowded conditions in which farmed fish live are not
only inhumane, but increasingly breed disease and foul the nearby waters
and endanger indigenous fish species. **Even I was surprised to learn that
70 percent of the farmed fish in the world comes from China, where
standards are often even more lax than they are in North America, and
that China is the fastest growing supplier to the United States. Bottom
line:** Continually seek local and international information on the health
and pollution status of fish populations. Because of this problem with

pollution I strongly recommend you make careful choices in the fish you eat.

The following chart comes from my favorite source of data on the health of the world's fish populations, the nonprofit Environmental Defense Fund website, www.edf.org/seafood. This organization continually monitors health advisories from more than 120 government and scientific databases to come up with an overall safety rating for each type of fish. Scientists at Environmental Defense Fund calculate recommended consumption levels based on methodology developed by the EPA. I like the way edf.org works with the data, telling you how many meals you can eat per month. Their assumptions are based on weight and portion size (which I've detailed below), so you can find a mix that's right for you. Mercury is particularly toxic to fetuses and young children, so the women's category is more conservative. Of course, pregnant women should avoid fish altogether.

YOUR MONTHLY FISH ALLOTMENT: A NUMBERS GAME

The number of times *per month* you can eat fish depends on what fish you're eating—if you stay within the 4+, you can have at least four meals, *total, per month.** Exposure is cumulative: Eating fish from a highly contaminated group (0–3) reduces the number of meals you can have overall.

Fish	Meals Per Month Women**	Men**	Health Risk
Wild Alaskan salmon	4+	4+	Low Level
Atlantic mackerel	4+	4+	Low Level
Shrimp	4+	4+	Low Level
Tilapia	4+	4+	Low Level
Farmed rainbow trout	4+	4+	Low Level
Pompano	4+	4+	Mercury
Sole	4+	4+	PCBs

Clams	4+	4+	Low Level
Farmed oysters	4+	4+	Low Level
Black sea bass	4+	4+	Mercury
Canned light tuna	4+	4+	Mercury
Mahimahi	4+	4+	Mercury
Skate	4+	4+	Mercury
Maine lobster	4+	4+	Low Level
Halibut	4+	4+	Mercury
Red snapper	4+	4+	Mercury
Eel	3	3	Mercury
Wild oysters	3	3	PCBs
Grouper	3	2	Mercury
Fresh tuna	3	2	Mercury
Chilean sea bass	2	2	Mercury
Flounder	1	1	PCBs
Atlantic salmon	1	1	PCBs
Swordfish	0	1	Mercury
Bluefin tuna (sushi)	0	0	Mercury, PCBs
Striped bass	0	0	PCBs, mercury
Bluefish	0	0	PCBs, mercury

* Source: environmentaldefensefund.org

** Note: Assumes 144 lb woman/6 oz portion; and 172 lb man/8 oz portion. Children have a lower threshold of tolerance and should eat less fish. Pregnant women should *not* eat fish.

The Air You Breathe

What sent my patient, Sam, to the ICU was exposure to the volatile organic compounds (VOCs) in carpet adhesive. VOCs are petroleum-based chemical compounds that readily evaporate—becoming caustic airborne toxins—from a vast array of products including paints and lacquers, paint strippers, cleaning supplies, pesticides, building materials and furnishings, office equipment such as copiers and printers, correction fluids, adhesives, permanent markers, nail polish and fuel. **VOCs are consistently higher indoors (up to ten times higher) than outdoors, and even our own EPA admits VOCs may have short- and long-term adverse health effects.** For several years the EPA has recommended that copiers and printers be placed away from where people sit. A number of states have issued more stringent VOC standards, causing some companies, like paint manufacturer Benjamin Moore, to reduce VOC emissions from all of their products. A growing variety of building materials and household products emit low or no VOCs, and it's worth doing your homework to track down these healthy alternatives. A good place to start is the website www.greenguard.org, which certifies low VOC-emitting products. In addition, Americans' tax dollars have been put to good use with the National Institutes of Health website of Material Safety Data Sheets (MSDS) for household products. This storehouse tells you exactly what health

NonToxic Is Chic

Interior designers often prefer the following for their natural look, but I like them because they are healthier for you. Ask for these when you renovate:

Soy-based paint remover
Milk and clay paints
Zero VOC paints
Venetian plasters
Low VOC glazes, lacquer, and sealers
Beeswax polish & wood finisher
Natural clay plaster finishes

hazards exist in household products: go to www.householdproducts.nlm
.nih.gov. Demand to see the VOC data on any products you use, and beware of blanket reassurances about the safety of these products.

If low VOC paints haven't hit your local store you might want to
point out to them that occupation as a painter has consistently been
associated with a 40 percent increased risk of lung cancer. Conventional
paints are typically loaded with VOCs that fly out of the can and enter
your respiratory system, wreaking havoc on your DNA. **The industry
has been quietly acknowledging the health hazards in paint, and a
number of companies have begun to offer healthier options.** One of my
favorites is AFM Safecoat paint, which contains zero VOCs, and is also
free of solvents, heavy metals, and formaldehyde and has almost no odor
during application. A number of other non-VOC paints are coming on
the market—take the time to find them.

Another major source of VOCs, carpet offgassing, can include a mix
of up to two hundred different chemicals including the probable carcinogen formaldehyde. The source of chemicals can be the carpet fibers, the
backing, or the adhesives used at installation. While offgassing can last for
weeks according to environmental scientists who measure such things,
there are also long-term concerns. Wall-to-wall carpet can harbor environmental toxins including fungal spores, bacteria, and dust-mite drop-
pings (researchers have found an average of 67 grams of dust per square
meter of carpet). There are numerous solutions:

- First and foremost, use area rugs whenever possible.
- Go for natural fibers—the rug itself should be cotton or wool
  (though beware of wools treated with mothproofing).
- Check the backing—latex and backing that's glued on, rather
  than sewn, can offgas a multitude of chemicals. Look for carpets with jute or other natural backings sewn on.
- If you must have wall-to-wall make sure the installers are
  using tacks, not adhesives. If they must use adhesive, ask for a
  nontoxic type such as that available at afmsafecoat.com.
- Last but not least, buy a high-quality vacuum cleaner with a
  certified HEPA filter to capture small particles rather than
  bringing them up from the floor then spewing them out the
  back end. Use it often.

The Way You Clean: Cleaning is an important way to reduce environmental toxins, but all too often it simply adds to the chemical burden. It's

a good idea to evaluate all of your cleaning products and habits for potential VOC exposure. The rule of thumb is to start with those products you're most in contact with—hand soap, laundry detergent and softener, shampoo, body wash and body lotion, countertop and surface cleaners—all can be sources of toxic chemicals.

Take a good look at the hand soap you use every day. I am opposed to antibacterial soaps. First of all, studies have shown it's primarily the length of time you scrub under running water that determines how clean your hands get (the amount of time it takes to get through one verse of the Happy Birthday song is just about right for a good handwashing). Second, there's mounting evidence that the antibacterial compound, triclocarbon (called triclosan on most labels) is a hormone disruptor that may be linked to rises in reproductive problems—and this chemical is not removed from the environment by water treatment plants. If you really need to sterilize your hands, use a 70-plus percent alcohol product such as Purell—now found routinely throughout hospitals.

Bottom line: Buy a simple handsoap without chemical or antibiotic additives. I'm also a big believer in using scent- and dye-free laundry detergent (residues of which can stay in contact with your skin all day and night). In general, stay hypervigilant about the products you are using at home. **Be aware that cleaning products are known to contain carcinogens, reproductive system toxins, allergens, and neurotoxic substances. Luckily, every day there seem to be new, gentler, and safer products on the market for keeping your house and your environment clean.** (A good place to look for such products is www.gaiam.com.) Learn about these cleaners of the future, and start using them; you will no doubt notice, as have I, that these healthier products smell better than their more toxic counterparts, and they tend to energize—as they sanitize—your environment.

A Word About Plastics

I predict you'll be hearing a lot more about the hazards of plastics in coming years. It is estimated that U.S. consumers use more than 10 million plastic bottles per *day*! A growing number of scientists are concluding that certain plastics can expose people to harmful chemicals—especially when used for storing and serving food. **Of major concern is a basic ingredient in many plastics called *bisphenol A (BPA)*.** Historically used to make Nalgene bottles, baby bottles, and food can linings—plastics that contain bisphenol-A are designated by the #7, which can often be found imprinted on the bottom of the plastic container. BPA has been found to leach from bottles into babies' milk; from can liners into foods; and from bottles into soda. **Scientists have identified BPA as a hormone disruptor, and have begun to establish a link between low levels of this chemical and some diseases on the rise in the United States, specifically obesity and diabetes.** In Japan, plastics manufacturers voluntarily discontinued using BPA, the Canadian equivalent of the U.S. Food and Drug Administration classified BPA as a dangerous substance, and manufacturers in the U.S. are beginning to discontinue its use as well.

Safer Plastics

Follow these recommendations for reducing exposure to toxins in plastics.

Seek out glass, ceramic, stoneware, wood, and stainless steel materials for kitchen equipment and food storage.

Avoid storing fatty foods, such as meat and cheese, in plastic containers or plastic wrap.

Use stainless steel or wooden utensils for cooking.

Check recycling codes and look for safer plastics such as #2HDPE, #4LDPE, and #5PP.

Avoid plastics that have been shown to leak hazardous materials into food: #3PVC, #6 PS, and #7.

Avoid putting plastic in the dishwasher.

Throw away plastics with cracks or cloudiness.

Use glass baby bottles or plastic bag inserts that are polypropylene or polyethyelene (#5).

Do not microwave foods in plastic containers.

Do not allow plastic food wraps to come in contact with hot food.

Follow expiration dates on canned foods, which typically employ plastic liners

Yet another ingredient in plastics, called *phthalates*, may be an even bigger problem. The United States is one of the few developed countries to permit the import of plastic toys made with this polyvinyl chloride (PVC) additive. This is a concern that's very well explained by author Mark Schapiro in his terrific book, *Exposed: The Toxic Chemistry of Everyday Products and What's at Stake for American Power*. He writes, "In the average home phthalates are everywhere—in shower curtains, shampoo bottles, raincoats. A component of that distinct 'new car smell' comes from phthalates in the dashboard. It's been found in umbilical cord and breast milk. Phthalates when ingested can impede the production of LH, a hormone responsible for triggering cells in the testes to produce testosterone, and for the normal menstrual cycle." Phthalates were banned in Europe eight years ago. You should try to avoid them as well. Here, suggestions for reducing your exposure to plastic residues.

Airplanes and Cars

Airplane and car interiors can be full of pollutants primarily due to the materials used for the interior finishes, which are made of plastics that outgas (particularly when temperatures rise), circulating particles of the plasticizers known as pthalates, which are known hormone disruptors (see above). In addition, by virtue of traveling at or above 30,000 feet in the atmosphere, airplane cabin air can contain high levels of ozone (in particular, narrow bodied planes rarely have ozone control systems). Ozone is a known respiratory system irritant (it's been shown that the more overweight a person is, the more likely it is that ozone will cause breathing problems). In one fascinating study in the journal *Environmental Science and Technology* researchers demonstrated that oils on your skin and hair can react with ozone, magnifying its deleterious effects. The take-home message of that study was that if you shower before a flight you may feel better afterwards. For all these reasons—and because of the numerous cleaning products used in between flights—airline cabin air can be particularly challenging for people with allergic, asthmatic, and other respiratory conditions.

If you have to fly every week for a living or spend a lot of time in your car, short of wearing a gas mask, you will want to follow the detox program at the end of this chapter and in the 21-Day Plan, include as many organics in your diet as possible, and make sure you reduce toxins in the other parts of your life that you have more control over.

Cosmetics

Mercury in mascara, lead in lipstick, coal tar (a known human carcinogen) in toothpaste, and mouthwash. Killer cosmetics may be the least of your health worries, but they present a hazard indeed. In fact, cosmetics present enough of a hazard that the European Union has taken steps to limit toxic chemicals in personal products. In January 2003 the EU banned the use of chemicals that are known or strongly suspected of causing cancer, mutation, or birth defects. Unfortunately, we have not taken the same steps in the United States and in Canada.

Short of going completely au naturel, there are steps you can take to reduce dangerous exposures. Carefully evaluate your sources of greatest exposure; products that you use over a large surface of your body—such as moisturizing lotion or bubble bath. Lipstick, toothpaste, and mouthwash, of course, come in direct contact with your mouth and gums, where they can be readily absorbed. On the following page a list of ingredients to avoid—check the labels . . . it's all about choices. Good news is that California and Massachusetts have passed legislation to ban the most dangerous ingredients in cosmetics. See www.safecosmetics.org for a list of companies that have voluntarily removed the worst offenders—or buy European cosmetics.

Heavy Metals

Poisonous elements—mercury, lead, cadmium, and aluminum—that are ubiquitous in nature (though in infinitesimal amounts), heavy metals have accumulated to significant concentrations in the environment as a by-product of industrial manufacturing processes. The EPA has determined that all of us have the ability to have low levels of these heavy metals inside of us without damage. But, as is the case with so many pollutants, those studies have not taken into account cumulative industrial exposure to multiple chemicals (which everyone alive today has experienced) nor has the EPA taken into account individual differences in the body's heavy metal detox mechanism. **The main systems responsible for maintaining energy—nervous and cardiovascular systems and the mitochondrial respiratory chain—are damaged by heavy metals.** Toxic effects in the nervous system include growth and developmental delays,

COSMETICS *NOT* TO DIE FOR

Here is a list of cosmetic ingredients that contain potential health hazards. These have been banned in Europe, and in some states of the United States. I'd avoid them.

Ingredient	Might Be Found In . . .	Potential Health Hazard
Triclosan	Antibacterial soap	Hormone disruptor
Coal tar FD&C Blue 1 and Green 3	Dandruff shampoo, anti-itch cream, toothpaste, mouthwash	Probable carcinogen
Diethanolamine (DEA)	Moisturizer, bath products	Hormone disruptor
Toluene	Nail polish	Nervous, reproductive system toxin
1,4 Dioxane (PEG)	Bath products	Carcinogen
Formaldehyde	Bath gel, nail polish, hair dye	Immune, respiratory system toxin
Artificial fragrance	Multiple products	Hormone disruptor
Parabens	Multiple products	Hormone disruptor
P-Phenylenediamine	Hair dye, foot powder	Nervous system toxin, allergen
Lead	Lipstick, hair color creams	Nervous, reproductive system toxin
Mercury	Eyedrops	Nervous system toxin
Hydroquinone	Skin lightener, moisturizer	Probable carcinogen
Pthalates	Nail polish	Hormone disruptor

Source: Environmental Working Group's Skin Deep database, www.cosmeticsdatabase.com.

reduction in cognitive functioning, and diminished function of the cardiovascular system. They also interfere with the generation of antioxidant and detoxifying molecules. The ability to excrete these toxins, particularly mercury, is highly individual. Most people's natural detox mechanisms can clear slightly elevated levels of mercury. For higher levels of mercury, a prescription chelating agent may be needed. I routinely test for heavy metals for anyone who is experiencing unexplained fatigue—and I recommend you do so too.

Boost Your Detox System

Here is my detox program, which consists of the following key elements:

Reduce exposure to toxins

Increase detox foods that support the body's natural detox mechanisms.

Nutritional supplements (when indicated) to boost the body's natural detox.

Saunas to release toxins stored in fat tissue.

One-day juice cleanse to clean the slate.

Consume more clean water to mobilize toxins.

Gut rehabilitation (when indicated) to improve the gut's detox ability.

I. Food

In Chapter 2 we covered many Power Foods that are maximally beneficial for healing the body and generating energy; a crucial part of helping your body generate more energy is helping it spend less time and effort detoxifying. Some of the most important foods that help make the job of detoxifying more efficient are:

- **The Brassica family (cruciferous vegetables): broccoli, cauliflower, kale, and Brussels sprouts.** Yes, this incredibly powerful vegetable family, which we all know is good for us but everybody loves to hate, also happens to be important for detox. Just take one member, broccoli, as an example; these little green trees (as my eleven-year-old daughter likes to call them) contain numerous potent phytochemicals:

Indole-3-carbinol, sulfurophanes, and *glucosinolates* to name some of the biggies. Indole-3-carbinol (which is only formed after crushing or during cooking) helps the liver break down old estrogen into harmless forms that can be eliminated. The harmful estrogen metabolites have been identified by researchers (Eleanor Rogan and others) as a major factor in stimulating the breast's estrogen receptors, predisposing women to breast cancer. Cruciferi's *sulfurophanes* increase Phase II detoxifying conjugators in the liver and elsewhere as well as performing tumor-destroying functions. That's a lot of power from little green trees and their knobby cousins.

- **The Allium family (sulfurous vegetables): onions, leeks, chives, garlic, shallots, and ramps.** Think of this as the vegetable underground working (in a highly complex way) to liberate your body from toxins. These members of the Allium family (which happen to be lilies) are rich in sulfur, a major component of detoxifying conjugators. The family name comes from allicin, released by crushing or cutting the garlic bulb (which loses its beneficial properties within hours of exposure). Onions also have quercetin, one of the most powerful phytochemical antioxidants: it quenches free radicals and acts like a natural antihistamine for people with allergies.

- **The thistle family: artichokes, dandelions, and burdock.** Ancient and ubiquitous healing plants, members of the thistle family have been shown in research to enhance the flow of bile, thus aiding in liver detox. Milk thistle in particular has been shown to help protect the liver from food-borne toxins (including poisonous mushrooms). Both artichokes and dandelion contain inulin, which helps regulate blood sugar.

- **Green tea.** As discussed in Chapter 2, green tea is a Power Food: it is one of nature's best antioxidants. Green tea also has been shown to induce Phase I and Phase II detox enzymes and conjugators, thus lending a powerful hand to your body's detox mechanism.

- **Fiber.** Speeds removal of toxins from the gut by binding them and preventing them from being absorbed in the first place.

- **Nuts/Seeds.** Provide essential fatty acids to reduce inflammation that produces toxic by-products requiring extra energy to neutralize. Pecans and walnuts also contain beneficial ellagic acid (see red berries).

- **Seaweed: arame, hijiki, kombu, wakame.** In addition to numerous vitamins and minerals, seaweed contains alginic acid, which is thought to bind heavy metals in the intestines, and cause them to be eliminated.
- **Spices: turmeric, ginger.** These potent antioxidants and antiinflammatories also enhance Phase II liver detoxification.
- **Herbs: Rosemary, oregano, parsley.** These herbs are powerful antioxidants with antimicrobial properties as well.
- **Red berries:** Among the numerous benefits of berries is ellagic acid—found in many red berries, particularly raspberries, and some nuts (see above). Ellagic acid has been shown in research to increase Phase II liver enzyme activities, enhancing their ability to target so-called reactive intermediaries, lending crucial support to the liver's detox mechanisms.
- **Yogurt.** Yogurt is terrific for gut health, helping to reset the immune system. The lactobacillus culture in yogurt has also been found to be highly protective against the toxic effects of the carcinogens found in fried meat.
- **Red wine.** Resveratrol in wine and dark grape skins has been shown to inhibit damage caused by the heavy metal cadmium. In addition to inhibiting many other cell-damaging free radicals, it may be one of the most important anti-aging phytochemicals.
- **Whole grains.** In addition to many health benefits bestowed by the critical nutrients in the grain's germ, whole grain (higher fiber) diets increase elimination and decrease absorption of environmental toxins compared to refined flour diets.
- **Citrus fruits.** In addition to copious amounts of vitamin C and antioxidants, citrus oils contain limonene, which is said to increase the level of glutathione S-transferase, one of the most important Phase II conjugators.
- **Water.** The simplest way to help your body flush toxic by-products is to drink copious amounts of clean, filtered water that will allow the kidneys to better eliminate the detoxified conjugated products of Phase II detoxification. Lack of water—dehydration—also makes it harder for both nutrients and toxins to move through the ground substance that is in between cells—such as that area between the gut cells and the blood vessels that all absorbed substances need to traverse.

II. Nutritional Supplements

There are important supplements to consider taking to help support the liver's—and nearly every cell's—ability to identify, detoxify, and remove toxins. All of these have beneficial effects on many functions in the body. The list below is a guide to which nutrients are most beneficial, based not only on their importance for detoxification support but also on their ability to help with other health issues—and on their ability to reduce energy expenditures (increasing net energy) by freeing up resources from detoxifying. These supplements should not be taken all together. Usually one or two at a time will suffice. The selection depends on your global health issues and general nutritional and detoxifying needs. It is important to discuss with your health care provider the best combination of activities, foods, and supplements for you. Note that some very important nutrients (such as the omega-3 fatty acids from fish oil and flax) are not on this section's list as they are not specific for detox (see Chapter 2 for these).

NUTRITIONAL SUPPLEMENTS FOR NATURAL DETOX		
Function	**Name**	**Why should you consider taking this?**
Liver Detox	**B Vitamins**	If you need support for your nervous system in addition to your liver
	Minerals (copper, zinc, selenium)	To increase the body's ability to make its own natural antioxidants, and increase efficiency of energy-generating processes
	Antioxidant vitamins (C,E, carotenoids)	If you are exposed to a lot of toxins or if you do not eat a wide range of fruits and vegetables
	NAC (N-acetyl-cysteine)	If you have heavy metal exposure or breathing problems
	SAMe (S-Adensyl-Methionine)	If in addition to needing help detoxing the liver, you have depression issues or joint inflammation

Liver Detox	**MSM** (Methyl-sulf-methane)	Present in sulfurous foods, but you need more to help not only with the liver, but with general inflammation, especially joint problems
	Glycine	Critical amino acid for phase II detox, improves recovery of the liver after alcohol-induced damage
	Lipoic acid	Helps support circulation (especially in diabetics) in addition to the liver
	Milk thistle	Supports the liver, protective against both natural foodborne and industrial toxins
	Bitters	Promotes better digestion in addition to increasing flow of bile and enzymes within the liver
	Schizandra	Ancient Chinese remedy for detoxifying, especially within the liver; often combined with other Chinese herbs for broader use
Gut Repair	**Prebiotics** (Beta-Glucan, Inulin, Fructo-Oligo-Saccharides)	If you are having intestinal problems and you are taking probiotics: supports growth of beneficial bacteria and helps inhibit pathologic ones.
	Probiotics (acidophilus, bifidophilus)	Helps digestion, intestinal function in general, and the immune surveillance within the intestines
	L-glutamine	Supports repair of the intestinal lining: also critical for nervous system protection
Heavy Metal	**NAC/glutathione**	Important nutrient for helping remove heavy metals once they are within the body

III. Saunas

Used historically in many indigenous cultures (Roman, Russian, Scandinavian, Turkish, Mayan, Inuit, and Native American) for literally thousands of years, the use of saunas as a detox tool has recently caught the attention of scientific researchers—particularly since the 911 disaster at the World Trade Center left so many people loaded with industrial toxins. While every cell and especially your liver and gut are designed to remove circulating toxins, the more serious long-term problem with toxic body burden is that chemicals tend to set up long-term housekeeping in your fat cells, which are very slow to detoxify—if they ever do. These unwelcome visitors then become like the neighbors from hell, causing all manner of damage to DNA. The hope—one that is beginning to be borne out by research—is that taking a sauna can help move toxins out of fat cells.

The idea is to raise the core body temperature, and basically to sweat out the gunk. **Scientists have been able to determine that mercury, dioxin, antibiotics, and even heroin and cocaine can leave the body through your sweat glands—but that doesn't tell us whether or not those toxins have been liberated from fat cells.** In some interesting research on PCBs, scientists have demonstrated that concentrations of PCBs in fat tissue were reduced with saunas. An additional study suggests that the skin's sebaceous (oil) glands—which discharge when you perspire—are an excellent excretory system for PCBs—which argues heavily in favor of having a good sweat.

The jury is still out on whether or not saunas enhance the release of toxins from interior fat cells. The practice is not harmful for healthy (nonpregnant) people, though, and has other benefits such as stress reduction, improving circulation (lowering blood pressure), and muscle relaxation. I recommend a good sauna whenever possible, but your health care provider needs to give you the OK before considering sauna for regular therapeutic use. There are precautions to consider, including health issues that may prohibit their use, such as severe chronic disease, pregnancy, heart disease, and while using certain medications. And because saunas naturally dehydrate, proper hydration and electrolyte balance are essential before going in.

Overall, I think saunas will be found to be increasingly helpful in detox programs such as those currently in place for 911 rescue workers. In the meantime—if your health allows it (which is the case for most of us)—take saunas regularly and enjoy.

IV. Juice Cleanse

My basic rule of fasting is *never water alone*. You need nutrients to aid in detox; which is why I refer to the day without solid food in the 21-Day Plan as a *Cleanse*. **This is not a fast that denies your body nutrients and caloric energy, but rather it allows your digestive tract to rest while providing maximal nutrients, minimal sugars, sufficient calories, and zero pollutants.**

Like saunas, periodic, brief fasts have been used beneficially for thousands of years in indigenous health systems, and I recommend them, having reviewed the research and experienced a number of different fasts. The most basic beneficial outcome of fasting is in starting with a clean slate. Not only does fasting rest your overworked gut, but especially if you introduce maximally healthy nutrients (with vegetable juices, probiotics, fiber, etc.) fasts can promote detoxification, reduce inflammation, improve overall health, and dramatically increase energy.

For this program, I ask you to follow the juice regimen for just a single day, but juice cleanses have been shown to be effective and safe for as many as three days. In one series of highly convincing studies conducted in Scandinavia, patients with severe rheumatoid arthritis were placed on a supervised juice fast for one week, followed by a vegetarian diet for a month. By the end of the period, patients had dramatic improvements in every parameter measured for their illness—there was a decrease in pain, stiffness, and use of medications along with a sense of improved energy and overall well-being. Even more astounding, the measurable improvements lasted for up to six months, even after patients went back to their former less healthy diets. In a different kind of study, researchers looked at the effects on heart health of the religious practice (in this case Mormon) of fasting for a day every month by evaluating 515 elderly people in Salt Lake City, Utah. **Those who reported fasting once a month were 39 percent more likely than nonfasters to have a healthy heart. One theory for the beneficial effect, which is backed by animal studies, is that periodic withdrawal of food might resensitize the insulin-producing beta cells.** By improving insulin metabolism fasting may have an effect on better heart health.

Important new research by English gerontologist Alan R. Hipkiss and others highlights one of the key mechanisms by which periodic fasting may not only protect your DNA but also improve your ability to generate energy and increase life span. This happens by the activity of internal anti-aging molecules of the family called sirtuins (SIRT 1–7). While most of the initial research has been conducted with animals, the mechanisms relate closely to the same processes and chemicals occurring in humans. Episodic fasting not only improved the ability of the mitochondria to withstand damage and more efficiently generate energy, but facilitated other mechanisms that significantly extended the life of the cell.

The key to a successful cleanse is in providing essential nutrients (including calories) and drinking sufficient fluids. Providing nutrients with freshly made juices is a key to maintaining energy levels and providing support for your body's detox mechanisms. One of the biological processes of fasting is mobilization of substances for detox in the liver and throughout the body. This vigorously activates Phase I liver detox, producing many oxidative (free-radicalized) intermediary by-products. This then necessitates a highly active Phase II to clear the toxic by-products. If you don't drink juices to provide abundant phytochemicals rich in antioxidants and key nutrients for making Phase II conjugators— and particularly if you start out nutrient depleted—a fast can actually make you feel toxic as Phase I buildup overwhelms Phase II. Because the Phase II conjugates need extra replenishing during a cleanse, I recommend fresh juice every two to three hours made from a rainbow of vegetables and fruits, with an emphasis on dark greens, including the deeply detoxifying Brassica family (see my juice recipes in Part Three). Drinking water or other non-caffeinated minimaly sweetened beverages in between these juice "meals" aids in flushing out neutralized toxins, staving off hunger, and preventing blood pressure drop.

The payoff of the one-day juice cleanse usually comes the next morning when you wake up feeling more energetic and "clear." It is essential to make careful choices as you transition back onto solid food. If you are suffering from severe chronic disease, diabetes, or are pregnant, consult your physician before undertaking the juice cleanse.

V. Gut Optimization

As we've discussed, your gut is your first line of defense against most toxins. Just about everyone can treat his or her gut better, but particularly if you suffer from irritable bowel or other digestive systems, here's what you do: chew better; eat mostly vegetables, fruit, and fiber; provide healthy bacteria such as the probiotic cultures found in yogurt. You chew your food better so that the gut has to do less work breaking down food; and certainly eating fiber is a simple solution—the more fiber you eat the easier it is for the gut to clean itself. But encouraging the growth of healthy bacteria is a bit more complex.

The healthier your gut bacteria, the healthier you will be overall— this is a maxim understood for centuries by many cultures that have cultivated the making of yogurt as a sort of art and medicine. Recently, scientists have confirmed that having an abundance of unhealthy bacteria produces inefficient digestion, and can release toxins that inflame the intestinal wall and leak into the general circulation, causing fatigue and other symptoms (including worsening inflammatory conditions such as rheumatoid arthritis). Most recently, scientists have uncovered evidence connecting specific species of bacteria in the gut to being overweight: certain bacterial species are able to extract calories from otherwise indigestible food, and are thought to be one link to the obesity dilemma. Establishing healthy gut bacteria also strengthens the immune system and helps keep the intestinal wall barrier system intact.

So how do you get the good bacteria? Eating yogurt loaded with sugars and additives (as are the majority of yogurts sold in supermarkets) will not help. Reglarly eating plain, unsweetened yogurt, preferably from nonhormone-treated animals, or taking a probiotic supplement (acidophilus or bifidophilus) are important ways to build your gut's flora. You can add a touch of honey, if you'd like. People who suffer from milk allergies can use goat yogurt, now widely available, at least in most health food stores. I also love my yogurt with a little cucumber and some walnuts or flax meal. As your gut begins to feel better, and you wean yourself off sugary varieties of yogurt, you will start to understand why plain yogurt has been considered a part of good nutrition around the globe for many thousands of years.

What Not to Do

Colonics: There is no published information that colonics aid in detoxifying the body, though you will often see them included as part of non-medical detox regimens in health spas. A colonic removes about four feet of stool from the large intestines, which can result in a feeling of relief—of course it would, since you are lighter with an empty colon when you finish. But within a couple of days the colon fills up again. Since the small intestines—not the colon—are primarily responsible for removing toxins, extracting the contents of the colon really cannot reduce your toxin burden. Cleansing can only happen from altering what you put into your body, and fine-tuning your detox mechanisms with food and supplements—not from a colonic flushing out the lower portion of your intestines.

Purges (emptying the digestive tract): A purge should only be conducted under medical supervision, for example, in preparation for a colonoscopy. While healthy people who experience temporary constipation can take an occasional laxative, they are *not* meant for regular use. Chemical laxatives (including herbal senna and cascara) result in dependence. A full purge (removing every piece of matter from mouth to anus, excuse the graphic description) can be occasionally helpful: Some of my patients report that precolonoscopy purges result in improvements in bowel problems. The detox regimen in this program can do the job without the purge.

Coffee enemas: Yes, you read that correctly. Coffee enemas are used in many so-called detox clinics in the United States and elsewhere. They are purported to help the liver detoxify. I would steer clear of them. While recent scientific literature does give some support for coffee's ability to enhance the liver's detox mechanism, there are many other foods, practices, nutrients, and herbs that can do the job without hooking yourself up to an espresso machine—or as in the case with coffee enemas, introducing coffee into your rectum.

Chapter 4

Power Exercise, the Energy Factory

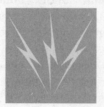

PATRICK HAD BEEN A HIGHLY MOTIVATED, productive construction manager in his late twenties, but had spent the last four months battling a difficult viral infection. For several weeks tests had shown that the virus had completely abated and that he was in a prolonged recovery phase, but he continued to complain of fatigue and uncharacteristic sluggishness.

Through this period he had remained mostly sedentary, afraid to exercise for fear the energy he would expend while working out would somehow reactivate his illness. Formerly lackadaisical about his personal health habits, the illness had brought Patrick to a newfound awareness of the importance of leading a healthy lifestyle—except that he was still avoiding exercise.

While excessive exercise (pushing yourself to exhaustion) can suppress the immune system, moderate exercise actually strengthens the immune system and helps the body generate energy. I finally convinced Patrick to start a cautious exercise program. He started with light aerobic walking and 30 crunches every other day. Within only one week he had more energy than he had had in months, and within two weeks he felt, for the first time, that he was putting the illness behind him. A month later he was more invigorated than he had ever been, with his new-found love of exercise.

NOTHING RAISES YOUR ENERGY FASTER and more effectively than exercise. The simple act of moving can jump-start your metabolic machinery. **Recent research shows that exercise has a direct, immediate effect on energy—if you do nothing more right now than stand up and hop up and down for three minutes you will feel a surge of energy and you will feel more alive.** Kindergarten teachers have known this for years, but now even the top medical researchers have shown on a molecular level that exercise—just a moderate, brief bout—increases the level of energy producing chemicals in your cellular energy factory, the mitochondria. This power surge happens everywhere in your body from your biceps to your heart to the parts of your brain that control memory and intelligence. When you exercise, you're not just training your muscles, you are also training your DNA. That's an amazing thought—that you can actually change the DNA that you inherited—and in such a simple way. Studies show that, with moderate exercise, the mitochondria literally grow in size and become more efficient—it's like trading up your cellular batteries from triple AAA to lithium. This all means that the more you move the more energy your body will make—that's why movement was a key factor in Patrick's recovery.

I hate even to use the word exercise because so many people feel they've heard it all before—and that they've tried and failed. Statistically, most gym memberships are dropped after the first two months—you join for the New Year and then quit going when you simultaneously get the flu and have to do a last-minute rush job on your taxes. But being fit is not about barbells and fancy treadmills. It is not a club you join and abandon. Moving your body to a point of raising your heart rate is a fundamental aspect of physical and mental well-being, one of the most efficient methods your body has of generating energy. There are many ways to exercise, from simple walking to dancing to yoga or whatever else activates your body and raises your heart rate. What matters most is *not how* you work your muscles and raise your heart rate but that you do so *consistently*.

The human body is like a self-winding watch—it's designed to generate energy when you move. When you activate your muscles, everything is geared toward revving up your molecular machinery: Oxygen utilization becomes more efficient; sugar is processed better; fat and calories burn faster; brain cells regenerate quicker; you think more clearly; your heart gets bigger and stronger; the balance of your nervous system shifts toward the calming aspect (parasympathetic); and your emotional happy switch gets turned on by the release of neurotransmitters like serotonin and endorphins. **Forget everything you think you know about exercise, I want you to see physical activity as a means to reconnect with your body as it was meant to be—a wellspring of pure energy.**

To be blunt: You shouldn't be sedentary until you're six feet under. If you need motivation, go watch the group that leads the New York City marathon every year—they are wheelchair athletes paralyzed from the waist down but they have incredibly powerful upper bodies. If they can train for and finish a 26.2-mile race using only a fraction of their muscles to propel their bodies, you can start to move too! My simple program of basic movement and core training, along with specific energy exercises and a dose of sports psychology, is designed to give your body exactly the activity level it needs to achieve optimal energy. It works best if you just take it one step at a time.

How Exercise Generates Energy

The ancient Greeks were the first certifiably exercise-obsessed Western culture, but scientists of all eras have recognized that humans were designed to be continuously on the move. Your genome is the same as your hunter-gatherer ancestors', whose active lifestyle of roaming around procuring (then later harvesting) food dominated human history up until the twentieth century. The sedentary lifestyle that's causing so many health problems today began to take hold with the advent of commercial farming and mass-produced cars; then television came along to keep us glued to our seats; and now we're up against a vicious triumvirate with the rise of computers, the Internet, and video games. I know people feel they're exercising with their Nintendo Wii games, but waving your arms in front of your TV set is not exactly the same as taking a brisk constitutional in fresh air.

Quite simply, you are not designed for a life without exercise; humans are supposed to move every day—whether that means walking for twenty minutes, pulling weeds, or going to the gym. This is not at all unique to people, most animals traverse vast distances daily relative to their size. Research from the Salk Institute showed that if you put a running wheel in a mouse's cage it will run 4 to 5 kilometers every night, and will eventually become a better problem solver than its neighbor without a wheel. The reason for this need to move is complex—it's certainly a genetic imperative that insures finding food, but energy creation also seems to be at the molecular heart of the issue. **As little as thirty minutes of brisk walking causes measurable increases in the production of energy-generating substances, in the transport of energy within the cell, and in the transmission of energy between cells.** By this measure, exercise is like plugging into the grid—it creates energy (as long as you don't overdo it).

The O_2 Factor

Oxygen is a crucial raw material of energy production. And the extraordinary ability of exercise to increase the oxygen supply to your cells makes exercise the OPEC of your body's energy needs—when you exercise the raw material of energy floods the market. With exercise your lungs become more efficient at extracting oxygen from air; the heart pumps more blood and blood vessels dilate, which increases oxygen delivery; hemoglobin releases a considerable quantity of reserved oxygen when body temperatures rise; and with time new capillaries actually grow. When you don't exercise, you're practically suffocating your cells—you're not maximizing your oxygen reserves or your energy supply.

Some of the most groundbreaking—yet elegantly simple—science on the biology and benefits of exercise has come from a *brain research* lab at University of California at Los Angeles. The director of the UCLA Neurotrophic Lab, Fernando Gomez-Pinilla, Ph.D., has been leading methodical studies about the influences of exercise and diet on the brain—specifically on how those lifestyle factors can aid in recovery from spinal cord and brain injuries as well as help reverse Alzheimer's and even the deleterious effects of a diet high in saturated fat. Gomez-Pinilla's research has led deep into the fundamental mechanisms of exercise physiology, which in turn has allowed his team to unlock some of the secrets of energy creation.

Since the early 1990s scientists have known that the body's ability to generate energy (in the form of the molecule ATP) nearly doubles within five to ten days of starting a training routine, but it took the ingenious scientists at UCLA to begin to understand why this is true. In 2006, they were able to demonstrate that exercise significantly stimulated genes to produce more of the energy-balancing factor (mitochondrial uncoupling protein 2) responsible for producing energy (or ATP) as well as for reducing the free-radical by-products of energy production. **Their research showed that moderate exercise can both turn on the energy switch and clean up the pollution generated by energy production. This happens throughout the body.** But they went even further and demonstrated that the same energy-balancing mechanism switched on by exercise also activates proteins responsible for making the brain better able to think, via a mechanism called synaptic plasticity (synapses are the connections between brain cells and when they're plastic, it means that they can grow and improve). Exercise accomplishes this by boosting brain-derived neurotrophic factor (BDNF), a molecule responsible for shaping the old gray matter or brain cells. Exercise is so powerful, researchers found, that BDNF can be elevated for a full day following a session of moderate exercise.

By this measure, exercise would be considered a miracle drug if you could bottle and sell it, but it's right at the tips of your toes. Just take a brisk walk, and this miracle cure is yours.

With exercise, as in all aspects of your life, what begins at an energy level—with thought or intention—translates to the molecular level and then reverberates throughout your body. **When you exercise, you make more energy-generating mitochondria and they work better; you also train your muscles to burn more sugar calories for the same amount of effort and to produce more enzymes that metabolize fat like a lot of little Pacmen zipping around eating up flab.** As muscle grows and fat begins to dissipate, your cardiovascular endurance and energy levels rise and it becomes easier to exercise.

Deeper breathing makes an important contribution to the exercise-energy equation. Intriguing research from Alan R. Hipkiss, a pioneering anti-aging researcher, demonstrates that aerobic exercise regenerates the principal enzyme (NAD) responsible for both supporting the basic operation of mitochondria and retarding mitochondrial aging. The studies suggest that aerobic breathing regenerates this crucial mitochondrial enzyme by reducing reactive oxygen species (free radicals). In other words, a moderate aerobic workout—that doesn't overstress the respiratory system—renews energy-generating mitochondrial structures and can even reverse some of the effects of aging discussed in Chapter 2—not all bad for a "therapy" that's absolutely free and helps you lose weight to boot!

Tired Muscles?

For years we thought muscle fatigue and soreness were due to lactic acid buildup, but it turns out an entirely different mechanism may be at work. Investigators at Columbia University recently identified calcium leakage as the culprit. It's long been known that muscle contraction occurs when calcium enters into the muscle cell; when the calcium moves back out, the muscles relax. The latest research reveals calcium is actually stored in tiny packets in the space between cells and released when the muscles need to contract. However, for some people the packets of calcium start to leak. When this occurs, the calcium's effect is diminished. Without fully loaded calcium packets, the muscles get less calcium when they need it and they contract less efficiently. Making matters worse, the escaped calcium builds up around the muscle causing an enzyme to be released that actually damages muscle tissue. This is basic research; we don't yet have firm recommendations about how to plug the leaks, but because the findings have exciting implications for heart muscle fatigue many scientists are searching for more answers. Stay tuned.

The Depression Connection

A growing body of research points to exercise as a spectacular energizer when fatigue stems from depression. The runner's high is a widely recognized phenomenon, but even I was surprised with the latest findings from investigators at Duke University. **The study pitted moderate exercise against Zoloft for beating depression—and exercise won hands down!** In a cohort of older patients with major depression, Zoloft initially worked faster than exercise to relieve symptoms, but at the ten-month follow-up the group that walked or jogged on a treadmill for ninety minutes a week was significantly less depressed than the medicated group. Exercise elevates all of the same neurotransmitters targeted by antidepressant medications (serotonin, dopamine, noradrenaline), but this and other studies support the use of exercise instead of prescription antidepressants for many people. This is cheering news, indeed, given that exercise is a "therapy" with few side effects—especially if you keep it moderate enough to avoid injury.

Many studies show that treating depression improves your energy-generating capabilities. While there are certainly people who do need psychotropic medications to stabilize their emotional lives, for many people mood dictates their energy levels, and a sure, healthy path to a better mood is regular exercise. In my experience, many people ready to get off of antidepressants have succeeded by incorporating a regular exercise program (along with other healthy lifestyle changes) into their tapering-off schedule. (A note of caution: Chronic overexercising to the point of exhaustion can make depression worse, and individuals on antidepressants should not taper or stop their use without a doctor's supervision.)

How Much Is Enough?

> "If anyone is compelled by any movement to breathe more,
> that movement becomes exercise for him."
> *Greek physician Galen, c. 166 AD*

This isn't the first time I've looked to the past for healing wisdom, but it really is incredible to me how perceptive Galen's comment was almost two thousand years ago. He was speaking at that time about what we now call aerobic exercise, which is increasing oxygen supply to your cells and revving up your metabolism through movement and breath work. In reality, the question of how much is enough depends on your goals. In my practice, the bar is set atop two pillars: Prevention and energy generation. With exercise I want you to prevent chronic illness and increase your energy supply. This requires three aspects of activity: Revving up your metabolic machinery with movement and deep breathing; activating your core muscles with attention to your posture; and, finally, increasing your strength. You can achieve these goals in a number of ways without becoming a gym rat. In this chapter and the 21-Day Plan I offer a foolproof method for getting in touch with your inner athlete. At the very least we will jog your genetic memory back to a time when you had to move to survive!

Revving Up the Machinery

After reviewing most of the literature and working for decades with patients, I clearly see that the simplest and best remedy for fatigue is a straightforward prescription of aerobic activity: You need ninety minutes a week of movement that raises your heart rate to 70 percent of its maximum capacity (60 percent if you're unfit). **If you move your body to the extent that your heart beats noticeably faster, your breathing is more rapid, *and you can still hold a conversation,* then you are in the right zone.** I'll even settle for you to commit to cumulative ten-minute bouts of this kind of activity that adds up to thirty minutes in a day, three days a week. Dancing like crazy to iTunes for ten minutes at a time will do it. I'd be very happy if you were to do a continuous, thirty-minute, aerobically active workout—if you can sustain that routine over the long term. The key is for you to come up with a heart rate-elevating activity (or range of activities) that you can—and will want to—perform for ninety minutes a week for the rest of your life.

Any movement (even parking farther from the mall entrance and walking the few extra steps) will improve your health, but you must raise your heart and respiratory rates in order to challenge your mitochondria to produce more ATP and to increase your energy. **The difference between regular motion and motion that will create more energy is the difference between strolling the supermarket aisle and walking at a brisk pace up a gentle hill.** Walking briskly (at the pace of a jog without the pounding) is enough, whether you're on a sidewalk, a treadmill, or a nature path in the woods. Biking (free or stationary) is great, swimming, jumping rope, walking stairs, doing jumping jacks to your favorite song, running gently in place—all of the above are acceptable ways to rev up your machinery and generate energy molecules. What matters to me and most all the exercise experts in the world is that you reach your magic number for producing results: 70 percent of your maximum heart rate, which is 220 minus your age multiplied by 70 percent (see 21 Day Plan, Day 5 for more details). That's somewhere between walking at a normal pace on a flat surface and running so that your heart is pounding and you can't catch your breath.

The beauty for novices is they are guaranteed to get results. Studies of sedentary middle-aged men with heart disease showed that measures of fitness improved by 50 percent when they began a fitness routine, while similar training in normally active, healthy adults improved by only 10 to 15 percent over the same period. One patient of mine is a restaurant owner who has had a very tough time with weight. He and his wife had been exercise averse for years. Then one year a friend gave them a Christmas present of two weeks with a trainer, a gift he told me about initially with an attitude of disdain. I didn't see them again for six months until one day I ran into them in the park in their exercise clothes. They told me they were too cheap to waste the gift—and knew their friend would find out if they didn't use it. So in January they took the plunge. After their first half-hour walk they passed up a crème brûlée that night. After the second walk they invested in good sneakers. In the end the two weeks were a revelation to them. **He said, "I noticed the difference in my energy right away, and almost felt sad for the years I'd spent depriving my body of what it needed."** Six months after that, at his next checkup, he had shed fifty pounds and said he felt "like an eighteen-year-old again." The key here is that your best motivation is going to be the real results you will experience almost immediately.

Moving to the Next Level

Once the 70 percent target heart rate begins to feel too easy, you have two choices for upping the ante—lengthen your workout or increase your intensity. The smart move is to increase the target gradually, say, to 75 percent of max for one week, then 80 percent the next week. (Athletes can push their target heart rate to 90 percent of maximum, but regular folks shouldn't.) If you're a walker, one simple way for you to increase target intensity is to add ankle weights, which can increase the energy expenditure of walking to values usually observed for running (handheld weights also increase the intensity, but pose a downside risk of raising blood pressure and putting a strain on posture). Taking a hill or the stairs a little faster will do the same, but with less consistency than ankle weights.

It's often tempting to just keep on trucking for longer and longer periods, but that's not the most efficient way to intensify a workout. Some elite athletes train by running up to 150 miles a week, but unless you're looking for a new full-time job as a runner, I give you permission to stop an aerobic workout after 30 minutes. Adding an interval training session to your aerobic routine dramatically increases your metabolism for hours after a workout. With interval training (short bursts of exhaustive activity separated by brief rest), you burn more fat than you would by just lengthening your jog or brisk walk. A good interval workout—if your joints can handle it—is to sprint all-out for forty-five seconds, then rest for sixty seconds and repeat three or four times. With interval training you can rapidly improve your aerobic capacity, and you will find you're able to carry on a conversation while exercising at a much more vigorous pace than you were able to before challenging yourself with intervals.

Overtraining—It is possible to get too much of a good thing: Jacqueline had been coming to me for years, always complaining of low energy and susceptibility to colds. She slept only five or six hours a night and kept an intense job as an ad executive. Six days a week she started her day at 5:00 a.m. with 90 minutes of intense exercise. For years I had been nearly begging her to reduce her exercise level and get more rest. She felt that it was only the exercise that kept her going, and was mortified at the idea of putting on a pound with less exercise. Finally she had to travel to Canada for two weeks, staying in a small town with a hotel that had no gym; and it snowed heavily nearly the whole time she was there. A couple of days she got outside to run early, but after a few days gave up and slept more—and felt an immediate difference in her energy. I got a call a month later to tell me that she had not had such high energy in years: after returning to NYC she tried my advice, exercising moderately (down to sixty minutes four days a week), and felt terrific. Thank goodness for inclement weather.

A subset of my patients, like Jacqueline, overexercise and suffer fatigue as a result. If you get up too early and exercise too much, or you don't take enough rest days in between exercise sessions it's possible that you're overtraining. Rather than rejuvenating you and increasing your energy, too much exercise can produce a state of energy depletion and unwellness. Over-exercising also produces way too many cell- and mitochondrial-damaging free radicals. It depletes the body's energy-reserve (glycogen) stores, leading to anaerobic (without oxygen) rather than aerobic (with oxygen) metabolism—which is very energy inefficient. These processes lead to a degradation of the cells' ability to function and create energy. **It's documented that too much exercise with inadequate rest increases susceptibility to infections, decreases the body's ability to heal, alters sleep patterns and hormonal patterns and increases circulating**

levels of the stress hormone cortisol. Studies show that overtraining actually undermines performance. If you've been pushing yourself hard and feel you've hit a wall in terms of your performance abilities, try getting more rest: it's what overtrainers need most. You may find that your fitness miraculously improves—even as you sleep!

Activating the Core

Raising your heart rate is the nuts and bolts of energy-generating movement. Then there's what I consider to be the more intellectual part of the package—core training. Core training—that is, strengthening and engaging the muscles of your abdomen and torso—has become something of a fitness fad in the past decade. **But in my experience with increasing energy in my patients, core work is essential, and it's a wonderful way to combine conditioning with raising vital energy—or a deep sense of inner strength—which Eastern traditions refer to as Qi or prana.**

You may have been in a yoga session and heard the instructor holding forth on the second and third chakras (according to Ayurvedic medicine these energy centers are in the general vicinity of your lower abdomen and solar plexus). This area is the seat of the core muscles, which are coordinated by a collection of nerves that stretch the length of the spine from the chest down, with powerful connections throughout the body. The core includes the deepest muscle in your abdomen, the grandly named transversus abdominus. The TA is like a weight belt, it attaches at your lower back on either side of your spine and wraps around your abdomen, clinging to your rib cage at its uppermost edge and to your pelvis at its lower most edge. This is the muscle that characteristically atrophies with a sedentary lifestyle (and stretches—or sometimes even splits in half—with pregnancy), resulting in a protruding stomach and an aching back. Sitting on top of the transverse abdominus is the rectus abdominus, the muscle stretching across the front of the abdomen, which in peak condition is the "six-pack" that power lifters strive for and elite athletes naturally develop by logging training time. **Engaging the full core is what allows seemingly miraculous athletic performance.** Tiger Woods doesn't swing the golf club with his arms alone; he swings with his core. Same thing can be said for a true home-run hitter. And the same should be said for each one of us. When you sit, stand, or walk, you should engage your core to support your back and take chronic, energy-draining strain out of your everyday activities.

You can can do this formally with yoga, Pilates, tai chi or, in the case of my program, crunches and push-ups along with attention to the core during any activity. (See the 21 Day Plan, Day 2 for the best way to do a crunch.) Say hello to your core when you lean over the sink to brush your teeth or put away groceries—hold in your stomach muscles, engage your transverses abdominus, breathe deeply and slowly, and feel the energy rising from your solar plexus. **When you move with a properly engaged core, it's like igniting the spark of energy that comes from completing an electrical circuit.** You don't have to call it Qi or a chakra, but you will see that finding and activating your core gives more power to your activity and to your life. In addition, developing core skills—whether or not you go on the extent to become a yoga or Pilates devotee—provides the balance that centers the spine, protecting you from lower back and neck injuries that can become truly debilitating over time.

Hollywood's Secret Core

Excellent posture is one factor that separates the gods and goddesses who walk the red carpet on Oscar night from the rest of us. But movie stars are usually not born, they are made. They *learn* to engage their core—often with the help of countless yoga or Pilates classes or by studying the Alexander Technique, a system developed by a Shakespearean actor in the 1920s. Alexander technicians describe their mission as reducing unnecessary muscular force applied to the body. I like to think of good posture as taking the strain off your spine—banishing the dreaded shoulder slump with your neck flexed forward, vulture-like. When you stand, your neck and spine should be in a straight line at a 90-degree angle to the ground; visualize your body as hanging from a string attached to the crown of your head. The best way to achieve such stellar alignment is to engage your core: Get a grip on your abdominal muscles; use your diaphragm to initiate breaths; tuck your butt slightly under your pelvis; move your shoulders back by pinching your shoulder blades closer and downwards; and feel that string pulling your head up-ward. Here's a good exercise that will help reshape your body in the mold of a softer version of a Marine Corps sergeant or red-carpet diva: While sitting (you can do this periodically at your desk or anywhere), straighten your spine; hold your arms straight down; palms facing forward so that you are forced to bring your shoulders back and down; now twist gently at your waist, keeping your shoulders and chest in a horizontal line while your neck remains in a straight vertical line with your spine. Breath from your diaphragm, not your chest. Practicing in front of a mirror is a powerful help. Most of us have no idea what our posture looks like, which also separates us from movie stars, who have to endure seeing themselves on the big screen.

Increasing Your Strength

In my experience, strength training inhabits the absolute lowest realm of most people's exercise existence, and yet it's a key anti-aging activity that is easy for you to perform. **Strength training is an ideal way to realize the potential your body has for creating energy. By building muscle, you build more energy factories.** Regularly giving your muscles a resistance challenge is crucial for avoiding chronic musculoskeletal problems, and it allows you to burn more calories per pound—it keeps your metabolism physically young. Strength training also builds healthy bones throughout life, and—along with core work—helps stop you from aging into a hunchback. Most people think of bone as an inert, steel-like structure forged in childhood, but this fails to recognize the secret life of your skeleton. Bone is a dynamic, living part of you—it's composed of connective tissue, cells, and blood vessels within a calcium matrix. Your body needs constantly to deposit layers of calcium to maintain the integrity of your skeletal matrix, and the best way to encourage continual remodeling is to apply the healthy stress of weight-bearing exercise.

The marvelous thing about strength training is that beginners have the most dramatic results. In general, previously sedentary people can improve muscular strength by 40 percent, while an elite athlete would only improve strength by 2 percent in the same period (of course they're

Push-Up Reality Check

Research shows that strength builds quicker when you increase *load* rather than repetition. If you have never been able to do more than a couple of push-ups at a time, here's how to get stronger: Increase the challenge throughout the session, with your last push being hardest. For beginners, start your push-ups from a standing position. Place your toes about 24 inches from a wall; place your hands flat against the wall with arms stretched straight out, and slowly bring your nose to the wall by bending your arms, keeping your core engaged, and body in a straight line like a plank. Now push away from the wall until your arms are straight again. Do this a dozen times; rest; then move onto the floor for two rounds of bent-knee push-ups—straight spine, core engaged. Finally, do one perfect all-out push-up, on your toes, body straight as a board. Next time, end with two perfect push-ups. Soon you'll be up to six or more.

starting at a much higher level). It is entirely possible to double the size of your muscles with intensive strength training. (This increases the size and number of mitochondria, both increasing your energy generation, as well as allowing you to burn more calories, since muscles are highly active metabolically and more muscles than fat means better ability to use calories from food.) Bottom line: Your muscles are starving for attention, and they respond relatively quickly when you give them a challenge.

Strength training doesn't have to be pumping iron. It can also be part of your core workout, or the central focus of, say, a yoga practice. In my program, both push-ups and core crunches accomplish strength training together with core work. The key to getting stronger is to provide gradually more intense challenges so that your last lift is the most difficult of the day—for example do bent-knee push-ups, but make the last a full push-up; or do tricep pulls with a one-pound weight, and on the very last one use a five pound weight. But make sure to allow your muscles to fully recover after a session. Every time you do a weight-bearing exercise you are producing slight, microscopic injury to the muscle tissue. The process of repair is what actually thickens and strengthens the tissue. A day or two of rest for each muscle group is essential for allowing the remodeling process that produces stronger muscles.

As you progress—on the road to mini-Mr. or -Ms. Universe status—it is increasingly important to vary your routine. There are so many muscles in the body that working only a few eventually creates imbalances and injury. Once you've mastered the sit-ups and crunches of my program, go ahead and explore other routines. While weight and circuit training are O.K. I prefer exercises that unilize multiple muscle groups, mimicking normal daily activities. I glean terrific tips from the monthly magazine, *Men's Health,* which has a regular "Fitness" section with new ideas for strength training. But let's not get ahead of ourselves. First try to master six perfect push-ups at a go. Then you can entertain dreams of glory.

Gym Toys 101

If you've ever taken a peek at the strength-training section of a gym you've seen quite a few toys—sort of looks like the Polar Bear cage at the zoo. While I'm not a big fan of buying stuff for exercise—most stationary cycles in people's homes turn mysteriously into clothing racks—some strength toys can be useful for working on those hard-to-reach and long-neglected-muscle groups.

- **Bands:** Basically massive rubber bands that come in different tensile strengths to provide resistance. Hold the bands in front of you, core engaged, and stretch the ends of the bands in opposite directions to exercise the triceps and upper back muscles.
- **Balls:** You can pimp your push-ups with an exercise ball. Push up with your hands on the ball to improve balance, or with your feet on the ball and hands on the floor, core engaged, to really ratchet up the level of difficulty. Sitting on a ball and trying to remain stable while doing any exercise—such as moving hand weights—engages the core, improves proprioception balance, and intensifies any exercise.
- **Weights:** Handheld weights are still the standard for strength training. But I'm not taking about hulking up a 50-pound weight, which is invariably done with horrendous postural adjustments. Simple one- to five-pound hand weights are

perfectly adequate training tools. I prefer exercises that mimic normal activities. Take a two-pound weight and, with your your core fully engaged, simply go through the motions of loading the car with groceries—lift and reach—or of putting away a carry-on bag in the overhead compartment—lift the weights from shoulder height to up over your head.

- **Balance Boards:** These add the element of balance to your strength training. New to the scene are microelectric balance boards, which provide a nearly infinitesimal electric vibration that requires your nervous and muscular systems constantly to work for balance

- **Jump Ropes:** The sine qua non of aerobic and resistance training—jumping rope provides aerobic, core, and upper body training. But skipping rope is extremely rigorous—most people new to aerobic training will be exhausted after a couple of minutes.

Why are ancient martial arts so powerful?

Yoga, tai chi, and other martial arts are the best means I know of for connecting your energy circuits. Such exercises have been developed by masters of these arts over thousands of years to gain access to energy sources—through mind, muscle, and breath control. In the West, we love the fantasy of superhuman power in martial arts movies like *The Matrix* and *Crouching Tiger, Hidden Dragon* (or even Jackie Chan). These stories actually contain a seed of truth; while you're not likely to achieve wingless flight, martial arts challenge the body completely and yield results unlike any other exercise system. Also, learning the mysteries of martial arts almost always requires studying with a master—a situation that is both cinematic and conducive to getting better results. Working with ancient martial arts requires controlled breath work and focus—at their essence they are meditative and energy generating movement exercises.

One of my favorite real-life martial arts tales comes from a Qi gong experience I had a number of years ago. A very dear friend of mine, a dedicated runner in her early thirties who'd always considered herself to be fit and regularly jogged three miles around New York's Central Park reservoir, came with me to a rare class given by one of the great qi gong masters visiting from China. We stood stock still, breathing, and occasionally lifting our arms—following the movements of a five-foot-two-inch 85-year-old man wearing sweatpants and a T-shirt—for forty-five minutes in a dingy little New York walk-up studio. I was fretting that my friend would find this typically subtle Chinese practice (similar to Tadasana, or the mountain posture, in yoga) to be unbearably tedious. I myself was struggling—muscles quivering, sweat pouring down my back—and trying to hide it, when all of a sudden the master stopped the class and abruptly told someone to sit down. I turned and saw that my friend was on the verge of passing out! The master chuckled softly and had her put her head between her legs until the dizziness passed. It turns out the seemingly mild practice of just a stationery Qi gong had been incredibly vigorous for this healthy young woman, who was reduced to a quivering pool of sweat while the elderly Master Wu stood there fresh as a daisy.

Try as I have to find a scientific explanation for the vigor of these subtle practices, the research is incomplete. In any case, Western scientific experiments are not necessary in order to validate systems that have been practiced successfully and with excellent health results in Asia for thousands of years. In Chapter 1, *Power Mind,* I detail some of the science that has examined the beneficial effects of Eastern practices like yoga (the most extensively studied of these practices). In one session, for instance, yoga has been shown to lower blood pressure, improve digestion, and reduce hostility, among other effects. Over the long term, yoga can reduce the time it takes your heart and vascular system to recover from stress, improve the way your cells respond to sugar, and activate a host of antianxiety and antidepressant neurotransmitters. From my observations as a scientist and practitioner, studies of the other martial arts like tai chi and qi gong would likely yield similar results. In fact, they have already been shown definitively to improve balance in the elderly—which reduces their likelihood of falling and sustaining debilitating injuries that reduce their lifespan and enjoyment of life.

On a strictly physical level, practicing the martial arts activates a vast range of mechanisms. They can involve the entire structural framework of the human body—bones, joints, ligaments, muscles, tendons, nerves, the cardiovascular, respiratory, and digestive systems. They can also engage the mind in a deeper, more focused, and eventually contemplative state. You can derive enormous benefits from regular physical practices at the beginner's level.

Here are some basic guidelines for those who want to start a martial arts or yoga practice.

- Find a teacher who closely monitors alignment: What shocks most people when they first try yoga is that it's a *weight-bearing exercise* requiring a tremendous amount of strength. The key is to practice with proper alignment so that the bones are in a correct position to carry the load, and the best way to insure that is to take small classes or preferably private sessions when you first begin.

- Start simple: Unless you're a stretching fanatic, for most people the most difficult part of starting a yoga, tai chi, or qi gong practice is that they lack range of motion and balance. But these practices will increase your range of motion and stability in ball and socket joints such as shoulders, hips, and knees by focusing first on seemingly simple postures. First, you'll practice the basics before you begin to exert additional pressure on your joints and muscles with more challenging positions. Your teacher will proceed slowly with good reason.

- Go soft and slow: Postures that promote lengthening of muscles that have become chronically shortened because of high heels, sitting at your desk or on your couch, or concentrating your exercise regimen on walking or running, are a major cause of moaning and screaming among yoga and martial arts initiates. Classes that move too quickly and push too hard can exacerbate pain and tightness rather than help you work through them. On the bright side, muscles are relatively responsive and quick to strengthen and stretch with repeated gentle practice. The payoff: Lengthening and strengthening also improves your balance and physical groundedness and centeredness as your muscles begin to assert a more symmetrical pressure on the skeleton.

- Always engage the core muscles: The "airbag" effect—contracting abdominal muscles on the exhale with exertion—is probably one of the most powerful secrets of martial arts (weight lifters use it, too).

- Be prepared for exercise, not just relaxation: A properly executed posture will combine the actions of muscles, tendons, joints, skeletal and nerve groups in ways that no other exercise can. This synergy is the key to a good workout. Yes, yoga definitely counts as exercise.

- Breathe consciously: No discussion of yoga or martial arts would be complete without mentioning the use of breath. A proper session will actively awaken control of the accessory (or helper) muscles of breathing—the muscles in the lower back, abdomen, shoulder blades, mid back, sternum, and pectorals that make your ribcage work like a bellows to pull air into the lungs. By activating these muscle systems you draw more oxygen deeper into the body, which increases the oxygen supply in your blood and to all of your organs, and provides fuel for your cells to create more energy.

• Focus your mind: Tai chi is derived from qi gong, which is a set of purely meditative and healing exercises. Yoga is the same. Martial arts exercises—as should be the case with all exercise as well—should be done with your mind clear and focused only on the work you are doing. Mental tension and stress should melt away with exercise; with martial arts, achieving a meditative state is a key goal.

Martial arts fully involves mind, body, and spirit. As part of my program, I highly recommend you take some introductory courses in an Eastern physical art—whether yoga, tai chi, qi gong, or another system. You'll gain something from learning any of these techniques. You may find yourself connecting with a practice and decide to use some aspect of it for the rest of your life. For instance you may use the controlled breathing of tai chi at work, or the stretches of yoga as part of a warm-up or cool-down session. However deep you go, you will most certainly erase the element of boredom that can creep into the necessary human pursuit of a physically active life and significantly increase your energy.

Beyond Oxygen: The Benefits of Breath Work

When you begin to explore martial arts with a master, you will learn that breath work operates on a level far beyond the evident material or physical reality of a practice. In most every Eastern tradition breath work is spiritual work. In yoga, the most powerful type of breathing is called pranayama, and its practice seeks to unify body and mind. *Prana* is a Sanskrit word that translates roughly to life-force and *ayama* translates roughly from Sanskrit to the storing and distribution of life-force or energy. Practitioners of pranayama consciously move energy by controlling their breath—as do tai chi and qi gong practitioners.

Many people mistake breath work for deep breathing, but deep breathing implies a forced tensing of muscles. Pranayama-style breathing is the opposite of tension—it is a state in which the mind observes the smooth flow of inhalation and exhalation of air, with nothing to impede the flow—even though you hold your breath briefly in between the inhale and the exhale. The key, however, is that you retain the indrawn breath without straining to hold it. This retention is the point at which the energy or spirit of the breath is distributed, and it's a crucial moment in pranayama.

People sometimes tell me they get a little panicky with breath work. This may be because they're so unused to breathing deeply or rhythmically outside of a stressful situation that they associate the initial efforts of breathing with fear and tension. I suspect they may also get tripped up by their expectations that they'll master the practice quickly or fear of failure that comes with attempting to learn something new. Helpful words of wisdom for the novice come directly from B.K.S. Iyengar, the great Indian-born yogi who developed Iyengar yoga, a healing system that's practiced around the world. In his book, *Yoga: The Path to Holistic Health*, Iyengar writes, "If you fail after a few cycles be content with the knowledge that you have practiced three or four cycles with awareness and attention. Do not turn away from failures. Accept them and learn from them." In Western psychological parlance, Iyengar's tolerant perspective is known as suspending judgment—a practice I heartily endorse, especially when learning any new techniques. Allow yourself to learn and make mistakes. Allow yourself to feel uncertain and don't be afraid of this brief period of uncertainty. You will become more comfortable as you practice. You're learning a great tradition that will be good for you. Allow yourself to be a student of this new way of creating and managing your energy.

Think, Eat (and Be) Like an Athlete

I'd like to put to rest the myth of the buffed versus the buffed-not that pervades society. We place our athletes on pedestals, creating legends around them and their regimens (and even their equipment!).

Everyone holds the potential for getting into shape. You can improve your fitness. If you're used to sitting all day, and tomorrow you walk a mile, you'll be more fit because of the activity and more fit to do it again.

All of your activity contributes to your fitness, just as all of your inactivity contributes to being sedentary. Every extra step you take counts towards a more fit you. Some people are further along the fitness continuum, but the reality is we all have an inner-athlete.

The crucial difference between you and, say, an Olympic rower—or even a movie star getting ready for a part—is the amount of time spent working out. While athletes often have great incentives for working up a sweat, they're not all born with a burning desire to go to the gym. Indeed, there are countless tricks for getting athletes to exercise more and perform better.

Creative Visualization—Viewing yourself as athletic may very well be one of the most powerful tools you have for becoming athletic. All top athletes use visualization techniques before and during competition to enhance their performances, but only recently have neuroscientists begun to understand why this works. An intriguing study at the Cleveland Clinic, Department of Rehabilitation Medicine and Biomedical Engineering, showed that thinking about exercise actually got people in better shape. **Simply visualizing a muscle contraction—without actual exercise—strengthened muscles by as much as 35 percent over a twelve-week period of visualization.** The muscles didn't actually grow in size, but the act of visualization strengthened the brain's signals to the muscles and signaling the muscles is an important first step in conditioning.

You can use this power of the mind to wake up your muscles to overcome whatever mental obstacles are stopping you from getting out and moving. The two keys are to make your imagery as realistic as possible, in full color and detail—and to visualize in the present tense. Try this: Before you go out for a walk, see yourself power-walking right down to the seams of your leggings, see your fine posture, your broad chest, your powerful strides, your arms swinging, your muscles rippling, and repeat an affirmation in the present tense: "I am fit" or "I am strong." Now, go for your walk.

Tunes—Using music has been an open secret in sports psychology ever since Rocky Balboa ran up the steps of the Philadelphia Museum of Art to the chords of "Gonna Fly Now." Athletes still use that song to get themselves psyched up. The shrinking of MP3 players to lightweight, portable sizes has solidified the marriage of music and sports. So effective is music in enhancing performance that MP3 players have been officially banned from marathons by the sport's governing body, USA Track and Field. Similarly, top swimmers commonly use tempo timers—basically water-proof metronomes that maintain the beat, more or less, of Justin Timber-lake's "SexyBack"—for training, but they are illegal in elite-level racing because the driving beat provides a competitive edge.

But of course you can use music to enhance and even jump-start your athletic performance. **Numerous studies confirm that people exercise longer and more vigorously to music.** One of the most important elements is tempo, which research shows should be between 120 and 140 beats per minute—within the range of most people's target heart rate and most commercial dance music. Very conveniently, iTunes now has a Nike Sport Music section, which includes training CDs from athletes like Serena Williams and Lance Armstrong (who suggests working out to Weezer, Keane, and Audioslave). There's even a new Nike + iPod that comes with a motion sensor that allows you to record, download, and monitor the progress of your training sessions. Check it out. Or make your own action-packed song list. And know that absolutely nothing separates you from Rocky Balboa. Lance Armstrong, on the other hand, may in fact be from another planet.

Warm Up—Have you ever had that feeling in the first five minutes of an exercise session that you can't possibly continue? That's because you haven't given your body a chance to warm up. You wouldn't think of starting your car on a 10-degree day and hitting the accelerator to the floor without first letting the engine warm up. It's the same thing with your body. When at rest your muscles are not at their most efficient; a full 70 percent of the oxygen in your blood is unused and kept in reserve for strenuous activity. But blood flow does not adjust instantaneously to a sudden increase in effort. The ultimate risk is that people in poor cardiac health can trigger a life-threatening event by exercising too quickly before the metabolic machinery has been primed for action.

A gentle warm-up—even just lightly hopping up and down before starting a brisk walk—causes your body to begin to deliver blood and oxygen more efficiently. Hemoglobin releases oxygen more readily as your body temperature rises—it's like using a fuel injector to the carbure-tor. Nerve transmission becomes faster as you warm up and the muscles utilize and create energy more efficiently as your metabolism quickens. All of these factors can explain why you may feel horrible at the beginning of a workout—or why you breathe so heavily if you suddenly sprint to catch a bus. But if you take a moment to warm up gently from your initial cold phase, you'll begin to allow the athletic you emerge from the sedentary you. You'll see and feel the difference.

Nutrition

As all elite athletes can attest, your nutrient needs increase as your exercise increases. Most particularly, exercise uses B vitamins, antioxidants, and carbohydrates in abundance. For the moderate exercise recommended in the 21-Day program, a rainbow diet full of fruits and vegetables should be adequate, but if you fall short of that, a multivitamin may be a good idea.

Here are a few tips to ensure you don't use up your energy stores with exercise. First and foremost, be sure you are adequately hydrated before you exercise. Drink at least a pint of water an hour before you exercise. Sugar-packed energy drinks are unnecessary except in extenuating circumstances, for example, if you're running a marathon or you have arrived from sea level to an 8,500 foot mountain and plan to hit the slopes hard. The way to get quick energy is to take it on board beforehand: Eat a primarily complex carbohydrate–based food one to four hours before exercise. Don't overeat—exercising on a full stomach is counterproductive to both your exercise performance and energy (not to mention digestion).

Supplements

When you start to significantly ramp up the intensity and duration of exercise to higher aerobic levels and greater resistance, there are specific supplements that may benefit energy and performance. If you are under a doctor's care for a medical condition, consult your doctor before taking new supplements.

Vitamins and minerals: As we have seen in Chapter 2, many vitamins and minerals are important for energy generation in both the cell's Krebs cycle to extract energy molecules from sugar, and within the mitochondria to produce ATP batteries from these molecules. Arguably the B vitamins are the most important with regard to exercise (B6, for example, supplies the central mitochondrial enzyme NAD), and calcium and magnesium for muscle recovery. A well-rounded plant-based diet can supply these, but for endurance and highly stressful events, taking a mixed vitamin/mineral supplement is a good idea.

Creatine: This is an important food nutrient for exercise performance. Creatine is a protein that is part of all muscle fibers and important as a building block for an energy reserve system in cells called phosphocreatine. Creatine supplements have been the subject of many studies, and has been shown to improve performance and muscle strength at a dose of 20–30 grams (one ounce). It can help decrease recovery time, increase lean body mass and strength, improve hydration of the cell, and increase performance both for aerobic and resistance training. (Precautions include the risk of intestinal cramping and even muscle cramps with high doses and prolonged use. Inadequate hydration increases risk of creatine side effects. People with kidney disease and people taking kidney-stressing medications should not use creatine.)

D-Ribose: Ribose is one of the intermediate sugars created within the cell on the way to creating ATP from oxygen and glucose—it is about halfway there in the Krebs cycle just outside the mitochondria (see Chapter 2 for more on this). Taking ribose (usually 20–30 grams) can provide a quick burst of energy. It minimally affects insulin levels. But it is not long lasting, and is probably best used only *during* a workout. (Precautions are minimal if used as recommended occasionally with exercise.)

Pyruvate: This simple sugar, like ribose, is an intermediate sugar downstream from glucose on the way to creating ATP. A number of research studies show that using it (5–10 grams/day) can help cells draw in glucose, increase glycogen stores, and improve performance, especially in endurance events. Pyruvate's effect is roughly equivalent to carbohydrate loading before exercise, or using carbohydrates during exercise. (Precautions are minimal as with ribose.)

Citrate: Taking citrate (found as sodium, calcium, or magnesium citrate) can reduce fatigue by reducing acidity, thereby reducing potassium accumulation inside cells. Another way to promote alkalinity is to eliminate sodas and adopt a more plant-based diet; that will naturally favor a more beneficial alkaline internal environment.

N-acetylcysteine (NAC): This amino acid discussed in Chapter 3 for detoxification also helps decrease the tendency for fatigue from exercise in two ways: First, NAC helps reduce free radicals and clear toxins better; and second, it plays a role in decreasing potassium accumulation in muscles, by helping produce more efficient ATP-driven pumps for balancing the cells' potassium and sodium levels.

Zinc: Low level supplementation with this mineral can help increase exercise stamina as shown in a 2005 study from the USDA Human Nutrition Research Center. A small amount, 5 mg (less than the daily recommended level of 11 mg) was shown to reduce carbon dioxide buildup, help clear lactic acid, and increase stamina. (Precaution: as with all minerals too much can be toxic. With zinc the safe intake level is set at a maximum 25mg/day. Studies with exercise have measured benefits with lower doses. Taking extra zinc may necessitate adding copper, as zinc inhibits copper absorption.)

Fenugreek seed: Surprisingly, this plant seed has been shown to increase the ability of the cell to replenish glycogen after exercise by up to 60 percent. This is due to an amino acid not normally present in human's muscles (4-hydroxyisoleucine) present in fenugreek. This amino acid also may be an important nutrient for regulating blood sugar and insulin. Dosage is 30 grams (one ounce) per day. (Precautions: do not take fenugreek seed if you are taking anticoagulants—blood thinners. Also, fenugreek can lower blood sugar, so diabetics on medication and hypoglycemic individuals should use this supplement only with close supervision by your medical doctor.)

Marine algae extract, astaxanthin (a carotenoid in the same family as lycopene and beta-carotene): In multiple published studies from Japan, this sea plant extract has been shown to allow cells' metabolism to be more efficient—burning fatty acids for fuel more than glucose. By this, it also may help reduce body fat. It also has been shown to reduce damage from free radicals. This supplement illustrates the nutrient power of the seaweed and algae families that nutrition scientists are just beginning to explore. (Precautions include the need to know your source: algae is harvested from the sea and may contain some micro-contaminants such as other forms of algae. People with immune suppression, including AIDS, should avoid it.)

Eight Simple Energy-Generating Exercises

Brisk walk: If I had to choose one energy-generating activity to recommend above all, it is walking. Walk at a pace brisk enough to increase your heart and breath rates; maybe tackle a few flights of stairs while you are at it. As you walk, actively engage your core, monitor your posture, be aware of the range of motion in your hips and thighs, and breathe consciously, working your ribcage like a bellows. You might look a little strange to the casual observer, but you'll feel so much better when you are finished. With a little practice (and creative visualization), you may even give the impression to others that you are expert enough to be counted in the ranks of professional walkers—after all, racewalking is an Olympic sport.

Breath Work: Inhale quietly and slowly, allowing your abdomen to rise, to the count of 4, pause holding the air lightly to the count of 4, exhale slowly, allowing your abdomen to contract, to the count of 6. Repeat four times. The simple act of slow, deep breathing can be incredibly energizing—and relaxing (see Breath Breaks in the 21-Day Plan).

Seated Warrior (Virasana): This is a very simple stretch and a phenomenal way to expand your breathing capacity (if you have trouble with your knees or back, do this sitting in a chair, not on the floor). Kneel on the floor, shoulders back and down, neck and spine in a straight line perpendicular to the floor. Lower your buttocks to your feet. Raise your arms in front of you to shoulder level, tightly interlock your fingers, palms facing you. Now rotate your wrists and forearms so that palms face out, fingers away. Maintain your posture. With fingers clasped and palms facing away, raise your arms until palms face the ceiling. Keep your shoulders pinched back, sternum lifted, chest expanded, relax throat and neck. Look straight ahead, body and neck in a straight line perpendicular to the ground—no tilting. Breathe evenly and hold the posture for one minute or as long as it's comfortable. With time you can extend this to five minutes. Bring your arms gently down to your sides. Place palms on the floor, kneel, stand up first with one leg, placing hands on knee for leverage.

Downward-Facing Dog (Adhomukha Svanasana): This simple yoga posture definitely gets your circulation going, but it's not recommended for individuals with high blood pressure, frequent headaches, or who are pregnant. Stand with your feet hip-distance apart, core engaged, head in a straight line with your spine. Take an abdominal breath. Bend from the waist until your palms touch the floor (it's OK to bend your knees). Place your right foot back about four feet from your hands. Now place your left foot alongside your right so that your butt is in the air, heels on the ground, and you are in an inverted "V" position (again, it's OK to bend at the knees if it's uncomfortable to straighten your legs all the way). Straighten your spine (no hunching over). I like Rodney Yee's description in his book, *Moving Toward Balance*, "Practice with bent legs, emphasizing the lift of your sitting bones . . . Feel the integration between the length of the sides of your waist, the opening of your chest and the extension of your arms." B.K.S. Iyengar further recommends tightening muscles at the top of the thighs and pulling in the kneecaps. Just hang out there for a moment, breathing quietly, arms and back straight, heels on the floor. Now bring your right foot back close to your hands, then your left foot, and slowly stand.

Qi Gong Energy Ball: With this exercise, visualize yourself holding a large ball of energy, move slowly and focus on breathing—your arms should move with very little effort, almost as if they are moved by an invisible energetic force. Feet are parallel, knees slightly bent, butt tucked under, arms at your sides. Take a deep, abdominal breath in and out and continue to breathe consciously throughout the exercise. Begin by allowing your arms to float slowly up, shoulder-width apart, palms facing each other as though you're holding a giant beach ball of energy, waist high in front of you. Bend your arms at the elbows, bringing the imaginary ball closer to you. Now slowly rotate wrists to face palms away from your body and push the ball away until your arms are straight, stepping forward onto your left foot (knee remains slightly bent). Allow arms to float wide apart so that you make a T, bring arms gently down to sides with palms facing each other as you step left foot back to its original place. Float arms upward again, in front of you, holding the ball of energy. "Lift" the ball over your head and let go, now allow your arms to slowly float back down to your sides, breathing quietly, core engaged, butt tucked under, shoulders down and back. Repeat, this time stepping right foot forward.

Hopping: Jumping rope is the best, full-fitness, aerobic energy-generating exercise, but it's not always convenient to whip out a jump rope. You can hop up and down just about anywhere—next to your desk, standing in line at the bank, waiting for a train. Hop thirty times; finish by standing for a moment with good posture and taking four slow abdominal breaths.

Push-ups and **core crunches** (see above).

Rock out with your iPod: No explanation necessary. Freeform dancing is not only fun, but allows you to log an aerobic workout without the psychic pain.

Chapter 5

Power Rest, How to Recharge Your Battery

FREDERICA CAME TO SEE ME feeling as though she "could no longer function." In her mid-forties she'd developed insomnia and had become so chronically exhausted it was beginning to ruin her life. She was exceedingly short-tempered with her family, had begun to develop headaches, indigestion, and more frequent colds than ever before. As a result of her problems, however, she had tried to observe some good health habits—she had become more conscious of eating a well-balanced diet, exercised regularly (sometimes too intensely), and cut out any stimulants after noon. Even so, she was still exhausted by 8:00 p.m. Most nights she could fall asleep around midnight, but invariably woke up at 4:00 or 5:00 a.m. (sometimes known as The Hour of the Wolf, when our greatest fears tend to surface if we're awake). She would toss and turn, rarely going back to sleep. She was lucky if she got six hours of sleep on any night. It had become a vicious cycle, possibly accelerated by barely perceptible hormone shifts of middle age.

She had tried her regular physician's prescription sleeping pills (which he had given her only after he'd performed many batteries of tests to determine that she had no underlying illness), but they either left her feeling badly hung-over, or they wore off after four hours. She reported that her doctor's attitude was, "Hey, I'm more tired than you. Get over it." Over-the-counter and health food store supplements, and even prescription hormones, seemed to have no effect whatsoever.

It was clear to me Frederica was suffering from stress-induced insomnia. This is the sleep problem I most commonly see. The cure would not be found in a sleeping pill, but in getting better control of her mind and thought processes, and in addressing possible underlying nutritional issues. I asked her to limit alcohol intake to one glass of wine with dinner (processing a heavier load of alcohol can cause early hour awakening), and placed her on a multivitamin with B-complex.

Frederica then began the real work of learning how to help her body sleep. I taught her how to do progressive relaxation exercises at bedtime: starting by contracting muscles in her neck and jaw, and gradually working her way down to her toes—focusing on the exercise and letting random thoughts go. This helped her drift off into a more peaceful sleep, and she didn't get stuck in her prior habit of allowing fears and anxieties to flood her mind just before falling asleep. When she woke up in the early hours of the morning, she practiced dream remembrance: As soon as she was conscious of beginning to wake up she was immediately required to lock onto her dream. No matter how scary or weird the dream was, she had to stay in it in order to block the old habit of ruminating on her worries as soon as she woke up. More than half the time, she reported, this dream remembrance allowed her to go right back into the sleep cycle. If she lost the dream or awakened without memory of one, she immediately started either the progressive relaxation exercise or a breath-focused meditation. By the end of the first two weeks, she was clocking in seven or eight hours of sleep most days. Her energy soared.

FREDERICA'S STORY IS VERY COMMON — sleep deprivation is at epidemic proportions in the United States—a recent study found that 71 percent of Americans are sleep-deprived and get less than eight hours per night. Much of this national sleep debt has been rung up by choice—people just don't want to turn out the lights. Before the electric light bulb was invented, people slept an average of ten hours a day.

Today Americans sleep less than seven hours on average, and a number of factors including stress, medications, and habitual snoring often degrade the quality of that sleep. The incidence of insomnia, trouble falling or staying asleep, is rising (in part due to the aging population—yes, older people tend to have more sleep issues). As a consequence, sleeping pill sales are at an all time high. One study put the national price tag of treating insomnia at $13 billion. Clearly, it's time for people to start getting proper sleep.

Scientists have only recently begun to explain what every mother in the world knows: sleep plays an important role in overall health. Inadequate sleep is now associated with heart disease, diabetes, and obesity among other chronic diseases. Recent investigations show that eight hours is optimum for proper healing and cellular rejuvenation, and that—even more surprising—the most powerful healing occurs between the eighth and ninth hours of sleep. Bottom line: Just about everyone should make an effort to get more sleep, and more regenerative rest.

You probably don't have time to catch up with lost sleep by napping in the middle of the day—God bless the cultures that encourage a siesta—but you no doubt can make some adjustments in your habits to allow a better quantity and quality of regenerative rest at night. I'll share some very simple and practical—nonpharmaceutical—ways to improve your sleep in this chapter. As you start resting more, you will see that more and deeper sleep buys you considerable energy.

Healthy, Regenerative Rest

One of the comments I frequently hear in my office is, "I don't need a lot of sleep." A corollary of this is the oft-repeated phrase, "I don't have enough time to sleep." As gently as I can, I break the news that adequate, regenerative rest (there is such a thing as nonregenerative sleep, which I'll get to in a moment) is a critical foundation of health as well as an important source of abundant energy. Let's take a look at what science knows about sleep.

Why We Sleep

There are three main reasons to sleep: to conserve energy by slowing down metabolic processes, to regenerate tissue, and to clear out toxins. Slumber is a time of semi-*hibernation*, when the body's neurological and hormonal systems operate mostly at low levels that conserve energy: body temperature is allowed to drop, so there's less work in generating heat; there's no new food to digest; blood pressure decreases; heart and breathing should be steady and slow for the majority of sleep time. This slowdown allows for *regeneration*; it gives time and resources for the cell's surface receptors and internal processes to recoup, repair, and replace. Sleep is also a time of *detoxification*, when the body is able to clear out energy-draining molecular by-products that accumulate during the day as a result of high levels of activity.

By putting all systems on low power, sleep offers your body time and energy to carry out a full range of maintenance duties: rebalancing hormones (for example, replenishing cortisol and insulin supplies), strengthening the immune system, consolidating memory, and repairing overworked areas of the body. **While you slumber, your brain's immune cells get to work producing a crucial substance called interleukin 12, which is necessary for processing memory as well as for conferring immunity to disease.** During the day, the natural ebb and flow of the body's processes create cell-damaging free radicals (by-products of normal metabolism) that tend to multiply in the presence of toxins such as heavy metals or excess sugar. Sleep's metabolic slowdown allows the body to clear out these harmful substances, preparing the detoxification systems for the demands of the next day's activities. Sleep improves cognitive functioning; both napping *and* a full eight hours of sleep have been shown to result in better performance on tests. Sleep may also actually help restore energy levels in the body by clearing the cells of a sleep-inducing molecule in the brain called adenosine (see box).

Sleep makes you smarter, gives you energy, and builds immunity. And that's just a few of its benefits.

The emotional repair that also occurs while you slumber awards good sleepers with better energy. When you sleep, levels of serotonin, the emotion-regulating neurotransmitter, decline. This low level is not terrific if you wake up in the middle of the night, but the decline is felt to allow cell surface receptors of that happy molecule to resensitize and become better at keeping mood swings at bay the next day. **This refreshing of chemical receptors in the brain explains why most people have a brighter outlook in the morning, and why you should try not to think worrying thoughts at night when your brain chemistry may be more vulnerable to dark scenarios.** (Relaxation exercises help dissipate negative thoughts that tense your body and keep you awake.) Sleep depriva-

A Sleep-Energy Connection

Recently, scientists have begun to piece together a picture of sleep as an energy-restorative state. In a cunning bit of biological multitasking, a compound called adenosine—the backbone of the energy molecule adenosine triphosphate (ATP)—can put you to sleep when its levels rise in the brain. The accumulation of adenosine as a result of energy expenditure during the day is thought to trigger slow brain waves that make you sleepy at night. The body actually prevents itself from overexertion by using a component of its energy-generating molecule to induce sleepiness. Then, when you sleep, your body gathers sleep-inducing adenosine from inside cells and in between cells, and uses it to replenish the energy. This molecular recycling routine is key to sleep's ability to rejuvenate your energy supply.

tion has even been shown to have a profound effect on your ability to form moral judgments. Going without sleep impairs a person's ability to integrate emotions with logic, which is a necessary skill for moral reasoning. The good news is that having a high level of emotional intelligence prior to sleep deprivation helps when it comes to making moral decisions in a state of exhaustion. In one fascinating study, sleep deprivation resulted in an elevated expectation of a higher reward for risky behavior in one part of the brain, and activity in the part of the brain having to do with expectation of loss was diminished. (You might want to inquire about your financial adviser's sleeping habits!)

Dreaming is not well understood, but it is another means by which sleep addresses emotional balance. In dreams, you try to work out the day's anxieties and stresses, another way in which sleep is a time for emotional repair.

All of the wonderful things sleep can do for you depend on getting a good night of it. As you'll see in the following section, good sleep is not only a function of quantity—how much you get—it is also a function of quality, or what kind of sleep you get.

What is a good night's sleep?

In the hundreds of university sleep labs in the United States, where people's brains are wired to scanning machines and oxygen monitors while they dream of faraway places, researchers have learned that sleep is an incredibly dynamic operation. In healthy young adults—whose brainwave patterns have been used in sleep medicine as the model of what's normal—there are two states of sleep: *non-rapid eye movement* (NREM), which constitutes 75 to 80 percent of overall sleep; and *rapid eye movement* (REM), which constitutes most of the remaining 20 to 25 percent (brief periods of waking contribute about 5 percent of sleep time). **Sleep is *initiated* with the dominance of non-rapid eye movement, with its four distinct stages; and sleep *culminates* with a dominance of rapid eye movement, a mentally active form of sleep that allows you to wake up relatively alert (unlike reptiles, which are paralyzed by a state of torpor upon awakening, which may sound eerily familiar to some).** Throughout the night, the body cycles between the two states, and to get a good night's sleep you need enough of both, which is known in the medical business as having good sleep architecture.

Like a deep-sea diver, your consciousness descends through the stages of non-rapid eye movement toward the deepest and most restful fourth stage called *slow-wave sleep.* Then your brainwaves take the plunge into rapid eye movement—where the body is almost completely paralyzed but the mind is active with *vivid dreaming*—before ascending back to the lighter stages. **In eight hours of sleep, your brainwaves should submerge into vivid dreaming and then resurface again every ninety minutes—or about five times a night.**

As you alternate between the two states of sleep, your body alternates between two states of nervous system control. For the most part, NREM sleep produces slow alpha and delta brainwave activity on a brain scanner (electroencephalogram or EEG), and it is governed by the calming, parasympathetic portion of the nervous system that produces a steady heartbeat and breathing rate with low energy expenditure. By comparison, the vivid dreaming of REM sleep produces vigorous brainwaves—equal to and sometimes even more intense than waking daytime activity—and it is governed by the stimulating or sympathetic nervous system, which causes quickening of your heart and breathing rates as well as a rise in blood pressure and energy expenditure. For a good night's sleep sufficient to rejuvenate the mind and body and give you better energy for the next day, you need go to bed early enough to leave time for a full menu of both states of sleep.

The biochemical mechanisms for initiating and maintaining sleep are extraordinarily complex and involve a wide range of neurochemicals and receptors within the brain as well as chemical modulators (thyroid, cortisol, cytokines) coming to the brain from throughout the body. Some of the important substances within the brain that are critical for proper rest include melatonin, produced by the pineal gland at the base of the brain, which is the master regulator for the body's sleep-wake circadian rhythms; and orexins, recently discovered peptides present in many regions of the brain that help maintain wakefulness. Maintaining healthy sleep cycles also depends on having balance between two receptors found throughout the brain that induce sleepiness and alertness. The NMDA (N-methyl-D-aspartate) receptor provides stimulation to nervous system cells helping keep you alert during waking hours; and the GABA (gamma-aminobutyric acid) receptor sedates the cells. During waking hours you want NMDA to predominate, and of course you hope for the opposite GABA dominance when you are ready for sleep. But while biochemists play with the complexities of these sleep systems to find new prescription drugs for inducing sleep or maintaining alertness, the mechanics of getting a good night's sleep are really quite simple.

When you go to sleep and _how long_ you sleep determines whether or not you get a healthy, full run of all the states and stages of sleep—you need eight hours with more than half of that under your belt before 4:00 in the morning. Slow-wave sleep predominates in the first third of the night. At around 4:00 a.m., when your circadian rhythm (your body's internal biological clock) brings your body temperature down to its lowest ebb, rapid eye movement begins to predominate; and the deepest stage of slow-wave sleep can fade away altogether. With a full night's sleep, as sleep time is extended the amount of vivid dreaming (REM) sleep increases. If you occasionally stay up until the early hours of the morning you will get short-changed on slow-wave sleep and have a less regenerative rest.

I like to think of non-rapid eye movement as the shutdown mode of your own personal software—it is the required first part of sleep. Rapid eye movement represents a shift to an altered state of dream-consciousness that usually follows the shutdown state, and thrives in the low body temperatures of the wee hours of the morning. Quite simply, sleep is a journey through different states and you need to take the time to fully realize that journey in all its states.

Unhealthy, Energy Draining Sleep

If it's true, as Tolstoy said, that unhappy families are each unhappy in their own way, then poor sleep is the unhappy family of the human genome—everyone seems to have his or her own unique way of not sleeping. There are, in fact, many causes of poor sleep, but by far the most common are stress and the normal changes of aging. Many other functional problems, like sinus conditions or chronic pain, can destroy sleep as can lifestyle choices like alcohol over-consumption. Making matters worse, poor sleep can magnify problems like chronic pain and stress, creating a vicious cycle and wasting precious energy.

Over a period of about five years even sleep doctors were losing sleep over the definition of insomnia, which had been described traditionally as difficulty initiating or sustaining sleep, or early awakening. But there was a growing group of people with daytime complaints often associated with insomnia—fatigue, trouble concentrating, and moodiness—who were not reporting that they had trouble with sleep. The sleep medicine community finally decided to include daytime symptoms that usually stem from sleep loss as part of insomnia, so, now, the realm of conditions related to trouble sleeping has expanded. You don't have to be lying awake counting sheep to qualify as having a bad night's sleep: your sleep can be very poor if it is constantly disturbed, for example, by heavy snoring. Below I cover a number of conditions that are known causes—but too often go unrecognized—of poor sleep. No matter how you miss out on sleep, however, your energy will be worse off.

The consequences of poor sleep range from total exhaustion to major health problems. With deprivation your body becomes inefficient at making energy: it dissipates a lot of energy as heat, resulting in a sort of energetic spinning of wheels. A protein in the energy manufacturing mitochondria called mitochondrial uncoupling protein-1 (UCP-1) is over-produced during sleep deprivation. This molecule disconnects—or uncouples—the machinery within the mitochondria, forcing it to burn the nutrients within as heat rather than transforming them into other more useful forms of energy. It's the somnolent equivalent of burning the furniture when you start to run out of firewood!

Mounting evidence suggests that sleep problems are intimately related not only to lack of energy, but to illnesses such as breast cancer, obesity, diabetes, immune deficiencies, and especially heart disease. In one fascinating study from the University of Chicago Department of Medicine, sleep deprivation crippled the effectiveness of a flu shot! **Sleeping for four hours a night for six days reduced healthy students' immune system response to flu vaccines by 50 percent compared to volunteers who had normal sleep.** Amazingly, it took between three and four weeks of normal sleep for the young volunteers to develop a healthy vaccine-conferred immunity to the flu after just one week of reduced shut-eye. Never underestimate the value of good sleep habits!

Just take a moment to consider your heart. Thanks to the venerable Nurses Health Study (an ongoing multicenter investigation that's followed 122,000 nurses for more than 30 years), we've learned that getting just *one less hour of sleep* per night (**for example, shifting from eight to seven hours on a regular basis) significantly *increases* the risk of heart disease.** A similarly significant study in Japan showed that a drop in sleep time from eight to five hours just two nights a week can help trigger a heart attack in people at risk for heart disease. Not only does a proper night's sleep protect your heart, even napping helps. I was encouraged to learn from a recent study of 23,000 people by investigators in the Department of Epidemiology at the Harvard School of Public Health that three half-hour midday naps per week dramatically reduced (by 37 percent) the risk of suffering a heart attack and dying (as long as the nap doesn't come right after a big meal, which actually increases the risk of a heart attack)! Even the occasional catnap (just one or two a week) lowered the risk of heart-related death by 12 percent. Who wouldn't trade a catnap for a heart attack if given the chance?

Still not convinced you should give up late-night TV? With all due respect to Jay and Jon and Dave and the rest of the late-night jokesters, consider that a good eight hours sleep is even thought to be important for weight control. In a recent highly publicized study, researchers at Columbia University, Mailman School of Public Health, Department of Epidemiology analyzed sleep habits and the body mass index (ratio of weight to height) of more than 9,500 people and found **those who slept for only five hours each night were 60 percent more likely to be obese than those who slept for seven or more hours per night.** Scientists at the University of Chicago have produced a series of studies showing that sleep deprivation leaves its mark on metabolism and hormones, specifically leptin (released by fat cells and signals satiety) and ghrelin (produced by the stomach and signals hunger). In one study, after two sleep-deprived nights, participants' blood levels of leptin dropped by an average of 18 percent and their ghrelin levels soared by 28 percent, which helps explain why lack of sleep makes you eat and put on weight.

When you miss an entire night's sleep, your body goes into recovery sleep mode the following night in which it makes up for lost sleep by spending lots of time in slow-wave sleep, sometimes skipping rapid eye movement altogether. If your sleep is disrupted frequently in a single night the body also tries to recover by increasing time spent in slow-wave sleep. But with a night of fitful rebound sleep you get short-changed on vivid dreaming sleep, and are likely to wake up groggy without the help of the REM phase to activate your brain cells.

Jet lag is a study in rapid eye movement chaos. **REM sleep depends on your circadian rhythms, and jet air travel across time zones is a sure way to wreak havoc on your body clock.** To experience a full REM cycle you have to get significant sleep between 4:00 a.m. and 8:00 a.m., when your circadian rhythms produce a 24-hour low in body temperature. When you fly east across time zones you start your day at a time when your body is supposed to be in the active dreaming cycle (for example your wristwatch says 8:00 a.m. but your body clock says 5:00 a.m.). You get shortchanged on mentally active sleep and start your day straight out of slow wave sleep, which feels quite sluggish. On the flip side, if you fly westward across time zones, you might fall asleep at the bottom of your circadian cycle when your body "thinks" it's about 4:00 in the morning. In that case it's possible to go straight into vivid dreaming without passing through restful slow waves.

A jet-lagged night of all REM or no REM can leave you feeling pretty strange. A walk in the morning sun at your destination can help reset your biological clock (see *Light Therapy*, below) so you don't feel as out of sync. Taking an extract of the body-clock regulating hormone, melatonin (see *Nutritional Supplements*, below) two hours before bedtime in the new time zone has also been shown to help you dissipate the effects of nagging jetlag.

The body usually recovers on its own from the occasional bad night's sleep or trip across the Atlantic. Trouble starts, however, when the states and stages of sleep are chronically mixed up, or when you just don't get enough night after night.

Bad Sleep: The Causes and Cures

Poor sleep can be a function of inferior quality (having your sleep stages out of sync for any number of reasons), or inadequate quantity (getting too little sleep, which cuts off sleep stages), or it can be a function of both, which is absolutely the worst-case scenario. No matter what the cause, however, you can get your sleep problems under control and it is vitally important that you do so. I find that the best way to encourage my patients to practice better sleep habits is to let them know exactly what conditions and choices have a negative impact on sleep.

Aging—It turns out that the definition of normal sleep goes out the window as we age. Much of the trouble has to do with shifting hormones at midlife—for men, too!—that affect the amount and type of rest you get. Chronic conditions that often come with age such as arthritis, sinus congestion, and acid reflux can also disrupt sleep. With age, there is a decrease in growth hormone and evening elevations of the stress hormone cortisol as well as an increase of the immune system messengers called inflammatory cytokines (especially interleukin-6)—all of which negatively affect sleep and reduce the amount of time spent in the more restorative stages 3 and 4 of non-rapid eye movement. This means that older people are predisposed to have problems not only with sleep quantity but sleep quality—with inevitable consequences for both their health and energy.

Some of the trouble with aging can be addressed with better stress management. **By age forty, levels of the stress hormone, cortisol, tend to be elevated for most people, which scientists now believe may be a result of that hormone not reaching its low point at night.** Managing stress during the day so that you are able to get to sleep earlier and sleep longer may promote beneficial declines in cortisol at night. In some cases sleeping more can be seen as an anti-aging potion—circulating testosterone levels in healthy men are known to decline with advancing age, but when men sleep longer they are able to make more testosterone. Which just goes to show sleeping is not for sissies!

One of my favorite observations from sleep medicine labs is that people of a certain age (65 and up) tend to believe that their sleep is *worse* than it actually is. Much of the trouble has to do with attitude. With meticulous psychological surveys, scientists have determined that whether a person views getting less sleep as insomnia or merely accepts it as a normal part of aging depends largely on his individual attitude about growing old. One of my longtime patients who cruised into her seventies with abundant energy once told me that she had learned to accept getting less sleep as "No big deal." I'm not suggesting you ignore a sleep problem, but I am encouraging you not to become one of those folks of an advanced age who sit around complaining about sleep—that's a sure energy-draining activity.

Stress—Unbridled stress causes difficulty falling asleep as well as sleep disruption (waking in the middle of the night with trouble getting back to sleep). People wracked with stress can't turn off the worry: when they lie down their minds race; or when they wake up in the middle of the night, their worries take hold and keep them awake. Researchers have begun to follow the destructive path of the stress hormones and other biochemical messengers that keep your neuroendocrine system hyperactive, even into the middle of the night.

Stress per se doesn't necessarily keep you awake, but worrying about stressful things can keep you awake. And because sleep deprivation mimics the effects of stress by elevating stress hormone levels and activating anxiety-promoting areas of the brain, you set up a vicious cycle: you're stressed so you can't sleep; then the lack of sleep makes your stress worse. You quickly become perpetually exhausted. Unremitting stress has also been shown to trigger nightmares, increasing demands on your nervous system. This is why I strong recommend night-time relaxation exercises in the 21-Day Plan.

The many negative effects that unbridled stress produces in your nervous system can have serious consequences during sleep. **The early morning between 4:00 and 8:00 a.m.—when rapid eye movement (REM) is at its peak—is the time of day with the highest incidence of heart attacks (and this doubles on Monday mornings).** This is largely due to stress-induced declines in your heart's ability to handle the shift from the calming, parasympathetic nervous system dominance of non-REM sleep to the stimulating, sympathetic nervous system dominance of REM sleep. As your nervous system starts to wake up, a stressed heart sometimes just can't take it. Clearly, cardiovascular problems need to be diagnosed early and treated by a specialist. Along with proper treatment, a conscious stress reduction program coupled with regular moderate exercise will help to protect the heart during times like the early morning when nervous system shifts require healthy flexibility of the heart muscle.

One further caveat has to do with managing stress when you actually do wake up. If you wake up, jump out of bed, and go straight into panic mode over your work responsibilities it can be tough on your ticker. This is why I strongly recommend you start your day with the two-minute meditation, the Early Morning Wake Up Call, detailed in the 21-Day Plan (see Part Two). Starting your day with your stress under control will keep it in better control all day and give more consistent energy.

Sleep Apnea—Sleep apnea is a condition in which breathing stops for at least 10 seconds at least 15 times per hour during sleep. It's often accompanied by loud snoring and is considered to be a major cause of exhaustion during the day. Short of your spouse guessing that you have the condition, daytime sleepiness is one of the biggest symptomatic tip-offs to sleep apnea. **On the extreme end, sleep apnea can cause you to wake abruptly gasping for air.** In some cases it does not wake you but continues to cause blood oxygen levels to decline—often significantly—throughout the night; suffocating the heart, the brain, and all of the body's cells. Each spell sets off alarms (*take a breath!*) making it all but impossible to move beyond the very lightest stage of non-rapid eye movement sleep—forget about vivid dreaming! Studies of apnea demonstrate that it's associated with dominance of the sympathetic nervous system, which places stress on the heart, too.

The causes of sleep apnea are varied. It has a strong genetic component (if a parent has apnea, you have a 40 percent chance of getting it), most likely due to inherited traits in the anatomy of the neck and pharynx that make it harder to keep the airway open during sleep. It's more common in men and its frequency rises with age. Drinking alcohol and sleeping on your back can trigger the problem. By far the most common cause is obesity, which increases the risk of developing apnea by more than 1000 percent! Excess body weight puts pressure on the throat and prevents it from opening enough to facilitate breathing. Up to 70 percent of people with obesity have sleep apnea. Having an underactive (hypo)thyroid can be a hidden cause of sleep apnea, and when treated, sleep apnea often also clears.

The symptoms of apnea are pretty far-ranging, from frequent awakening, daytime exhaustion, poor memory, and loud snoring (about 10 percent of habitual snorers have apnea). The health consequences can be devastating, including a significant increased risk of hypertension and heart attacks. For example, many people who have uncontrolled high blood pressure—for which medications seem not to work well—actually have sleep apnea as the cause. A continuous lack of oxygen during sleep can precipitate an acute heart attack. If you have any of the symptoms of apnea you should consider being evaluated by a sleep medicine specialist—hopefully before you have a heart attack.

If you have sleep apnea, it is possible to receive a prescription for a continuous positive airway pressure device (CPAP). This device is placed over your nose and mouth and produces positive pressure (like a vacuum cleaner on reverse) that forces open your airway and causes more oxygen to flow into your upper airways and lungs. By stopping the drop in oxygen levels and frequent wakening, the device allows your body to pass through all the cycles of sleep. CPAP has been shown to conserve sleep energy and improve daytime energy levels. Oral appliances—which you can obtain from a dentist—to reposition the jaw muscle and tongue and increase the airwave space can be almost as effective as CPAP in moderate apnea; and people tend to prefer the less invasive nature of an appliance compared to the CPAP device. Surgery should be the last option, and would only be useful for anatomical defects of genetic origin.

Before going for these big-gun prescription devices, however, there are a few changes you can make in your sleep habits that may reduce, or even resolve, sleep apnea.

- Lose weight. It is dramatically beneficial for sleep apnea; a 10 percent weight loss produces a 26 percent reduction in apnea.
- Reduce alcohol intake, especially later in the evening. Alcohol can over-relax the muscles in the throat and pharynx and contribute to their collapse.
- Elevate your head by 30 degrees (pillow specialty stores sell wedges to place under your head) to reduce the force of gravity on your throat.
- Switch to sleeping on your side instead of your back, again to avoid the forces of gravity. Use a pillow as a bolster to hold onto and help keep you in the side sleeping position.
- Tenacious back sleepers can try the sleep ball technique, in which you actually attach a tennis ball to the seat of your pajamas to prevent you from sleeping on your back.

Snoring—Scientists are undecided about the health consequences of general non-apnea snoring. Light to moderate snoring is not caused by any abnormality, but rather originates from vibrations of tissue in the throat and air passageways. Your own snoring episodes can cause blood pressure to rise (not to mention what it does to your spouse), but snoring is not considered a cause of daytime hypertension. My primary concern is what snoring does to your ability to get a good night's rest: The resistance that snoring produces in your airways can cause frequent arousal and fragmented sleep. It can throw off the normal balance of calming, parasympathetic nervous system domination during sleep. Snorers have an increase in stimulating sympathetic nervous system dominance during sleep, which consumes energy and can lead to daytime fatigue.

Snoring solutions are the same as for sleep apnea. Try reducing alcohol intake and changing your sleep position before making the bigger financial and lifestyle commitment of obtaining a prescription device like the CPAP. Sometimes helpful is a surgical procedure called a uvulectomy, removal of the small punching bag (uvula) that hangs at the back of the throat to prevent it from obstructing the airway.

Chronic sinus congestion—The common cold or chronic stuffiness from allergies can pose a real challenge to a good night's sleep and can even lead to sleep apnea. You really do need the full cooperation of your nose to get adequate oxygen during sleep. A stuffy nose reduces the capacity of your major air passageway; and it forces you to work harder for air, which can make it easier for the back of the throat to collapse. Scientists even believe nasal congestion can block receptors in the nose that signal the brain that it needs air. A bout of a cold virus is not a big deal, but if you're routinely stuffy, I highly recommend working with an ear, nose, and throat doctor to determine the cause of chronic congestion and eliminate it. A 1998 study at Penn State University's Division of Allergy showed that targeted use of nasal steroids (like Nasonex) to quell inflammation improved sleep and reduced daytime fatigue for people with chronic sinus congestion. But there are remedies you can try short of using steroids.

Amazingly, the simple little device called a Breathe Right Strip—a stiff Band-Aid that sits on the bridge of the nose and physically pulls the nostrils open—can be a big help for congested sleepers. More permanent remedies—such as identifying subtle food allergies—that target the source of congestion are key. By following the elimination diet of the

21-Day Plan, you may find that congestion starts to clear up, as wheat, dairy, and other allergies can cause chronic sinus congestion. Getting acupuncture and chiropractice treatments from experienced practitioners can often help chronic sinus problems.

Gastro-Esophageal Reflux Disease (GERD)—The reflux of stomach acid into the esophagus—which is increasingly recognized as the cause of a wide range of problems including chronic sinusitis, asthma, bronchitis, and chest pain—does much of its dirty work during sleep and can be a major factor in sleep apnea. In a November 2007 study at Chicago Rush Medical Center's Department of Ear, Nose, and Throat Medicine, **correcting the hyperacidity of GERD significantly improved sleep apnea, sleep quality, and daytime fatigue of 70 percent of patients.**

The classic conventional remedy for GERD is acid-blocking medications. These certainly work. I recommend using antacids to get the problem under control if it's bad, and then targeting the causes of acidity. If necessary, have an endoscopy by a gastrointestinal specialist or ear, nose, and throat doctor to rule out significant anatomic abnormalities. Remedies other than antacids include elevation of the pillow, so that by decreasing the force of gravity, stomach acid doesn't backflow into the esophagus; and eliminating night-time acidic foods (especially tomatoes), spices, caffeine, and alcohol.

Chronic Pain—Chronic pain is a double-edged sleep sword: it can interrupt sleep, which degrades pain-inhibition processes in the brain, making pain worse the next day. Sleeping less doesn't affect pain as much as sleeping poorly does. A 2006 study at Walter Reed Army Hospital found that **pain reduced the quality of sleep in 55 percent of patients, poor sleep worsened the pain, and a poor quality mattress magnified both problems.** Evaluate your mattress (see below) and don't just live with pain. There are a number of avenues to explore including working with a pain specialist (often resulting in the use of stronger pain medications), a physical therapist, hypnosis, acupuncture, and working to reduce inflammatory elements of the diet (see Chapter 2).

Inflammatory Conditions—In conditions like arthritis, autoimmune diseases, multiple sclerosis, Lyme disease, even during a bout of influenza, the balance between proinflammatory and antiinflammatory chemicals (especially cytokines such as interleukins, TNF-alpha and others) that are produced by white blood cells of the immune system plays an essential role in regulating how well you sleep. These chemicals are produced during infections as important signaling messengers, but in chronic inflammation a steady stream of them can wreak havoc on your sleep and energy. In a study of elderly folks, higher evening levels of pro-inflammatory cytokines (especially Interleukin 6) were related to getting less sleep. A very slight increase was associated with an increased waking time of about 20 minutes. Obesity also results in a chronic inflammatory state—visceral fat is highly active in producing harmful cytokines that can interfere with sleep.

The single most important solution for reducing inflammation is lifestyle change: reduce weight and stress, exercise and sleep more, and eat an antiinflammatory diet (see Chapter 2). Cut out sugar and processed foods especially, reduce meat consumption, and incorporate anti-inflammatory foods such as fish oil, spices, and herbs.

Alcohol—If you're having problems with sleep or insomnia, you should consider cutting back on alcohol. When you drink alcohol as long as five hours before falling asleep, it can make sleep apnea or snoring worse (even if you don't normally have those problems). Alcohol triples the tendency for restless limb movement that causes frequent awakening. When you drink, you can fall asleep quicker and get to a deeper, slow-wave sleep faster (you pass out), but as the alcohol is metabolized by the middle of the night (usually after the first two 90-minute sleep cycles), sympathetic nervous system activity increases, which produces fitful sleep (you wake up in the middle of the night with a parched mouth, feeling lousy). Alcohol increases your deeper sleep at the beginning of the night and causes more restless sleep in the last portion of the night, so it can have an overall negative effect on sleep. While a glass of wine with dinner is ok. *Bottom line:* For anyone having trouble sleeping, imbibing a couple of nightcaps is not the cure.

Caffeine—America's favorite drug, the chemical stimulant caffeine can contribute to insomnia—even in your morning cup of Joe. The half-life of caffeine is three to six hours, meaning that if you have a cup at noon, a quarter cup's worth could still be in your system at midnight (as it could if you drink a larger dose, says, a two-cup sized Grande, at 6:00 a.m.). Caffeine has been shown to block the adenosine receptors. (As discussed in the Box above, accumulating adenosine during daytime is one of the triggers for getting to sleep at night.) Studies have shown that caffeine blocks this mechanism and disturbs proper sleep. As with its distant cousin, amphetamines, caffeine can cause significant withdrawal symptoms when eliminated—fatigue and headaches can develop after stopping even a one-cup per day habit. If you have insomnia and consume daily caffeine, wean yourself off slowly and stop for two full weeks to see if you sleep better and have more overall energy. The Power Up! 21-Day Plan walks you through this process.

Medications—It is truly shocking when you look at the list of medications that negatively affect sleep. **Insomnia is a commonly listed side effect of numerous prescription and over-the-counter drugs; they can cause a wide variety of disruptions in the sleep cycle including nervous system overstimulation in the early stages of sleep and nightmares in the later stages (see box).** Drugs affect the chemicals called neurotransmitters, which govern brainwave activity. Pseudophedrine (in Sudafed and other cold medicines) is a good example of how medicines affect sleep; many people using it regularly suffer unwittingly from debilitating over-stimulation—including insomnia from even a small daytime dose of decongestants. Antihistamines in cold remedies, on the other hand, actually make you drowsy. Many of the most commonly prescribed medications in America are on the list of drugs that affect sleep (unbeknownst to patients and, usually, their doctors, as well) including blood pressure medications, antiseizure medications, antihistamines, decongestants, and antidepressants. This is just one of many reasons that my goal for all patients is to reduce the number of medications they take by implementing lifestyle changes whenever possible.

Nightmare Medications

Here's a short list of drugs shown in clinical studies or case reports to cause nightmares: antibiotics (such as Cipro and Zithromax), antidepressants (especially SSRIs like Prozac), cardiovascular drugs (especially certain beta blockers like Inderal or Toprol), and certain antiinflammatories (like Naproxen). Bad dreams may be a small price to pay for curing a bad infection or stabilizing your heart rate, but just knowing these drugs can cause nightmares you may feel less anxious when the boogieman shows up in the wee hours.

Sleeping Pills—Sleeping pills are useful when acute stress or health conditions occasionally interfere with falling or staying asleep. They can also be used to reset the circadian rhythms of your biological clock when you're traveling. They become a problem when people use them chronically. First of all, sleeping pills do not guarantee healthy sleep architecture or complete elimination of daytime sleepiness. To do that, you need to treat the underlying condition and get to the source of the problem that causes insomnia (i.e., daytime anxiety). You will not get a magic, permanent fix from a pill. The quick-fix mentality can actually lead to a worsening of the sleep problem over time and to the appearance of other problems related to lack of sleep. Polypharmacy—the prescribing of multiple medications, often for the same conditions—has been an increasing problem, occasionally with tragic consequences, from the 1962 death of Marilyn Monroe to 2008's Heath Ledger.

A brief synopsis of medicinal sleeping aids contains two broad categories: those that leave you drowsy in the morning and could become habit forming, and those that produce addiction and/or dependency. The former group includes soporific antidepressants (tricyclics such as Elavil and SSRIs such as Paxil), the newer melatonin receptor agonist Rozerem, and OTC antihistamines (Sominex, Benadryl). The other group contains solely prescriptive sleeping medications that can be addictive—such as barbiturates (phenobarbital, Seconal), benzodiazepines (Dalmane, Valium, Klonopin), and narcotics (codeine, hydrocodone)—or can produce dependency such as Ambien, Sonata, and Lunesta.

I am not dismissing the use of prescription sleeping pills: I prescribe them myself sometimes (though rarely compared with most other physicians). Judicious occasional use of these powerful medications can be helpful for acute distress or jetlag, and are necessary for others with more severe medical conditions or severe sleep disorders, especially when overseen by a sleep disorders specialist. But there are many other ways, detailed in the following section, that sleeping problems can and should be addressed.

My Favorite Sleep Remedies

Make an effort to maintain a consistent pre-bedtime routine. This can include turning off stimulating activities (including electronic gadgets) at least an hour before sleep; utilizing relaxation rituals, such as breath work

and progressive relaxation techniques (see below). Keep a regular, reasonable schedule—get to bed as close as possible to the same time every
night (ideally by 10:00 p.m.) and wake up at roughly the same reasonable
time each morning. Sleep docs actually do call this consistency "good
sleep hygiene." Of course, everyone knows that mothers are the best sleep
hygienists in the world, but what follows are my best tips that *even* your
mother may not know.

A Good Pillow—This is an easy change that can make a huge difference.
The first thing I tell everyone to do is evaluate the pillow situation. A pillow is supposed to support your head so that your neck, airways, and
spine remain in a natural position with good alignment throughout the
night. A very convincing 2001 German Sleep Medicine Lab study found
that changing to a medium-firm pillow (the firmest was of no advantage)
significantly improved both non-REM and REM sleep for people who
have trouble sleeping without other underlying conditions or causes.
Bottom line: A pillow should support your head, not bury it.

Pillows also frequently contribute to allergies, which is a big no-no
when it comes to getting a good night's sleep. A crucial first step in improving sleep is to scrutinize your pillow for allergens, the source of
which can be the filling (down and feather allergies are very common) or
it can be dust mites inside the filling. I highly recommend that you exam-
ine the range of nonallergenic foam pillows on the market and get one.
When you find one that suits you, place it inside a dust-mite blocking pillow protector that goes under the pillow case (www.greenguide.com is a
great source for information on pillow allergies). But you also want to
toss your pillow in the dryer every few months to kill dust mites. Change
your pillow every couple of years as its unwavering service of eight hours
each day gives it a relatively short life span.

A Better Mattress—When it comes to mattresses, observe the Goldilocks
imperative (not too hard and not too soft); medium-firm is your best bet.
If a mattress is too hard it bites back and can cause pain and even numbness (limbs falling asleep) at pressure points; likewise, if a mattress is too
soft it becomes more work to move around and can cause muscle and
joint strains. The best mattresses support all of your body parts equally;
even at the heaviest points, your hips and shoulders.

Unfortunately, couples often have different mattress preferences, primarily because body weight is a big factor in mattress support. Sometimes the issue can be resolved with a topper. You can actually have a

firmer mattress with a soft feel by purchasing a bed with large quilting on the surface or by using a cushioned mattress pad. Because people over the age of 40 lose elasticity in their skin, they have less tolerance for a firm mattress surface. Memory foams, the current darlings of the market, can bring harmony to the bedroom by adjusting for the individual body type, but many people find these mattresses to be exceptionally warm, which is especially unwelcome if you're suffering hot flashes.

Test Drive Your Mattress

Test driving in the store is important—after all, you're going to spend more time in your bed than you will in your car. In a terrific survey, *Consumer Reports* found that people who spent 15 minutes testing a bed in the store—spending at least five minutes on each side, especially in their preferred sleeping position—were more satisfied with their ultimate choice than quicker testers. And they were as satisfied as people who were allowed to take the beds home for a test sleep!

As much as I hate to break this news, a recent study from the Musculoskeletal and Human Physiology Research Lab at Oklahoma State University showed that price *does* make a difference. Changing from a cheaper to a moderately high-priced mattress significantly improves sleep quality. Another similarly rigorous study showed that **by switching to a better mattress (in this case an adjustable air-spring/box-spring combination) a full 95 percent of study participants with chronic low back pain reported reduction in pain, and 88 percent reported a better night's sleep.** This data was supported by a *Consumer Reports* survey that found more than two-thirds of people with high-end mattresses were "very or completely" satisfied with their purchase compared to one-third of conventional mattress owners. You may want to take a look at spending priorities: Spending less on bedding and more on the mattress could be a sleep-inducing strategy.

Light therapy—You can use artificial full-spectrum lights in the morning to help reset the body clock so you can get to sleep at a more appropriate time in the evening. In the past decade, pioneering research lead by Columbia University investigator Michael Terman, Ph.D. established that the circadian rhythms that help set your sleep patterns are highly susceptible to changes in exposure to light rays—whether from the sun or from bulbs that mimic the full-spectrum of sunlight. **By exposing the eyes to specially designed full-spectrum lights (10,000 lux fluorescent bulbs) for 30 minutes in the early morning, scientists have helped people get to sleep earlier and stay asleep longer.** It is thought that regular exposure to such light in the morning triggers a more advantageous nighttime release of melatonin, the hormone that governs your body clock, but the mechanisms are not fully understood. You may be more familiar with light therapy for its use in treating seasonal affective disorder (SAD), a type of depression that shows up in winter months and stems from sunlight deprivation. Studies have shown that a course of light therapy treatments can have a dramatically positive effect on both sleep and symptoms of depression.

Light therapy can truly work wonders for people who find it difficult to fall asleep before midnight and are sluggish in the morning. Rapid improvement in falling asleep earlier is often experienced after just a few days of 30 minutes of exposure to a light therapy box upon awakening in the morning (see www.cet.org for more information on the boxes). For people (even teenagers) with more severe insomnia, who regularly stay awake until 1:00 a.m. or longer, shifting sleep patterns can involve sensitive timing. So while the procedure can be done at home, it is a better idea to work with a sleep specialist to devise the treatment program for serious insomnia. The treatment also usually requires waking up a little earlier each morning, which takes real commitment. But if you are miserable from insomnia, it's worth trying.

On the research forefront are special dawn-simulating sleep masks with embedded lights that turn on gradually four hours before the end of sleep. One might think leaving the shades open will do the same thing, but bare windows raise the possibility that your bedroom will be flooded with ambient nighttime light, which poses its own set of problems that are conveniently the subject of the next discussion, *Dark Therapy*.

Dark Therapy—If exposing your eyes to light in the morning helps you fall asleep earlier and sleep longer, it should come as no surprise that blocking exposure to light at night can positively influence sleep. Scientists digging further into the sunlight-melatonin connection have discovered that the blue spectrum of light has the greatest impact on melatonin and circadian rhythms. If you are exposed to blue light late at night—from a computer or television screen or a digital clock near your bed—it can wreak havoc with your body clock making it harder for you to get to sleep and to get up in the morning. Keep your room pitch dark at night, covering all digital clock or DVD player readouts. Interestingly, a 2008 study from the Corvallis Psychiatric Clinic in Oregon showed that using amber-tinted glasses blocked the excitatory blue spectrum of light commonly encountered during television and computer viewing. Using amber glasses during evening screen-watching time had a significant effect in inducing and promoting a good night's sleep.

Behavioral Therapy—Here's the Catch-22 of sleep psychology: worrying about not getting enough sleep can stop you from getting enough sleep. Sleep docs have even developed a protocol of behavioral modification that's been shown to work 70 to 80 percent of the time for people who can't sleep because of excessive preoccupation with, or apprehension about, falling sleep. Here's the drill:

- Go to bed only when sleepy.
- Get out of bed if you haven't fallen asleep in 20 minutes.
- Curtail all nonsleep activities in bed (no watching TV, eating, planning, or problem solving).
- Arise at the same time every morning.
- Avoid daytime napping.
- Don't get attached to unreal expectations about getting a perfect sleep every night.
- Do not blame insomnia for all daytime problems.
- Do not catastrophize (imagine all the bad things that will happen as a result) after a poor night's sleep.
- Finally, if this chapter is making you worry too much about sleep, put it down and go out for a walk in the sunshine!

Relaxation Exercises—Throughout the night, your brainwaves are continually cycling between slow-wave activity of non-rapid eye movement, and fast-wave activity of rapid eye movement. Meditation and relaxation exercises can significantly help you get back into slow-wave activity if you are awakened in the middle of the night. For getting to sleep faster or for falling back to sleep in the middle of the night try meditation or relaxation exercises found in the 21-Day Plan as a way of hopping onto the slow-wave sleep train that pulls you into the deepest stages of regenerative rest.

Acupuncture—Acupuncture, discussed in Chapter 1 as an aid to relaxation, is a helpful adjunct for treating insomnia. Thousands of research articles attest to the neurochemical effects of acupuncture, which significantly elevates endorphins to block pain pathways, promotes the production of chemicals that reduce inflammation, enhances circulation, and reduces the activity of neuromuscular spasm. Inasmuch as acupuncture balances the nervous system and neurotransmitters, there's a logic for its use in promoting relaxation, which results in a better quality sleep. In China acupuncture has been used successfully for two thousand years to treat sleep problems, though this effect has yet to be studied in controlled trials that are considered the gold standard in Western medicine. In my own practice I use acupuncture as part of a comprehensive approach to insomnia in conjunction with other treatments based on the underlying causes of the sleep problem.

Nutritional Supplements

"One pill will make you larger, and one pill will make you small, but the ones your mother gives you won't do anything at all." People are always looking for the quick fix.

With sleep, lifestyle factors (proper diet, exercise, stress control, sleep hygiene, etc.) are the most important means for successful long-term regenerative rest. Short-term prescriptions can be very helpful for acute insomnia that occurs in situations with great stress. While nonprescription nutritional supplements are generally less powerful than medications, they can provide a very helpful nondrug transitional aid to get you to sleep better until you can make lifestyle changes. If you are under a doctor's care for a medical condition, check with your doctor before taking any new supplements.

Melatonin

While many hormones affect circadian rhythms (your biological clock), the master hormone for regulation of the sleep cycle is melatonin. This hypothalamus-produced hormone rises just before you fall asleep and falls through the night, hitting bottom about two hours before you awaken. (It is also a powerful antioxidant that enhances the reparative function of sleep.) As mentioned above in "*Light Therapy*," production of melatonin is very sensitive to sunlight and can be normalized by altering exposure patterns. Studies going back decades are very clear that ingesting melatonin extract can help reset the body clock and alleviate jet lag. Melatonin can also gradually help insomniacs feel sleepy at an earlier hour: take 1–3 milligrams two to three hours before the desired sleep time. While melatonin can help normalize an out-of-whack sleep pattern, it is not a sleeping pill.

Valerian (valeriana officinalis)

Valerian officinalis, a species of flowering plant in the Valerian family, is the closest you can get to an herbal sleeping pill—its sedative powers far outstrip chamomile. Valerian would no doubt be more widely used in teas if it weren't for its particularly unpleasant odor. Research suggests that constituents of valerian root affect enzyme systems that control neurotransmitter levels responsible for sleepiness. In studies valerian capsules have even been used successfully to help people sleep during a period of withdrawal from Valium dependency. (Due to its sedative effect, Valerian should not be taken before driving and operating machinery.)

L-theanine

This amino acid, as discussed in Chapter 1, helps reduce tension and stress. I commonly recommend theanine as part of a comprehensive program for insomnia.

Tryptophan/5-HTP (or, alternately, warm milk)

The amino acid tryptophan has been well studied and used for decades to induce a drowsy state, however, it is now only available by prescription in the United States because one contaminated batch from China caused serious lung problems 25 years ago. As a result, some supplement companies sell 5-hydroxy-tryptophan (5HTP), a different form of the amino acid. 5HTP is less effective as a sleep aid than tryptophan. Warm milk is thought to increase tryptophan levels, and is a natural way to use this amino acid to assist with sleep.

Passion flower (passiflora incarnata)

Research has shown many active compounds in passiflora that lead to calming and sedating effects in the nervous system. Some studies have demonstrated this herb's utility as part of treatment for anxiety disorder and for patients coming off narcotics. Due to its mild potency, passion flower is most often found in combination with other calming herbs, particularly valerian. (It has some potential adverse reactions, including dizziness; and people with cardiovascular disease should avoid passion flower because of certain potentially potent alkaloids.)

A Cautionary Note on Kava Kava

Kava is a South Pacific herb used in ceremonies by indigenous cultures for its psychoactive properties, one of which induces a sleepy, dream-like state, which made it briefly popular in the United States as a sleep aid and antianxiety treatment. But I do not recommend kava for two reasons: (1) ingestion of kava capsules has resulted in cases of liver toxicity and even liver failure, and (2) its psychoactive properties can cause emotional disturbances, especially in people with psychological conditions. Try something else.

Chapter 6

Power of Connection: Cultivate Spirit, Access Positive Energy

I HADN'T SEEN DAVID in five years. When I asked where he'd been, he told me this powerful story of spiritual rejuvenation:

David's soul mate from childhood and wife of twenty years died suddenly from an aneurysm. He was inconsolable in his grief. Depressed, he had developed back pain and headaches and was so fatigued that it became difficult for him to get out of bed. Knowing that grief was the source of his problem, he thought he could handle it on his own. But, after the second year of grieving, David went to his parents' house for the High Jewish Holidays, and by chance the family rabbi stopped by. The rabbi asked how David was and he reported feeling fine, but his family disagreed.

When his mother told the rabbi that David hadn't recovered from the loss, the rabbi asked only one question: "Did David sit shiva for his wife?" (Shiva is a seven-day period of formal mourning after the funeral that is observed by Jews. During shiva, friends and relatives visit the home to offer condolences.) Having not participated in his religion since childhood, David initially scoffed at the idea.

After some persuasion, David agreed to undergo the ritual

with the rabbi by his side, even though it was two years after his wife's death. For seven days David sat in his home as almost everyone who'd ever cared for him visited him and sat with him. As he received their healing energy and thoughts, David became connected on a deeper level than ever with his friends and family—and also, he felt, with all of humanity.

At the end of that week, David felt a dramatic lifting of his spirits, and experienced waves of energy he had not felt since his loss. The powerful process of opening to the love and positive energy of others' showed him how deeply his spiritual life could affect his health and vitality.

DAVID REGAINED HIS VITAL ENERGY by connecting with his roots, with the healing power of a religious practice, and with a community of people who cared deeply about him and his family. David's spiritual healing, and the subject of this chapter, is about gaining access to a deeper, permanent, vital energy that works on a more profound level than the daily mechanics of a healthy lifestyle. It is necessary to recognize that you do not begin and end at your skin in order for you—and anyone—to recover your energy and health. Spirituality, connectedness, and love—realizing that you are part of something universal and eternal—bigger than your flesh and blood—are vitally important for well-being.

Connection is important in my practice as a means for my patients to rebuild energy. I am not alone in this, connection has been increasingly recognized as enormously important in the practice of behavioral medicine, a field that includes doctors, psychiatrists, psychotherapists, research scientists, and nurses concerned with social and behavioral factors that affect health. Connectivity can be achieved in many different ways. Western spirituality emphasizes a personal connection with God; Eastern and Native American spiritual philosophies place emphasis on a connection with all of nature and on being part of a greater whole that includes a universal energy or spirit. You can be connected through a relationship to the absolute or to your community or to nature or to music . . . or to any greater energy or entity that transcends the nitty-gritty of daily life and gives meaning to your time here.

Behavioral researchers have mapped the landscape of spiritual connection and have shown that it includes: frequent interaction with the transcendent as a fundamental part of life; perceived divine love; the perception that life consists of *more* than physical states, psychological feelings or social roles; a sense of wholeness and internal integration; a sense of inner harmony; the experience of awe at the beauty of creation; gratefulness; compassion; mercy; and spiritual longing—the desire to be closer or in union with the divine. In a fascinating study of spiritual experiences, researchers at the Fetzer Institute and Columbia University were able to measure with a survey whether an individual *experiences* God's love versus whether one just *believes* that God loves people as a whole. The investigators suggest that *feeling* loved is the key ingredient in making the link between spiritual issues and health outcomes. I have found in my own practice that it's vitally important to take the spiritual temperature of my patients, so to speak, in order to help them achieve total healing and optimum energy.

Until forty years ago, physicians cared for entire families; they knew who a person was within the family and within the context of their community—and they got insights into people's health based on what was going on in their lives. The old-fashioned family doc was much more attuned to the emotional and spiritual shifts that precede illness. It was not unusual for him to spend time chatting, inquiring about his patients' lives, before doing an exam. A 1997 study in *JAMA* showed that the typical doctor interrupts a patient after just 23 seconds and steers the conversation in the direction he wants it to go—which may not lead to the deeper root of what's underlying a person's problems. While I appreciate the need for efficiency in health care, I maintain that the family doc was actually deepening his ability to make a diagnosis by taking the measure of his patients' spirit.

By emphasizing the role of spirit and connectedness I give my patients permission (which some of them feel they need in the face of the demands on their time) and encourage them to use the energy and practices of spiritual connectedness and community that allow them to heal themselves and to stay well. **Skeptics might chalk the positive results up to elevated endorphins or decreased cortisol (anxiety hormone) levels, but I maintain that remarkable stories of the healing power of love, connectedness, and spirituality are footprints of a deeper energetic process that is constantly at work within us and around us.** And this energetic process is beyond what we can possibly understand with the gizmos and machines of scientific method.

This chapter will explain why you cannot afford to neglect the spirit when you are seeking increased energy in life and in your health. Cultivating connectedness is a joyous pursuit. There are so many ways to engage in a dance of energy with the universe. In the 21 Day Plan, I incorporate exercises for cultivating the "Power of Connection," And you no doubt will invent many of your own as you begin to connect.

Being Connected

Even though it's difficult to subject spirituality and connectedness to scientific methods of analysis, researchers continue to try—and to make great headway. A wealth of studies demonstrates the importance of connectedness in numerous aspects of health: your nervous system, immune system, neuroendocrine system, cardiovascular system, and your very longevity all fare better when you have healthy connections to a deeper sense of self and to the world beyond yourself. In the sections that follow,

The Connected Body

Noted Duke University religion and spirituality researcher, Harold Koenig, M.D., reviewed more than sixty studies published in peer-reviewed medical journals in the United States over a thirty-year period that established a causal link between immune and neuroendocrine system health. The key connectedness factors included spirituality, religion, social support, and social participation. The following functions were all improved by being connected:

Immune response to vaccination

Function of immune cells

Antibody levels to latent viruses
(indicator of immune system stress)

Production of cytokines
(molecular defenders of the immune system)

Hypothalamic-Pituitary-Adrenal Axis Response
(the stress hormone response)

Production of pituitary hormone

I'll discuss the most important categories of connection that research and tens of thousands of years of empirical experience have shown to improve your health and increase your energy.

Spirituality

I have had the great privilege of taking care of a number of Tibetan Buddhist rinpoches (pronounced RIN-po-chay)—these are the holiest monks in the Buddhist tradition. They embody the essence of Buddhism—compassion for others. Their most fundamental goal in life is to relieve the suffering of all creatures. Their deep spirituality doesn't give them immunity to physical illness—even the Dalai Lama gets a cold every once in a while—but their advanced spiritual work does give them a unique perspective on illness and a certain amount of control over their bodies. I was deeply moved by the sheer power of will of one rinpoche, in whom, during one of his infrequent visits for a check-up, I discovered what I suspected to be a massive tumor in his lower abdomen that was causing his lower body to become hugely swollen. After consulting with an oncologist he decided to undergo chemotherapy and radiation. He had no fear of death, but he told me that his work was not complete, and he felt that he needed some more time. He decided to go to Washington, D.C., for his treatment where he had followers who could look after him. There he would also be in the care of a wonderful oncologist with whom, it just so happened, I had worked with (and last seen) in Tanzania some twenty-five years earlier.

Three months after the move I received a call from his astonished oncologist: the tumor and all of the swelling had vanished, and tests could find no traces of the cancer! The doctors had never seen anyone come in with such extensive cancer, and achieve not just improvement but what seemed like a cure. With his body strong enough, the Rinpoche announced he would return to India to complete his work. I was sad to see him go, but elated at his recovery. Six months later I heard through a member of his community in India that he had decided his body was "tired" and he needed a new one. (All Tibetan Buddhists believe in reincarnation). He made preparations, and on a full moon of a Kalachakra Ceremony (a high holy day for Tibetan Buddhism) he left his body. I was a little broken-hearted, and also amazed at the power of his spirit; he couldn't beat the cancer, but he could set a schedule for it.

It is quite difficult to fathom the depths of spirituality of a Tibetan rinpoche whose entire life is dedicated to cultivating compassion and wisdom. But on a more general level, spirituality has been increasingly recognized in medicine as a positive factor for health. Studies on the topic have been generated by some of North America's top medical schools, including Harvard, Johns Hopkins, Duke, and the University of Pennsylvania. Many of the studies have concluded that spirituality should be recognized by health care providers and caregivers as an important factor contributing to quality of life, which in general contributes significantly to better health outcomes.

This growing recognition of spirituality is a welcome development for most people. **Studies both at Johns Hopkins and the University of Pennsylvania show that the majority of people don't mind being asked about their spirituality in a doctor's office, and more than 90 percent of those surveyed felt that a spiritual outlook was important for physical well-being.** When our medical students at Columbia ask, "Is there a place for spirituality in medicine?" my answer is a resounding, yes. And for the sake of scientific method, upon which our magnificent but sometimes short-sighted medical system is built, let's take a look at the research that supports my position.

One of the trickier aspects of studying spirituality is defining it. Researchers require standardized definitions. In order to put transcendence to the test, investigators commonly use questionnaires that thoroughly explore people's habits, values, and attitudes toward spirituality. Intriguingly, one of the scales, the FACIT *Spiritual Well Being* scale, can tease out the differences in attitude between having faith versus having a sense of meaning and peace, which scientists have dubbed existential well-being. Another scale, the *Daily Spiritual Experience Scale,* is intended to measure a person's perception of the transcendent in daily life and his or her interaction or involvement with the transcendent in daily life. The idea is to measure experiences rather than beliefs or behaviors.

A recent (2007) joint study by researchers at Harvard Medical School's Massachusetts General Hospital and the University of California at San Diego used similar scales to study the effects of spirituality in twins, a subgroup of the population that helps scientists separate genetics out from behavior. Investigators looked at the association between spiritual well-being and health outcomes in 345 pairs of male twins with a mean age of 48 years from a national cohort known as the Vietnam Era Twin Registry (made up of twins who served in the military between 1965 and 1975). Overall, spirituality was shown to be associated with better general health, vitality, and social functioning. **And having a sense of** meaning and peace turned out to be the most powerful factor of all, associated with significant improvement in overall physical functioning, general physical health, mental health, social functioning, pain, and vitality. I cannot name any other single lifestyle factor that would cover so many bases.

Some of the power of spirituality can be attributed to its effect on mood. We know that spiritual practices such as meditation and prayer have a calming effect on the nervous system, but having a sense of spirituality is equally powerful. In an impressive study at the University of Colorado Department of Medicine, doctors looked at the effects of spiritual well-being in patients with heart failure. They found that greater spiritual well-being, and in particular *having a sense of meaning and peace,* was strongly associated with less depression. The study suggests that enhancing spiritual well-being may be a potential therapy to reduce or prevent depression and thus improve outcomes in people with heart failure. I have to applaud this study. For physicians to suggest in a peer-reviewed medical journal that spiritual well-being might be a beneficial therapy for heart patients is quite brave and an extremely important step in bringing humanity back to medicine.

A further connection between spirituality, depression, and energy is beginning to surface as researchers are refining ways to study spirit. **At Johns Hopkins School of Medicine doctors found that daily spiritual experiences in older adults with arthritis were strongly associated with less depression and increased energy.** This would not surprise a rinpoche because, according to Buddhist doctrine, meditation produces energy. For example, meditation produces mindfulness, which is considered a source of energy that powers awareness of what is happening in the present moment. With daily spiritual exercises, the Johns Hopkins arthritis patients were tapping a source of energy, and they were able to report back to researchers that they felt more energetic.

One of the most powerful studies of spirituality—which should make insurance companies stand up and say a prayer—comes from Harold Koenig, M.D., co-director of the Center for Spirituality, Theology and Health at Duke University Medical Center, and one of the giants in the field of research on spirituality and health. Over a 21-month period he and his team examined 811 people, 50 years or older, who had been admitted to Duke's Medical Center. Participating in organized religious activity resulted in fewer hospitalizations and shorter acute hospital stays. And when the researchers looked at people who needed to go from the hospital for longer-term care at a nursing home or rehab facility, those who had religious activities and professed a sense of spirituality had significantly reduced long-term care days. (The effect was strongest for African-Americans and women.) In this study, spirituality was a simple, side effect–free, feel-good way to reduce long-term care hospital stays. Spirituality would be a pharmaceutical gold mine if it could be bottled and sold.

Spirituality is a powerful healing tool, but it is underutilized. **The same people who tell me that they see themselves as spiritual, routinely admit in the next breath that they do *not* have a regular contemplative practice to cultivate that spirituality.** My response is to encourage them to engage in a daily practice—even if it's simply the two-minute meditation or prayer that I prescribe for them first thing in the morning (see the 21-Day Plan, Day One). You—and everyone—should cultivate your inner life by following the spiritual connection that is meaningful for you. Ultimately, I want you to go beyond a two-minute practice once a day, to cultivate a spiritual attitude. Try it, you'll feel protected and connected.

Prayer

By one estimate, 82 percent of Americans pray weekly. And despite most doctors' reluctance to broach the topic it appears that many people know instinctively that prayer belongs in health care. In a study published in the venerable *Archives of Internal Medicine* and conducted at the University of Pennsylvania, researchers found a strong natural bias toward the power of prayer to heal: of 177 people visiting an outpatient lung specialist, 51 percent described themselves as religious and yet a full 90 percent of the patients believed that praying can influence recovery from an illness.

I once broached the topic of prayer with a patient who was having a very difficult time in her life; her child had been diagnosed with diabetes just after she'd completed treatment for breast cancer. In my office, she looked depleted and miserable, having come to ask for treatment for a sinus infection. When I turned the topic to spiritual resources, and asked if she ever prayed, she replied, "Oh, yeah, you mean like for the placebo effect?" From her point of view, and for many people, prayer is a sort of turbo-charged version of the power of positive thinking.

Some intriguing studies strongly suggest that prayer works even if you *don't know* you're being prayed for, and even if you are not a fol-

lower of the religion of the person who's praying for you. One of the most widely acclaimed prayer studies was conducted several years ago at CalPacific Medical Center by physician Elizabeth Targ and her group. What was so unique about this study is it was double-blinded—meaning the patients didn't know they were being prayed for—and it utilized prayers by people from eight different spiritual traditions including Christians, Jews, Buddhists, and Native Americans. Advanced-stage AIDS patients (who at the time they volunteered for the study all had the same degree of illness [including similar T cell counts]) were assigned on a ro-tating basis to the prayer givers, each one receiving prayer from a different healer each week. The results were nothing short of astonishing. When compared to the people who didn't receive prayers, the prayed-for pa-tients had seven times fewer days spent in the hospital, and four times fewer new hospitalizations, sixfold reduction in new AIDS-related ill-nesses, two thirds fewer severe illnesses, one-third fewer doctors' visits, and significantly less psychological distress. What I like about this study is it managed to isolate the effects of prayer from the effects of believing in prayer, which removes the placebo effect from the equation.

The first major rigorous double blind study of prayer, published in a peer-reviewed medical journal in 1988, was conducted by Randolph Byrd, staff cardiologist at the University of California, San Francisco School of Medicine. In Byrd's study, 393 patients in the coronary care unit were prayed for by Christian groups. During their hospital stay the prayed-for patients had significantly fewer cases of congestive heart fail-ure, cardiopulmonary arrest, and pneumonia; and they required less medication and fewer intubations (insertion of a breathing tube). This was a real shot in the arm for those of us who felt frustrated in our efforts to have spirituality's positive role in health care acknowledged more.

In a follow-up study, published in the *Archives of Internal Medicine* in 2001, researchers examined the effect of prayer on 990 patients in the Coronary Care Unit of St. Luke's Hospital in Kansas City, Missouri. This study was triple-blinded; neither the doctors nor data analysts knew which patients had been prayed for; and the patients didn't know they were being prayed for. The prayers were given by a diverse group of peo-ple trained to pray for better recovery. The patients did not have the dra-matic outcomes of the Byrd study, but improved in every measurement compared to the non-prayed-for group.

This is not to say you've got to enlist a prayer group to maintain your health. Praying clearly also has physiological benefits for the person doing the praying. I'm fascinated by the studies that show that there are changes in the brain during prayer. **Electro-encephalograms (EEGs) show shifts in the brain's energy during prayer.** Brain activity measured with functional MRIs (fMRI), and PET scans indicate that different levels of brain functioning may be attained as a person gets "better" at praying. Herbert Benson established that brain-wave activity commonly shifts toward calming alpha waves during a relaxation exercise such as conscious breathing. But when people with advanced praying skills, like Buddhist monks or Evangelical Christians, are at prayer, their brain waves shift toward a frontal midline theta rhythm (Fm theta), which reflects intense mental concentration as well as a meditative state characterized by relief of anxiety—it's what people often call a flow state, when you're concentrating so hard on something that you think only a few minutes has passed when it's actually been a half hour. Other studies suggest prayer has immune-boosting, antiinflammatory properties due to the relaxation response's effect on the vagus nerve, which regulates feedback between the automatic nervous system and the immune system. Again, few drugs come close to having such sophisticated and highly desired effects.

As tantalizing as prayer studies are, I agree with visionary physician and philosopher Dr. Larry Dossey that evidence-based research is not the *only* avenue for bringing prayer and spiritual intention to medicine. In his book, *Healing Beyond the Body*, Dossey writes, "Unable to see how prayer *could* work, too many people insist that it *cannot* work." It's possible that studies of prayer by their very design interfere with the effects. When I was scientific adviser to the first conference on Native American medicine to be held in North America, we encountered resistance from the leaders of several nations who felt that to take their prayer practices out of context would destroy their efficacy. **One tribal elder explained to me that healing prayer is part of a holistic system, which includes community and social support, and sometimes involves specific dietary restrictions and herbs, sweat lodges, and movement exercises.** To some, taking out one element and subjecting it to some sort of scientific scrutiny was unthinkable.

Regardless of what tradition prayers come from, I think most rational people will agree that science will never "prove" *how* prayer works. Some scientists have attempted to measure the energy that people emanate while praying. Philosophies that believe in the efficacy of prayer, from Larry Dossey's theory of nonlocal mind to the Buddhist concept of collective consciousness, more or less boil down to the idea that when you pray you connect to the absolute—a larger energetic reality that is within you and also surrounding you, throughout the universe. This connection of personal to universal energy or consciousness is what allows your intention to effect change across space and time.

For me in my practice, and for my patients who pray, it's enough to know that prayer *does* work. We can cite research as well as evidence from thousands of years of practice by spiritual leaders and their religious communities but we frankly just know it in our hearts. I see no reason for the American medical establishment to continue to keep people's spiritual lives out of the consult room. The most rational reason to encourage a contemplative practice is that prayer is one more powerful tool in your healing armamentarium to increase energy and promote total well-being.

Religion

When I was growing up in a conservative town in Northern California my mother was consistently religious and had us attend services regularly at the local Episcopal Church. The leader of our church was an extremely charismatic priest, L. Douglas Gottschall, who had been canonized (an elite designation) by the archdiocese for his work in trying to uncover the location of King Solomon's mine and other sacred treasures in Africa and the Middle East. Canon Gottschall wore a ring on his left hand that he said he found during his religious treasure hunts. Every Wednesday evening, he used this ring as part of weekly faith healing services. As an acolyte, I often assisted him while infirm parishioners came to be healed. I grew accustomed to seeing very smart, respectable people from our community come in to be touched by the ring and healed. I actually saw someone come in barely able to walk with assistance and walk out with a nearly perfect gait. I was pretty mystified by this as a youth, but from what I now know about religion I am no longer surprised. **Religion can combine almost all of the connectivity factors: Social support, belief in a higher power, cultivating a spiritual practice, music, art, and community service are all wound up in one big powerful package.** Combine that with the force of a spiritually powerful person like Canon Gottschall, and you've got a major healing center.

Some of the benefits of religious involvement can be explained by healthier lifestyle habits. For example, Seventh Day Adventists and Mormons have been shown to have lesser cancer incidence and increased longevity linked to moderate lifestyles shaped by their religions. But some studies factor out healthy lifestyle habits and still show beneficial results from religious practices. Let's take a look at a few of the studies that argue in favor of following a religious tradition's centuries-old blue-print for getting connected.

In medicine, when we want the big picture we turn to epidemiology, which tells us the common tendencies in groups of a whole lot of people. A number of such studies have established the protective effects of reli-gious involvement. One study of 6,545 residents of Alameda County, Cal-ifornia, that went on for 31 years likened the general protective benefits of religion to the known benefits of high socioeconomic status; non-church attenders had significantly higher rates of death from cancer and circula-tory, digestive, and respiratory diseases. More recently, Duke's Harold Koenig and colleagues examined records of a nationwide cohort of 8,450 men and women age 40 years and older from 1988 to 1994, seeking asso-ciations between religious service attendance and mortality. **Incredibly, the statistics yielded up a dose-response relationship: At each level of increased attendance the risk of dying decreased—from no atten-dance, to less than weekly, to the lowest risk of dying for people who at-tended religious services more than once a week.**

In a 1997 study showing a beneficial dose-response relationship between religion and health, Koenig and his team at Duke enlisted 1,718 elderly persons and looked for a correlation between religious attendance and immune system strength (measured by circulating levels of an in-flammatory cytokine called Interleukin 6 [IL-6]). More non-church at-tenders had elevated levels of harmful inflammatory molecules than occasional attenders. People who attended religious services once a week or more were 49 percent *less likely* to have elevated IL-6 levels than were nonattenders. **Religion appeared to reduce inflammation and strengthen the immune system independent of mood**—something Canon Gottschall could have told us without the hard labor of scientific research.

In study after study the message is clear: having a religious practice is good for you. In one compelling study, elderly surgical patients who were both socially active and found strength and comfort in their religious faith were *14 times* less likely to die during the six months following sur-gery than their less religiously connected counterparts. Those who re-ported attending religious services at least every few months had about half the death rate of those who never or rarely attended services. Once again, greater frequency conferred stronger results.

Hundreds of published studies provide so much evidence supporting the power of religious practice to improve health and well-being that noted epidemiologist Jeffrey Levin—who has reviewed most of the research connecting religion and health—is an advocate of a new approach to medicine called *theosomatic* medicine. In his book *God, Faith and Healing*, Levin defines this approach to medicine as "a view of the determinants of health based on the apparent connections between god or spirit or faith in god—and the well-being of the body." The studies have shown religion to be as powerful and in many cases more powerful at extending longevity than some of our most powerful medications. If you are at all inclined to attend religious services regularly, I highly recommend that you do so.

Community

I live in New York City—giant metropolis of more than 8 million inhabitants; you'd think it might be a lonely place with such high potential for anonymity, but I am constantly amazed at how people manage to create their own special, meaningful communities. There are communities based on shared nationality and shared love of the arts; dog lovers find each other; fashion followers find each other, musicians, punk-rockers, artists, architects, furniture buffs, comic book buffs, philanthropists . . . you name the group, there's a tight-knit community of them in New York. Each of these microcommunities is a center of collective energy, and their ranks are continuously energized by including others.

The human instinct to gather together has powerful benefits. Pioneering cardiologist and bestselling author, Dean Ornish, has elegantly explained feelings of isolation can have significant adverse effects on health and energy. One simple but illustrative study showed that people with the fewest social ties (3 or less) had 4.2 times greater risk of catching a cold than those with the most (6 or more) social ties. You might think, OK, big deal so you've got a cold. But many other studies have shown that loneliness and isolation can significantly depress the immune system as well. One fascinating study compared the immune systems in people who simply had the *belief* that there was available social support for them to those who felt they had no support. **Those who had the perception of social support had a stronger response to a hepatitis B vaccination, producing more antibodies than those who felt they had poor social support.** Researchers may have hit on an explanation for this phenomenon. Investigators at UCLA's David Geffen School of Medicine found that feelings of isolation are linked to alterations in the activity of genes that drive inflammation, the body's first immune response. This hard scientific link between isolation and inflammation helps explain why loneliness has been associated with inflammatory conditions such as heart disease.

We are hardwired to be social animals. Highly sophisticated neural circuitry that connects your brain structures makes it possible to process others' verbal and nonverbal cues (and intentions). This is what author Daniel Goleman calls "neural WiFi." In his book *Social Intelligence*, Goleman writes, "The most telling news here may be that the social brain represents the only biological system in our bodies that continually attunes us to, and in turn becomes influenced by, the internal state of people we're with." When you have a positive supportive community, the good vibes, so to speak, resonate in your body.

The meaning of a supportive community can be extremely diverse. It can be a church or parenting group, a chorus or crossword puzzlers, quilters or knitters, cake bakers or community gardeners. I was once visiting friends in a tiny town in Colorado and a vintage car show came to town. Being an admirer of custom cars I wandered over and found a vibrant community in action of individuals who had come together over a mutual love of old cars. They sat all day in the blinding August sun in the high country of Colorado talking about their cars and their respect for what each had accomplished with his or her car. They have a tremendous love for the skill, patience, time, and effort it takes to lovingly restore these cars. After eight hours, they hopped in their cars and drove to another town to do it all over again. They felt fulfilled.

A common problem for people today is that they have many daily interactions that don't add up to a community. Too many people expend way too much energy negotiating energy-draining interpersonal relationships at work, and spend zero time cultivating supportive community relationships. Some companies have tried to improve this situation in the workplace, by having a company picnic or other system-wide social event to shift the energy of a working community to become more nurturing. These give employees a chance to interact on a more human level—to engender a closer sense of community to help change what is all too often a stressful, competitive, energy-draining workplace environment. Because most people have to spend the majority of their time in the workplace, we need to strive to create a sense of community at work.

With the rise of the Internet, some people feel as if they have forged new communities while sitting alone in the comfort of their living rooms. In some ways the benefits of web activities are similar to journaling— greater self-understanding, a raising of consciousness about issues on a personal and international level, a gaining of insights into events—with an interactive audience. My only concern is whether these relationships are authentic. You may be talking to someone impersonating the friend you want. **It's hard for anyone over the age of thirty to understand, but people who spend an inordinate amount of time in Internet communities lose important interpersonal skills and the scope of energy that comes with interacting face to face.** I feel that people are spending too much time shut up in their energy-draining, blue-light dominated computer world: I'd rather see you get out and enjoy the natural world and interact with real people whom you enjoy so that you experience the vital source of connecting with others' direct energy.

Intimate Relationships

Intimate relationships are based on love and we find them within the nuclear family, with a spouse or significant other, in extended families of close relationships, and with one or two close friends and confidantes. These are the people you can go to when the chips are down. In today's society the definition of family has shifted considerably from the nuclear family of fifty years ago.

Many characteristics of families have changed. There are now fewer with children under the age of eighteen (our population is getting older because the baby boom is over). The average age at marriage has increased, and a greater proportion of all births occurs to women older than thirty and unmarried (.5 percent in 1960 to 33 percent in 2000). More parents are devoting less time to their own children and more to their own parents. This "sandwich generation" is pulled in multiple directions with longer average workdays and commute times, and the intrusion of television and computers into family life eroding time spent together. The role of family life has shifted dramatically. But intimate relationships still play a central role in people's lives and health.

Intimate relationships should be a source of healing energy, but too often can be one of energy-draining negativity. For example, having caring parents is a good predictor of health in later life. **A Harvard study that looked at 35 years of people's lives found the vast majority (91 per-**

cent) of people who *did not* perceive themselves to have had a warm relationship with their mothers had diagnosed diseases by midlife including coronary artery disease, hypertension, ulcers, and alcoholism. Only 45 percent of participants who *did* perceive themselves to have had a warm relationship with their mothers had these same health problems. A similar association between perceived warmth and closeness with fathers predicted future illness. Other research has established that hostility in the marital relationship lowers immunity.

I strongly recommend that you cultivate mindfulness in your intimate relationships regardless of your family structure—whether you're part of a home that some would see as fractured or you're trying to recreate a *Leave it to Beaver* traditional family. This means that you bring a freshness to every encounter. Many people are locked into habitual knee-jerk responses to their loved ones that ultimately drain the energy out of the relationship. Think about the attitude—the energy you are projecting to your loved ones. You cannot change your teenagers' pubescent moods, but you can shift the energy that you bring to the relationship with your teenager or your spouse, sibling, life partner, or the people who you count among your intimate acquaintances. **As you change the energy you bring to relationships, the energy you receive will begin to shift. Your intimate connections should be a source of positive energy.**

I often recommend that my patients reach out for help in repairing their intimate relationships. Couples and families can find help in Couples or Family Counseling. The goal is for each person to understand the other and to feel understood, and to reach a point in which behavioral and attitudinal changes stop the habitual negativity in a relationship. Compromise is seen not as a giving in, but as a positive step to satisfying the needs of each person. The improvement comes not just from valuing all that has been, and all that can be, but in the sheer good fortune you have to be in a loving supportive relationship. The improvement that comes from changing attitudes, expectations, and behaviors within the relationship is most often a noticeable increase in positive energy, joy and health.

Giving Back

A patient and friend of mine, a corporate executive, spends one night a month supervising the men's ward of a homeless shelter. I asked him, isn't this a stressful, energy-draining activity? His answer was, "It's the opposite, it's uplifting." He's deeply moved by the stories he hears. He says there are so many good people there whom fate just seemed not to shine on. That night at the shelter is one of the most satisfying things he does with his life and in many ways it seems more important to him than his regular job. He doesn't sleep much on those nights, but he comes away more energized than if he had spent a weekend at a spa.

You don't have to do something quite as dramatic as spending the night in a homeless shelter, but there are simple things you can do that can help you give energy to others. You can help your neighbor move boxes or organize a lemonade stand to raise funds for your local animal shelter or volunteer your time to any charitable organization—there are as many ways to give back as there are people in need. The passion that comes from compassion is a potent form of vital energy.

Music and Art

The creative arts have restorative powers and some are formal healing therapies: music and art therapy, dance therapy, and expressive writing or journaling are increasingly recognized as powerful therapeutic tools. In a study in the venerable *Journal of the American Medical Association,* expressive writing was shown to significantly improve asthma and rheumatoid arthritis. The benefits of music therapy in particular have been well established with hundreds of published studies. Listening to music (most commonly music therapy is administered by listening to a CD or iPod) has been shown to improve fatigue, stress, pain, anxiety, depression, sleep, hypertension, exercise performance, and recovery. It's also been shown to improve biochemical parameters such as the production of substances that improve brain functioning, reduction of inflammatory cytokines and adrenaline. One enterprising study showed a savings of 20 percent in overall home hospice health care costs where music therapy was added to the treatment. Neuroscientist Daniel J. Levitin puts his finger on the beauty of music in his book, *This Is Your Brain On Music*: "When we love a piece of music, it reminds us of other music we have heard, and it activates memory traces of emotional times in our lives. Your brain on music is all about . . . connections."

Quite simply, the creative arts take us out of ourselves and help us share the energy of the universe.

Nature

I was visiting a dear friend in a coronary intensive care unit, one of the *least* natural places on the planet, and I saw an extraordinary example of the power of nature. I was his last visitor of the day, it was late, and visitors were no longer allowed in the unit. He'd just had a small heart attack and emergency coronary angioplasty, a procedure that requires manipulating the vital coronary artery. He was feeling pretty delicate. I really didn't feel like leaving him and I felt he didn't want me to go. A nurse came in and asked, "Would you like to be visited by a volunteer?" Seeing the expectant look on the nurse's face my friend gave a polite OK. With a huge smile she said, "His name is Red." **In walked a volunteer with an officially trained, hospital-credentialed therapeutic dog! My friend's face lit up. And I left knowing that his heart was a bit lighter, simply because of the unexpected canine visitor.**

If dogs are allowed in the CCU, you can bet there's been a good deal of research into canine therapy. Visits by dogs have been shown to decrease postoperative pain in children, to reduce depression and increase oxygen saturation in patients undergoing chemotherapy, and to decrease blood pressure and depression in nursing home patients. Therapy with other animals such as cats and horses has also been shown to promote healing. Horses are playing a greater role in both physical and psychological rehabilitation medicine. Studies have shown that equine therapy benefits people with multiple sclerosis, cerebral palsy, and spinal cord injury. Animals provide a wonderfully healing interface with nature.

The point is to remind yourself that you're part of something beautiful and much bigger than yourself, whether nature for you means interacting with your pet, visiting your favorite beach, or taking a walk in your local park. Supreme Court Justice William O. Douglas took a noontime walk every day in the woods. There he made most of his major decisions. It was a time to let his mind free of the complexities of the day, and let the answers come to him, like in meditation.

In one fascinating study, researchers told a group of residents in a nursing home to take more responsibility for themselves, including caring for a 99¢ plant. The control group was given a plant and told the nurses would take care of it. The group given responsibility for the plant was dramatically more engaged in activities in the community, they were more alert and had better moods. (A full 93 percent of the plant-caretaking group showed improvement, versus an actual decline in overall well-being of the control group.) I'm not suggesting you force yourself to start gardening even if you have a brown thumb, but there are many ways to get connected to nature, and the important thing is to start now, today, reaching out beyond yourself and interacting with the energy that's all around you.

Energy Medicine

As a physician I sometimes recommend that my patients see energy healers; which most physicians do not do. Over the years I have seen some remarkable turnarounds in people working with practitioners of qi gong, Reiki, and therapeutic (healing) touch in particular. All of these involve the transfer of beneficial healing energy from one person to another. Early on in my career I was skeptical of these practices, but my eyes were opened about fifteen years ago when a patient of mine with chronic Lyme disease—which caused her partial blindness, impaired balance, difficulty walking, and problems with concentration and memory—was healed by an energy practitioner. This woman struggled for four years with the disease, had seen a dozen specialists but had had no significant improvement in her condition for over two years. Out of desperation she turned to a qi gong practitioner she'd heard about through friends. Incredibly, after a one-and-a-half hour session her eyesight dramatically improved, she was able to walk unassisted, and had more mental energy than she'd had since the disease began. While the results did not produce complete reversal, the improvement was dramatic and far better than anything conventional medicine had provided. When I last saw her, she felt emboldened to discuss beginning to taper off her medications with her neurologist.

What happened here? Well, no one really knows. There have been attempts to measure energy emanating from renowned healers; from the cruder early days using photography to wonderfully inspired recent research from psychologist Dr. Gary Schwartz at the University of Arizona using highly sophisticated bio-photon imaging to measure energetic emissions from healers' hands. In one study examining the effects of Reiki for cancer patients undergoing conventional therapy, there was a significant decrease in fatigue, pain, and anxiety after seven Reiki sessions over two weeks. Another randomized, controlled study showed decrease in heart rate and blood pressure in patients after three Reiki treatments compared to control groups.

Probably the best studied energy practice is therapeutic (healing) touch, which for thirty years has been part of the nursing curriculum at top nursing schools such as Columbia and NYU. Therapeutic touch doesn't actually involve touching, it's achieved by a transfer of energy from the practitioner's hands to the receiver. In one powerful study therapeutic touch decreased pain, anxiety, and suppressor T lymphocytes (which help regulate a balanced immune response) in burn patients. Another study published in *The Journal of Holistic Nursing*, showed an increase in hemoglobin (red blood cell) levels in healthy students compared to controls. Numerous other studies, particularly in nursing journals, show benefits from the use of therapeutic touch in the hospital, particularly with pain and mood states.

My colleague Dolores Krieger, Ph.D., introduced therapeutic touch to nursing schools. I couldn't agree more with her belief that the ability to engage energy in the healing process should be at the core of health care. I would only caution you to find the best practitioner. One study showed that Reiki practitioners had poor results on days they weren't feeling well. This is definitely an area in which having a referral from a trusted source is key. If you are in a hospital where therapeutic (healing) touch is offered I highly recommend you take advantage, as nurses are the standard bearers of these traditions.

The Interconnected Web

I was fortunate enough recently to meet Edgar Mitchell, a visionary scientist, the sixth astronaut to walk on the moon (he shares with Alan Shephard the record for longest moonwalk) and founder of the Institute of Noetic Sciences. He is one of the few human beings who experienced a greater spiritual connectedness while hurtling through space. Looking at the beautiful blue Earth from his spaceship on the return flight, Edgar was overwhelmed with the intimate knowledge that he was connected to his home planet. **In a moment of deep insight, he realized that he was also connected with everything—his energy was entangled with that of everything and everyone—through time and space.** That experience led eventually to his founding of the Institute of Noetic Sciences, which conducts research into the healing power and the energetic nature of consciousness.

In Chapter 1 you learned about a neuropepetide web that interconnects parts of your body separated by space—it allows your thoughts to send chemical messengers that affect your digestive tract, your emotions to affect your cardiovascular system, your hormones to affect your moods—and vice versa. Researchers are beginning to redefine their view of all matter in terms of this underlying energetic web. While the neuropeptide web communicates by chemical reactions, physicists have been able to demonstrate that instantaneous communication between subatomic particles occurs on an energetic level at speeds faster than the speed of light.

Working on an infinitesimally minute level of the smallest known subatomic particles and the forces that bind them together, physicists performing experiments with particle accelerators (the massive tools they've designed to split atoms) have demonstrated that **the objects we perceive as matter—from your loved ones to this book you're reading—are actually made of collections or patterns of energy.** Quantum physicists have further established that this energetic matter seems to be infinitely mutable (it can be in two places at once and move backwards in time, which is termed *nonlocality*) and it is continuously interacting with other matter that enters its energetic field, becoming perpetually entangled with it even across vast expanses of space.

Where most of us see empty space separating one living thing from another, physicists have shown all these empty spaces to be filled with energy that allows for continuous sharing of energy and information across space. You and I have no problem understanding that energy can transcend space in nearly instantaneous time: when someone plays a violin, you can hear the music a hundred yards away—traveling over invisible waves at the relatively slow speed of sound. When you turn on a light bulb you accept with little fanfare that the light fills the room in an instant, but it did in fact have to travel at the speed of light, transmitting the energy of the light's photons from the bulb to your dinner table. One of my favorite examples of invisible, energetic information transfer in everyday life is of a remote control garage door opener: When you press the button, an electromagnetic signal travels seemingly instantaneously to a receiver that opens the door. I'd like you to accept this image of energy just as you accept that a violin string transmits sound energy. Your thoughts can conceivably emanate like the energy of the door opener to be received by others and visa-versa.

This new science of energy has enormous implications for healing, and at the same time explains many of the healing phenomena I have witnessed over years of practicing medicine. The energetic web that underlies all matter helps explain the beneficial power of belief in any cure to heal illness and also informs us how the destructive power of negative thoughts can do us harm on a physical level. The existence of this web also helps explain how my patient was healed by qi gong practice, why being in a supportive community can be so powerful, and why helping others can be so energizing. The discoveries of quantum physics strongly suggest that all of us have the power to affect not only our own health, but also each other through the interaction of energy—including the energy of thought and emotion.

This very real energetic web tying together all matter allows for a cause and effect relationship between consciousness (the energy of thought) and healing (the returning of physical processes to normal). The transformative power of our own thoughts and intentions and of the thoughts and intentions of others involves an energetic process that transcends space, in what Larry Dossey has described as "non-local mind." As a physician I have witnessed the benefits of *nonlocality*; I have come to see the value of tuning in to our energetic selves. I've come to think of this process as plugging into an *interconnected web* of energy that ties us all together and makes us part and parcel of the universe, of each other, and, perhaps, of the absolute.

PART TWO

21 Days to Optimal Energy

Power Up

Cleanse

Maximize

Power Up
Day-by-Day

WELCOME TO POWER UP DAY-BY-DAY. My 21-Day Plan for Increasing Your Energy and Feeling 10 Years Younger consists of three vital phases that will purify and maximize your body's energy-generating capacity. For each day you will find a one-page summary of the plan for that day, followed by more detailed discussions of various aspects of the day that may contain new or unfamiliar concepts. Here, a quick overview of the three weeks:

- **Week One:** The first step is to increase, or *power up,* your energy-generating capacity. This requires reducing stress and gradually eliminating alcohol, red meat, wheat, sugar, processed and chemically treated foods—all of which cause inflammation. You will eat nutrient-dense (primarily whole) foods every three to four hours to stabilize your blood sugar and provide blocks of energy. You will begin regular guided relaxation. You will breathe more (using breath work every day), and drink more water and other healthy fluids (12 ounces every two hours), rest more (closing in on the desired eight hours a day), move more (20–30 minutes a day), and remove toxins, including negative thoughts (with a daily stress log).
- **Week Two:** The second step is to reset your metabolism by *cleaning out* the toxins. During this recharge phase, I will guide you through a one-day juice cleanse that will dramatically re-

duce inflammation and enhance detoxification. You'll follow that with a gentle recovery day. You will eliminate foods that may bring your energy down via allergic or other adverse food reactions. You will regularly consume power foods such as greens, green tea, mushrooms, nonwheat whole grains, flax, berries, and fish. You will practice powerful yogic breathing exercises and incorporate massage and other body work designed to help flush out toxins and increase vitality. You will continue to sleep more, exercise moderately, maintain hydration, and manage stress better.

- **Week Three:** The third step is to move beyond lifestyle changes to more advanced energy-generating techniques to *maximize* your energy. Inflammation, glycation (sugar aging), and the level of toxins in your body will have all decreased dramatically. With your new habits, you will be extracting more energy from food, coping with stress rather than letting it undermine you, raising your pulse rate daily to use energy more efficiently, and getting superior sleep. You will be ready for deeper body work such as Reiki or acupuncture. If, despite instituting all of the above, your energy is still not optimum, I will discuss using supplements to further maximize your energy supply.

Check for Illness First

It's essential that you be screened by your medical doctor for an underlying cause of your fatigue before starting the plan. Certain parts of the plan—including the cleanse and the sauna, may not be suitable for people with certain conditions. See the introduction on page 15 for a discussion of what to look for with your physician.

Negotiating Change

Bad news up front: In order to restore your energy over the next twenty-one days I will ask you to eliminate red meat, sugar, alcohol, coffee, wheat, and processed foods. Why should you do this? Because these foods tend to cause allergic, inflammatory, insulin-related, and other reactions that put a strain on your natural energy supply. For some people, this is a wel-come challenge and change (the plan offers many enticing substitutes for all of the above) as they have been wanting a reason to cut out these foods that, they've intuited, are not doing them any good. For others, the elimi-nation of these longtime gustatory companions will seem impossible. Do you *have* to get rid of all of them? Not exactly, I'm willing to negotiate with you rather than lose the chance to bring your energy back because you're worried you won't be able to get off and stay off them. I will offer you a way to work the plan in increments.

My first recommendation for you if you can't go "cold turkey" on what I call energy-negative foods is that you **eliminate only one or two target offenders at a time.** There are two ways to choose the first to go: You can eliminate the items you consume the least of, which is the easiest (but less effective) route; or you can follow a classic allergy-elimination paradigm and stop eating the offenders that you consume most often. What you flood your system with on a consistent basis is likely to do the most harm and cause the most potent cravings. Removing that offender will yield the greatest results. Removing your most energy-negative food will likely provide you with the best motivation to continue to comply.

The biggest impediment is fear of crashing, particularly from sugar and coffee withdrawal. Some people really do feel their lives and personal energy will come to a screeching halt, or at least be terribly disrupted, if they don't get their accustomed stimulants. This brings me to my second negotiating tactic: **If you can't go off your energy-negative foods cold turkey, try gradual withdrawal.** In the 21-Day program, for instance, you gradually reduce coffee, and substitute green tea, which gives you a more gentle lift. You don't have to give up the taste of sweetness alto-gether, as you will have plenty of fruits and natural sugars in the plan, but refined (white) sugar is off the list. The upside is that, once refined carbo-hydrates are gone, the compulsion for sweetness often fades.

I'll take a small change in habit over no change any day. One patient began the program as she was moving to a vineyard in Italy! Drinking no alcohol was out of the question so I suggested she take one glass of wine with dinner every other day rather than her accustomed two or three glasses every night. She reported developing a more discerning palate by drinking less. She also found it easier to get out of bed in the morning and had fewer headaches.

The simplest way to negotiate change is to focus on the positive. Rather than think of the plan as some sort of Spartan regimen, think of it as a new experience. My patients often report that the plan expanded their horizons. Some patients have even planned ahead trips to Asia at the end of 21 days, after having been introduced to its multitude of flavors and energy practices.

I'll offer one more incentive; you do not have to be on the plan for a lifetime, and you do not need to cut out these foods forever. Cutting out wheat, for example, doesn't always make a difference. Go ahead, try it again after abstaining for three weeks and see how you feel. Moderation is your mantra . . . everything in moderation.

Week One: Power Up

"Reduced to our own body, our first instrument, we learn to play it, drawing from it maximum resonance and harmony."   Yehudi Menuhin

Day One

❑ Power Mind: Learn the Early Morning Wake-Up Call
❑ Establish an Evening Stress Log
❑ Take the Energy Quiz (page 13)

❑ Power Food: Organic Menu
❑ Eat Every 3–4 hours, Avoid Blood-Sugar Swings
❑ A Quick Look at Inflammatory Foods
❑ Increase water (drink five to six glasses per day)

❑ Power Exercise: Baby Steps

❑ Power Rest: 8 hours
❑ Meet the Sleep Plan:
   Eight Hours Sleep Four Nights/Week
   Asleep by 10:00 p.m. 2–3 nights

Early Morning Wake-Up Call

On the first morning of the plan when you wake up I want you to be aware that you are in the midst of a critical transition from sleep to waking—your hormones, neurotransmitters, muscle fibers, and blood cells are ramping up in preparation for meeting the challenges of the day. Awakening can be a stressful time, but you are going to transform this stressful moment of the day into an energy-generating opportunity. You will dissolve negative or worrying thoughts that can sap your energy and wreak havoc on your body throughout the day.

Before bounding up, sit on the edge of your bed, spine straight, hands relaxed on the thighs. Take three deep breaths—drawing from your abdomen to the count of 4, hold for one count and exhale from your abdomen to the count of 6. Now sit quietly focusing only on your breath. When thoughts of your day come into your consciousness, allow them to leave. Focus on your breathing. If thoughts persist try repeating a mantra to calm your frantic mind (love, energy, peace, are a few)—or use images (clouds, ocean, loved ones). Stay this way for at least two minutes, which is long enough to begin to elicit the relaxation response. See Chapter 1 for more on how this relaxation exercise benefits your health.

Do not fear that if you relax in the morning you won't perform as well at work. You will soon find out what neuroscientists know about meditation and breath work—it stimulates portions of the brain involved in mental focus. You'll find you have better energy and more laser-like focus with the Early Morning Wake-Up Call.

Relaxation Rx

The following conditions are significantly improved by regular elicitation of the relaxation response with controlled breathing, meditation, and other methods.

Anxiety	Hypertension
Asthma	Insomnia
Cardiac arrhythmias	Irritable bowel
Chronic pain	Low back pain
Headaches	Mild/moderate depression
Hot flashes	PMS

Ref: Herbert Benson, M.D., *The Relaxation Response*

Eat Every Three to Four Hours, Avoid Blood-Sugar Swings

For the 21-Day Plan you will eat every three to four hours to avoid a drop in blood sugar. Low blood sugar produces an immediate energy drain; not only does your body have insufficient sugar to manufacture energy, but the hormone changes required to compensate for lack of blood sugar cause energy expenditure.

A Quick Look at Inflammatory Foods

The organic menus of the 21-Day Plan eliminate all major inflammatory foods. When digested, certain foods—like alcohol, red meat, sugar, and artificial ingredients—turn into substances that promote the creation of inflammatory molecules. These molecules, consisting mainly of a class called cytokines, are part of the immune system and are beneficial to the body in the short term (for example, they help in attacking infections). But a steady diet of foods that promote inflammatory substances can worsen or even cause inflammatory conditions such as arthritis, asthma, heart disease, and chronic pain. Inflammation drains energy and can even cause weight gain. By following the menus of the 21-Day Plan you will significantly reduce inflammation. (See Chapter 2 for a more complete list of inflammatory foods.)

Increase water

During the 21-Day Plan you will drink 8-12 ounces of water every two to three hours. (Non-caffeinated, minimally sweetened beverages like herbal tea count toward this.) Inadequate hydration causes the body to extract water from nonvital tissues in order to shunt water to key organs (heart, brain, and kidneys). Such stopgap water management can produce a significant drop in overall energy. Scientists have even shown that insufficient hydration can have a negative effect on memory.

Finding Clean Water: You're going to be drinking a lot of water over the next 21 days, so let's make sure it's healthy. Tap water has become suspect in many areas. Out-of-date municipal water treatment facilities do not adequately remove many twenty-first century industrial chemicals that can contaminate ground water, streams, and reservoirs (larger municipalities tend to have more stringent standards). Well water has no over-sight whatsoever, and can easily be contaminated from local run-off for example, from lawn chemicals. Old pipes that carry water to you can leach contaminants and breed bacteria. Home filtration is by far the best, least expensive, and most ecologically prudent way to insure your water is clean. Your second best bet is high quality bottled (preferably in glass) water, which is still better regulated in Europe than the United States.

What's in your water?

Every municipal drinking water supply is different. Here are examples of water contaminants repeatedly detected in the United States, and the best type of filter to eliminate the problem. You can obtain a report on your own water supply by contacting your local water authority.

Contaminant	Common Source	Potential Health Effects	Best Filter
Chlorination by-products	Municipal water chlorination practices	Potential carcinogen	Carbon (filters particles down to a fraction of a strand of hair)
Lead	Plumbing, brass alloy faucets	Kidneys, nervous system damage	Carbon
Mercury	Crop runoff, battery disposal	Kidney, nervous system disorders	Reverse osmosis (filters particles down to a single atom)
Microbes	Animal or human waste	Gastrointestinal illness	Reverse osmosis
Atrazine	Run-off from use as herbicide	Promotes breast tumor growth	Reverse osmosis

Source: www.nsf.org

Shopping for a Water Filter: Water filters can be placed where the water enters the house or underneath the kitchen sink. Carbon filters are sufficient for removing most contaminants, but reverse osmosis is considered to be the best filtration technology, though it requires a small water tank under the sink. One of my favorite filter manufacturers is Culligan, but there are many quality brands: Look for NSF International certification on the package label of whichever filter you choose.

Power Exercise: Baby Steps

If you don't already have an exercise regimen, start powering up your metabolism simply by walking for 20 minutes, but keep in mind that you are working toward the Power Up Workout (Day Three). You may already have a regular exercise regimen, in which case keep it up! If you don't exercise (like approximately 65 percent of the population), I'm going to make it simple for you. Begin by taking a 20-minute walk each day. Studies show that walking is sufficient exercise to give life-extending benefits, whether it's on your way to the bus, at lunch time, on the way home, or an evening stroll. Begin to make it part of your life.

Establish an Evening Stress Log

My goal is for you to begin to pinpoint the stressful moments in your day. With that in mind, I'd like you to get a notebook and keep a stress log that will help you recognize the stressors in your life. On almost a daily basis people tell me they are fine when I ask about stress, and then wind up near tears later in the conversation when they start to talk about (and actually recognize) the difficulties in their lives. Stress is cumulative, which is to say that relatively small stresses can have great impact when stress is loaded upon stress on a chronic daily basis. With this log you will begin to see patterns of stress that you can address. Once you've identified and named the stressful moments in your day, I hope you can begin to let them go each evening and, eventually, address them in order to reduce them.

Write down the three most stressful moments of your day. These can include an encounter with a difficult person, upsetting thoughts, or horrendous traffic on your morning commute. The point is to note where and when your blood starts to boil. Note the time and place and nature of the stress. Rate on a scale of 1–6 the level of stress, and give yourself a grade for how you coped with it. Once you've put it down in print, that's where it should stay. Now let it go.

Meet the Sleep Plan:
Eight hours of sleep, four nights a week
Asleep by 10:00 p.m. Two or Three Nights

During the 21-Day Plan you will develop regular, healthy sleep patterns, which means that most nights you'll get to bed around the same reasonable time and clock eight hours of sleep. Tonight, you're going to try for eight hours. You've got nothing to lose and everything to gain. When it comes to sleep your body is just like your cell phone battery: If you don't charge it long enough, it runs out faster. The same goes for your body: inadequate sleep = inadequate energy. As folksy as this wisdom sounds, we now have solid scientific evidence about what the body actually needs to do while you sleep. It takes eight hours for the body to optimally repair and regenerate cells, lower blood pressure (by as much as 10 percent), and manufacture protective and functional hormones as well as other key chemicals you need for energy generation. If you don't sleep long enough and deeply enough, your body will be inadequately recharged.

Scientists have pinpointed eight hours as the ideal amount of sleep. Considering that the majority of Americans get less than seven hours of sleep, I'm going to be realistic and ask that you shoot for eight hours at least four nights a week. I've added in bed by 10:00 p.m. two or three nights a week because I know many people try to make up for sleep shortages on the weekends, but if that means sleeping from 1:00 a.m. to 9:00 a.m. I'm still not happy. Research shows that the hours of sleep before midnight are more productive in their repair and regeneration of cells than the hours of sleep after midnight. In Chinese medical terms, it's best to be sound asleep between 11:00 p.m. and 1:00 a.m., when the body's Qi energy replenishes itself.

Day Two

❑ Power Mind: Early Morning Wake-Up Call
❑ *Establish Breath Breaks**
❑ Evening Stress Log

❑ Power Food: Organic Menus
❑ *Eliminate Chemical Toxins with Organics*
❑ *Increase Chewing*
❑ *Juice Cocktails vs Dessert*

❑ *Power Detox: Identify Environmental Energy Drains At Home*
❑ Power Exercise: *The Power of Walking*

❑ Power Rest: Asleep by 10
❑ *Calming Bedtime Routine*

* Note: New concepts for you are *italic*.

Early Morning Wake-up Call

This morning as you transit from sleep to waking, I want you to feel the energy in your body as it moves from its dormant state to its active state. Highly trained Buddhist monks can control the energy in their bodies to such a degree that they can raise their body temperatures even while sitting outside in the winter. I'm not suggesting you aspire to monk-like power, though anything is possible! My goal is to make you aware of the energy you possess.

This morning as you practice the Early Morning Wake Up Call, become aware of sensations of energy in your body—move your fingertips together and feel a tingling or vibration, or look for a release of tension from your spine or facial muscles. Take just two minutes, or as long as you'd like, to begin to feel relaxed and energized.

As you make your way through the Power Up plan, I want you to practice the Early Morning Wake-Up Call every day. You can keep it simple, as I've set it out for the first two days, or you can try different focuses for your meditative time. For instance, try the focus of the Connectedness exercises—mindfulness, forgiveness, letting go of grudges. If you already have a contemplative or spiritual practice, take this morning time to deepen it. Simply using a mantra that evokes a higher power can magnify the benefits of the relaxation response. As you work with this exercise, find ways of making it your own and of making it meaningful.

Eliminate Chemical Toxins with Organics

Eating organic fruits and vegetables is the best way to begin eliminating toxins from your body and get cleaner energy from your food. A growing number of scientists and physicians in the United States and abroad, myself included, harbor deep concerns about the wide array of pesticides, herbicides, and other chemicals used to grow foods. Apples and strawberries, for example, carry an average of five different pesticides per piece of fruit. While the chemical industry conducts some research on the individual effects of pesticides, scant research exists on the effects of continuous exposure to numerous pesticides on a daily basis, which is the average exposure for people eating nonorganic, conventional foods. I want you to reduce this cumulative load of industrial chemicals by buying as much organic food as you possibly can.

If you want to prioritize your organic purchases, a quick rule of thumb is that produce and dairy come first, followed by meats and then all other foods. It's more important to purchase organic thin-skinned fruits and vegetables such as berries, peaches, apples, tomatoes, and almost all vegetables. (Onions are about the only vegetable that I don't insist on being organic because they rarely carry pesticides.) Thick-skinned fruits such as oranges, bananas, melons, and avocados offer less exposure to pesticides because their edible insides are more protected from chemical contamination by the thick peel. (For more on organics, see Chapter 3.)

Increase Chewing

During the 21-Day Plan I want you to practice chewing more, at least 12 times per mouthful. Chewing is the first step in the process of transforming your food into energy. Unfortunately, few people chew enough. Most of us inhale our food, which increases the amount of energy needed to digest it and reduces the amount of nutrients and energy you extract from it.

Here's how it works. Many of the enzymes in your pancreas are also present in your mouth. When you chew well, your food is predigested by the time it hits your stomach. With improper chewing, you throw large chunks of whole food into the stomach, which churns and acidifies the partially chewed food, but cannot finish the job. This leads to indigestion and chronic poor absorption of nutrients, especially when your stomach doesn't have much acid (as can happen most notably when taking acid-suppressing drugs). The undigested food is difficult for the chemicals from the gall bladder and pancreas to break down fully. The remainder of the digestion then falls to the intestinal bacteria, which are not entirely cut out for the work, and in the process create gas, bloating, and cramping.

Just like mom told you, wolfing your food is bad—it leads to low energy. Chewing more is an easy way to reduce digestive problems and receive more energy from your food. Another key benefit of chewing more is eating less: When you eat slowly and chew well, you absorb your food more efficiently and get the "all-full" signal faster.

Juice Drink vs Dessert

Your dinner menu today includes a juice cocktail, Papaya Fizz, and no dessert. The drink has healthy antioxidants and enzymes in the papaya, but it also contains a fair amount of natural fruit sugar—enough to give up eating dessert as well. Throughout the 21 days the dinner menus alternate between juice cocktails and dessert. Feel free to substitute either one, if you prefer a special drink with dinner each night, then skip dessert or have a small bowl of berries. If you prefer dessert, go for any one of the desserts and skip the cocktail.

Establish Breath Breaks

During the 21-Day Plan I want you to reap the benefits of the relaxation response that you elicit with the Early Morning Wake Up Call throughout the day by taking Breath Breaks. The breath is the best means you have for directly changing aspects of your autonomic nervous system, which functions without conscious intervention to regulate the activities of the heart, muscles, and glands. By simply breathing deeply and rhythmically, with intention, you can slow your heart rate, lower your blood pressure, improve your digestion, strengthen your immune system, and calm your nervous system.

Take a Breath Break every time you are aware that you are breathing. Do this frequently—sitting, walking, eating, while in a tense meeting. You will immediately feel the tension in your body release. You will be less tight, less hunched in the neck and shoulders. You will have a calmer mind, slower pulse—slower life and greater energy. Here's how:

- Inhale with a slow, deep abdominal breath (allowing your breath to expand your abdomen) to the count of 4.
- Pause, holding in this fresh oxygen, for one count.
- Exhale slowly (allow your abdomen to contract) to the count of 6.
- Pause for one count. (Repeat two more times.)

Identify Environmental Energy Drains at Home

For the 21-Day Plan I want you to identify and eliminate major sources of chemical toxins in your home that may very well be draining your energy. I think the best approach is to evaluate the pollutants in your home that might target your physical vulnerabilities—do you have asthma, eczema, a family history of cancer, recurring bronchitis, headaches every time you shower; or do you wake up with a stuffy nose every morning that goes away by lunch? Are you exposing yourself to respiratory, hormonal, skin, or immune system disruptors? You can make quick changes that will stop your home from sapping your energy.

Take inventory of possible environmental sources of toxicity listed in "Home Sweet Toxin," below, and seek out healthier alternatives. The amount of exposure you have to any given toxin is the key to your evaluation. Items you are widely exposed to are more important than those you are minimally exposed to. For example, when evaluating your personal care products, those that come in contact with large amounts of skin (i.e., moisturizer or bath products) should be more carefully scrutinized than those that come in contact with only a small portion of skin. You are likely to spend more continuous time in your bedroom than any

other room in the house, so first evaluate your bedroom for possible offenders. One exception to the dose/exposure rule: I have zero tolerance
for vinyl shower curtains, Teflon pans, and microwaving in plastic containers—get rid of them, now! (See Chapter 3 for more on environmental
toxins.)

Home Sweet Toxin

Your domestic haven could be making you sick and tired. Below are
some of the biggest offenders. I subscribe to The Green Guide (green
guide.com) and greenerchoices.org for useful information on making a
healthy household.

Products	Toxic Chemicals	Potential Health Risks	Healthier Alternatives
Mattresses	Polyurethane, formaldehyde, toluene, PBDE (flame retardants)	Respiratory disruptor, carcinogen, neurotoxin	Natural-fill (wool or cotton), untreated mattress or pillow topper.
Wall-to-wall carpets	Adhesives and stain-proofing agents can outgas formaldehyde	Carcinogen, skin irritant	Jute, wool, hemp, or sea grass area rugs installed with VOC*-free adhesives
Paints	Benzene, formaldehyde, toluene, xylene	Carcinogen, neurotoxin	Look on labels for no-VOC or low-VOC paints, and let dry ventilated for 72 hours. Pregnant women should not paint.

Cosmetics	Phthalates, parabens, preservatives, coal tar, triclosan, DEA, heavy metals, Sodium lauryl sulphate	Endocrine disruptor, carcinogen, antibiotic resistance, neurotoxin, skin toxin	Look for these worst offenders on labels and try to avoid them. For cosmetics, the organic claim is not regulated.
Cleaning products	Chlorine bleach, ammonia, acids, fragrance, DEA and TEA	Respiratory, eye, skin irritants, carcinogens, endocrine disruptors	Soap, water, baking soda, vinegar, lemon juice, and borax. Be mindful of ventilation.
Vinyl shower curtains	Off-gasses plasticizers for as many as 5 years	Endocrine (hormone) disruptor	Go for washable cotton, canvas, silk, or rayon.
Kitchenware	Teflon, PVC (plastic)	Carcinogens, endocrine disruptor	Cook with enameled cast-iron or seasoned stainless steel; microwave and store in Pyrex, not plastic.

* Volatile organic compounds (VOCs) are noxious gases emitted from certain compounds that can be inhaled or absorbed by the skin over time.

The Power of Walking

During the 21-Day Plan I want you to derive maximum benefit from 20–30 minutes of walking. First I suggest you make peace with the concept of walking. Take a moment to recognize how lucky you are to be freely mobile. Walking is a privilege and a joy and a way of knowing the world that many of us forego for convenience. Many of us don't walk well and, rather than holding our bodies erect when we walk (which we're designed to do), we simply allow our bodies to slump down upon our legs and feet, which are forced to drag around dead weight all day long. Let's wipe the slate clean and start over.

Think of these as the first steps of your new life. Imagine you're walking on sand, with your toes lightly pressing on the ground (this is why doctors have always recommended soft shoes for toddlers—humans should engage their toes when they walk). Set down your heel gently (there should be very little sound, and certainly no elephantine thumping). Feel the toes activated and the ball of your foot pushing off as your foot prepares to leave the ground. Keep your length of stride reasonable: Don't reach with your legs. Slightly rotate your pelvis under while tightening your glutes and abs (this will eliminate swayback and flaccid glutes). Spine position is erect, with your abdominals lightly contracted, chest expanded, shoulders back and down (not up). Your head should feel as though there is a string gently pulling you up from the crown, the muscles under your chin slightly tight, your head positioned to balance a book.

Feel the elongation of your spine. Feel the effortlessness of your body as it moves through space. Feel blessed that you have the ability to walk freely. Use this time to move and to relax your mind. And breathe as though you need the oxygen, which you do!

Calming Bedtime Routine

From a very young age, bedtime rituals are the first step toward getting a proper night's sleep. You need a calming ritual that begins to organize your nervous system, not stimulate it. Bedtime laggards, who stay up later than planned, are about twice as likely as early-to-bed types to be on the internet or doing work related to their jobs during the hour before going to bed. And 87 percent of the population reports watching television before bed. Be mindful of how a program will affect your stress levels. TV and most other electronic devices overstimulate the brain and make it harder to move into a sleep zone, which requires a lot of soothing alpha brain waves. Go for soothing evening activities that make your brain sleep-prone.

It's important to fall asleep relatively quickly, not tossing and turning when the lights go out, which is a sure sign you haven't prepared yourself properly for sleep. People who take 30 minutes or more to fall asleep are more likely to sleep less than six hours on weekdays; they experience at least one symptom of insomnia and report that they get less sleep than the minimum they say they need to function at their best. On average, it takes 23 minutes to fall asleep, which means ideally you should have lights out by 9:35 p.m., and begin calming activities by 8:30 p.m.!

The best activities for the hour before bed are: Practice relaxation exercises (see Days 3, 4, 5, 8, and 15), calm reading (no page turners), take a hot bath with lavender oil, listen to soothing music, or drink calming tea with chamomile and valerian.

Day Three

❑ **Power Mind: Early Morning Wake-Up Call** *with Sun Salutation*
❑ **Daytime: Breath Breaks**
❑ *The Two-Minute Energy Boost*
❑ **Evening Stress Log**

❑ **Power Food: Organic Menus**
❑ *Eliminate Wheat*
❑ *Why Drink Green Tea?*
❑ *Sugar Substitutes*

❑ **Power Exercise:** *The Power Up Workout in a Nutshell*
❑ *20-30 Minutes Walking*
❑ *30 Crunches, 20 Push-ups (bent-knee OK)*

❑ *Power of Connection: Establish Positive Emotional Actions*
❑ *Letting Go of Grudges*

❑ **Power Sleep: Eight hours**
❑ *Tips for Falling Asleep: Progressive Relaxation*

Sun Salutation

If you can add the incredibly powerful yogic asana, the Sun Salutation, to your Early Morning Wake-Up Call every day or every other day or once a week you will start the game on a better energetic plane. I'd like you to get instruction on Sun Salutations from an expert, but here is a detailed illustration of how to complete the posture one time. Classically, sun salutations are done in pairs, starting first with one foot, then the other. Most important, don't rush; feel the energy moving through your body.

The Two-Minute Energy Boost

During the 21-Day Plan you will give up your accustomed pick-me-ups—the cup of coffee or the candy bar—and learn to generate quick energy in much healthier, longer-lasting ways, through breath work and relaxation exercises. Your Two-Minute Energy Boost can be any movement—from a yoga posture to hopping up and down—that gets your blood moving. The key is to use exercises that you can do anywhere anytime, with minimal space and no equipment. You can even do them where others can watch you because they are unobtrusive; you may even give others the idea to do the same. Here is a list of the energy-generating exercises that I explained in detail at the end of Chapter 4.

Abdominal breathing
Seated warrior
Downward facing dog
Qi gong energy ball
Hopping
Rock out with your iPod

Eliminate Wheat

As you go through the 21 days I am going to have you eliminate certain foods that could be either directly toxic to your health and energy, or produce an energy drag via allergies and other processes. In my experience, wheat is the most sensitizing food—nearly 50 percent of my patients

Sun Salutation

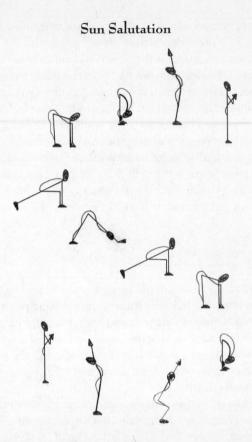

The Sun Salutation is an energizing combination of seven yoga postures, always performed in this order. You begin by placing one foot back, complete the series, then start again with the other foot. Before attempting this, spend time with an instructor or an instructional video to learn and perform it with good alignment.

become sensitive to wheat by age 40. This means that even though their allergy testing may be nonreactive, wheat produces subtle health problems—most commonly fatigue, but also other physical problems such as headaches, indigestion, and joint aches. Additionally many more people have subtle allergies to wheat, measurable either by skin tests or through blood tests—the latter creating a reaction that can occur up to three days after consumption. And the 5 percent of people with actual gluten-intolerant celiac disease can become quite ill after the tiniest bit of wheat. (See Chapter 2 for more information on allergy testing.)

The main troublemaker is the New World wheat hybrid that is most commonly used in North America for "wheat" in breads, pasta, and most all baked goods (even commercial oat bread routinely contains wheat as the main grain). In the menu plan, for the few times we include bread, we ask that you try one of the delicious Old World varieties such as kamut or spelt, to which most people are not sensitive. (And for celiac substitute with non-gluten grains such as quinoa, rice, potato, or corn.) Your body will tell you if cutting out wheat is the right thing for you. Either you will notice much more energy when you eliminate wheat, or you will feel immediately bad again when you reintroduce it after three weeks of clearing it out.

Why Drink Green Tea?

Health Benefits: Green tea one of the most powerful healing foods on the planet. All green and black teas come from the same plant worldwide, Camellia sinensis, but they are prepared with different processes that affect the healthful compounds in the leaves. Green tea is dried while black tea is fermented (oolong is partially fermented), and the fermentation process reduces some of the most important health-giving substances present in camella sinensis.

Green tea has catechins—some of nature's most potent antioxidants, which also may help keep your metabolism working at a higher level (potentially releasing more calories from fat). A cup of regular green tea does have some caffeine—10–30 mg, versus 100–150 for coffee—but the lift you get from green tea tends to be less of the roller coaster ride you get from coffee, largely due to the amino acid theanine present in green tea, which counteracts the effects of caffeine by promoting production of calming brain neurotransmitters. If you find that you are sensitive to the caffeine in green tea you can clear 80 percent of the caffeine while retaining most of the other beneficial ingredients by steeping your tea bag for one minute, then pouring out that tea and making a second cup of tea from the same bag.

Sugar Substitutes

Everyone is always looking for sugar substitutes. The problem I have with chemical, zero calorie sweeteners is they introduce yet more substances for the body to detox, AND they're actually associated with weight gain. Preliminary lab and animal studies show that when you eat non-nutritive sweeteners (perhaps even including stevia), the body's sweetness receptors—in the tongue and gut—send messages to the brain that result in a craving for more calories. I recommend you stick to low-glycemic agave nectar, or alternatively, use honey sparingly, because although you will be adding some calories with honey, at least you will also be adding beneficial antioxidants and other healthful phytochemicals and reduce the risk of confusing your brain into craving more sweets.

The Power Up Workout in a Nutshell
20–30 Minutes Walking
30 Crunches, 20 Push-ups (bent-knee OK)

Studies have shown that a brisk 30-minute walk three days per week gives you the cardiovascular benefits of more strenuous running or other more intense aerobic exercise. For example, it lowers blood pressure, helps repair the inside of the blood vessels, and reduces the inflammatory marker, CRP, the most powerful predictor of the risk of heart disease. Make sure to set three days a week aside to engage in aerobic walking. This is what is called *conversational aerobics*—your heart rate is raised, your metabolism increased, but you are still able to have a conversation while doing it, rather than feeling intensely winded. We will go more into how you can maximize the aerobic benefits of simple walking in Day 5.

Crunch Crunch Crunch

To jump-start your core you need to strengthen it; and the best way to accomplish this on your own, without the need for an instructor, is the core crunch—an improvement on the old-fashioned sit-up. Lie on your back; bend your knees so that your lower back presses against the floor. Rest your hands loosely against the back of your neck. Do not pull your neck up with your hands! Engage your abdominal muscles, and slowly roll your upper body off the floor, keeping your neck in a straight line with your spine. Stop just after your shoulders leave the mat. The secret to doing this most efficiently and safely is to treat your abdominal muscles and your ribcage as a single unit—and to breathe throughout the exercise. After you have elevated a few inches, slowly roll back down—without rounding your shoulders—then repeat. The motion should be smooth and slow, no jerking up and down, and no holding your breath. Do this until your muscles are just beginning to ache (for some people early on, just two or three proper core crunches can be excruciating!). Rest for a minute or two and do two more sets.

Work Your Way Into Proper Push-Ups

Research shows that strength builds quicker when you increase *load* rather than repetition. If you have never been able to do more than a couple of push-ups at a time, here's how to get stronger: Increase the challenge throughout the session, with your last push being hardest. For beginners, start your push-ups from a standing position, place your toes about 24 inches from a wall, place your hands flat against it with arms stretched straight out, and slowly bring your nose to the wall by bending your arms, keeping your core engaged, body in a straight line like a plank. Do this a dozen times, rest, then move onto the floor for two rounds of bent-knee push-ups—straight spine, core engaged. Finally, do one perfect all-out push-up, on your toes, body straight as a board. Next time, end with two perfect push-ups, and soon you'll be up to six . . . then on to 30!

Power of Connection: Establish Positive Emotional Actions
Letting Go of Grudges

I want you to keep your daily stress log so that you can focus on particular patterns of behavior that are counterproductive to you; holding grudges is a biggie. You need to be able to receive the positive energy of others in your community. What you project out is so often what comes back to you; ruminating on those who've wronged you is a sure to draw more negativity. Today I would like you to focus on how much and how often you hold grudges against others. Rather than thinking of the wrongs others have done to you, try thinking of what you can do to help others—it's a wonderful way to take your mind off yourself. Holding onto negative thought patterns will eat you up inside. I'm not suggesting you should become best friends with your nemesis, but let the negativity go.

Tips for Falling Asleep: Progressive Relaxation

This is a simple and effective way to release tension that's keeping you awake, shift the focus of your thoughts away from nagging worries, and at the same time say thank you to your body for all for the hard work of the day. Start with your toes: Inhale deeply and squeeze and scrunch your toes as hard as you can. Now exhale completely while releasing your toes, and say a small thank you to them for walking you through your day. Progress upwards through the major muscles of your body, contracting and releasing—thighs, buttocks, abdomen, then hands, arms and shoulders, and finally the face. As you move through your body, feel your limbs relax and begin to get heavier, and continue quiet deep breathing afterwards as you drift off to sleep.

Day Four

- ❏ Power Mind: Early Morning Wake-Up Call
- ❏ Daytime: Breath Breaks
- ❏ Two-Minute Energy Boost
- ❏ Evening Stress Log

- ❏ Power Food: Organic menus
- ❏ *Still No Alcohol . . . Why?*
- ❏ *Cutting Back on Caffeine*

- ❏ Power Detox: *Identify Environmental Energy Drains at Work*

- ❏ Power Exercise: Power Up Workout

- ❏ Power Rest: Asleep by 10
- ❏ *Tips for Nighttime Awakening: Dream Remembrance*

Still No Alcohol . . . Why?

I am asking you to avoid alcohol for these three weeks principally to let your body's detox machinery rest. As discussed in detail in Chapter 3, people are highly variable in their abilities to detoxify alcohol—and other drugs. For some, the buildup of toxic by-products (such as acetaldehyde) can produce considerable lasting fatigue. Some are very sensitive to the yeast and fermentation by-products contained in alcoholic beverages. But for everyone, abstention from alcohol and other drugs gives the detox systems (especially cytochrome enzymes in the liver) the chance to rejuvenate and work on clearing out some of the many other energy-draining toxic substances present in your body, such as pesticides, preservatives, and other pollutants. In addition, alcohol can affect sleep patterns, and sleeping for three weeks without any alcohol in your system should help give you more restful, energy-generating sleep. You will find a half-dozen nonalcoholic cocktails included in the menu plan. I recommend serving them in fun glasses and fulfilling the need to quaff without the alcohol.

Cutting Back on Caffeine

For the rest of the 21 days I'd like you eliminate coffee (or at least significantly cut back on it or switch to decaf). Too many people use caffeinated coffee as their energy drug—drinking it throughout the day to keep their energy up. Each time you drink coffee or high-caffeine beverages, you get a lift for a couple of hours, then are susceptible to a follow-up energy crash—leading you to drink more. Caffeine is a drug that can cause withdrawal symptoms, which means that the nervous system has become dependent on it. That dependence produces a yo-yo effect with energy going up and down. Cutting back on coffee will break the cycle of the yo-yo effect. Once you get past the withdrawal you can expect to have more consistent energy throughout the day. And, like alcohol, caffeine can affect sleep patterns, so getting it out of your system will give you a chance at a better night's sleep. I'm not recommending that you go cold turkey because I know this can be disruptive. If you know that you get severe withdrawal symptoms, taper your consumption by 50 percent each day and substitute regular green tea for the coffee you give up. By the fifth day of the plan shoot for cutting out caffeine altogether. Just give yourself three weeks to try it.

Identify Environmental Energy Drains at Work

Work can drain your energy, but usually we think this is due to difficulties with co-workers, or work that is too much or too stressful. All too often, however, the physical environment itself is an unrecognized work energy drain. Consider making the following changes.

- Get a HEPA air filter.
- Get an air-filtering plant such as a fern or large palm.
- Ask for any copy machine or inkjet printer to be removed from your immediate area (both can emit micronized particles of toner, considered air pollutants).
- Turn off overhead fluorescent lighting if you can, which is draining to the eyes. A better light source is natural light from a nearby window and a desk lamp that sheds light on your work without excessive glare.
- Get a glare screen for your computer.
- Consider using amber glasses (available at www.debspecs .com) that block the blue light from computers that can throw off your biological clock, disrupting your sleep cycle.
- If you're constantly on the telephone, use a headset to minimize nerve and muscle strain.
- If you're on the cellphone frequently, use an earpiece.
- Keep an emergency vitamin packet in your desk drawer for the times that you're exposed to sick co-workers or clients.
- Wash hands frequently, especially during cold and flu season.

Tips for Nighttime Awakening: Dream Remembrance

In my practice, waking up in the middle of the night is a far more prevalent problem than having trouble falling asleep initially. If you awaken in the wee hours, say, 4:00 a.m., dream remembrance may be a big help. At that hour, your brainwaves shift toward the vivid dreaming rapid eye movement (REM) phase. It's often at this time that people spring up to consciousness where stressful thoughts—that you haven't brought under control during the day—quickly commandeer attention and keep you awake. (For more on sleep phases see Chapter 5.)

As you get a glimmer that you are coming out of a dream and beginning to wake up, latch onto that dream, hold onto it and try to conjure every detail. Allow your mind to drift fully into the dream. In sleep medicine this is called rebound sleep, which is the natural tendency to go back into the stage you were in before waking up. By training your mind, you can take advantage of what your body really wants to do—sleep. If you lose the dream, use your morning meditation exercise to lock onto a state of mental relaxation that will keep conscious thoughts at bay. This is a mind game—your mind will try to bring in conscious thoughts (almost always incessant worries), but you have to keep them from entering center stage. By using your dream to distract from your worries, you keep yourself in sleep mode, which is where you need to be in the middle of the night.

Day Five

- ❑ Power Mind: Early Morning Wake-Up Call
- ❑ *Why Massage Matters*
- ❑ Daytime: Breath Breaks
- ❑ Two-Minute Energy Boost
- ❑ Evening Stress Log

- ❑ Power Food: Organic Menus
- ❑ *A Word on Weight*
- ❑ *Shopping for Fish*

- ❑ Power Exercise: Power Up Workout
- ❑ *The Power of Walking—Find Your Target*

- ❑ Power of Connection: Positive Emotional Action
- ❑ *Cultivating Forgiveness*

- ❑ Power Rest: Eight Hours
- ❑ Tips for Falling Asleep: *10-Minute Meditative Breath Work*

Why Massage Matters

I'd like you to have a couple of massages during the 21-Day Plan. Many people think of massage as a luxury, but it has powerful health benefits that put it closer to the necessity category. Massage therapists use hands, fingers, elbows, and forearms to manipulate soft tissues, targeting muscles, tendons, ligaments, joints, connective tissue as well as lymphatic vessels. Studies show numerous positive effects of massage include relaxation, improved sleep, and strengthened immune system along with relief of fatigue, pain, anxiety, and nausea. Massage is terrific for the circulatory system; it's been shown to lower blood pressure and heart rate. In one study at Massachusetts General Hospital, massage reduced diastolic blood pressure, calmed breathing, and reduced psychological distress and pain in patients undergoing cardiac catheterization. In another study, a back massage for spouses of patients with cancer resulted in improved mood, reduced stress, and increased the activity of natural killer cells (powerful immune defenders).

Massage can also be energizing. For fatigue, the deeper the massage the better. Shiatsu (deep tissue massage based on acupressure points that releases muscle tension) has been shown to significantly reduce fatigue after chemotherapy. And people with advanced kidney disease experienced a dramatic improvement in fatigue and depression after receiving acupressure massage (using strong finger pressure to target and release acupuncture points). Athletes have known for centuries that sports massage (a general muscle rubdown) relieves soreness and fatigue. The type of massage you get is less important than the often nearly intuitive ability of the massage therapist to locate and effectively release tension points (also known as trigger points) in your body. If you've never had bodywork you will be amazed at how energizing it can be, or if you're familiar with massage, think of this as permission to spend the time and money on your well-being. There are massage therapists who specialize in pregnancy massage, which is a wonderful idea, especially in the last trimester when muscles and connective tissue are under such stress. (Note: If you are being treated for a medical condition, especially if you're taking blood thinners, have significant musculoskeletal injuries, or vascular problems like tendency to clots, get permission from your doctor before having a massage.)

A Word on Weight

If you follow the 21-Day Menu plan you will be well within a healthy calorie range *and* composition. The increase in obesity in the last twenty years has been blamed on the quantity of what you eat—too many calories in the super-size-me era. But it's also a matter of the quality of what you eat. Refined carbohydrates significantly change the relationships between insulin, leptin, and many other hormones that control your weight and satiety. Recent research shows that eating fats that increase inflammation keeps you from losing weight. In my plan you won't go hungry, but you *will* eat a balance of complex carbohydrates, healthy fats, and lean protein, with an abundance of plant foods that will make the pounds fall off, even while you feel satisfied.

Shopping for Fish

Over the course of 21 days you will eat fish four different times, reaping the benefits of this source of rich antiinflammatory omega-3 fatty acids. For each recipe we have selected species of fish that are nearly free of mercury and other chemical toxins, and that are classified by multiple regulatory agencies as safe to eat four or more times a month (see Chapter 3). You'll see that each recipe works with more than one kind of fish, so that you can be flexible and select whichever safe fish is fresh and available on the particular day you shop. As I discuss in Chapter 3, wild fish is preferable to farmed fish because fish farming is a largely unregulated industry that can produce fish lower in healthy fats and higher in chemicals and additives (there are some exceptions—farmed shrimp, trout, and tilapia are all good choices). For updates on the safety of wild fish stocks, I recommend you check one of my favorite online resources—www.edf.org/seafood or the Monterey Bay Aquarium's Seafood Watch (www.mbayaq .org/cr/seafoodwatch.asp). If you frequent a good fish market, you will find your local fishmonger is an excellent source of information on what is fresh and healthy in your area—though even sometimes the most responsible fishmongers can't verify where the fish they sell comes from.

When it comes to being choosy at the fish counter I would follow Julia Child's lead as she wrote in *The Way to Cook*: "When you buy fish, open the package just outside the checkout counter (they rarely let you sniff before you choose it) and take a very careful, unhurried whiff. If it smells fishy or chemical or not right in any way, take it immediately to the store manager, give him a whiff, and get your money back." She also recommends placing fish on ice in the fridge (double-bagged in Ziploc baggies to keep water out). This is timeless advice from a master. In my recipes, culinary nutritionist Stefanie Sacks further recommends that before you cook it, you first wash your fish with lemon and salt, then rinse with water and pat dry with a paper towel. Following all of the above, you should have a non-fishy, delicious fish-eating experience.

The Power of Walking—Find Your Target

For the first couple of days I had you out taking a brisk walk, but now I'd like to get a little more scientific about exactly how brisk—and how aerobic—that walk is going to be. After many years of working with patients to get them into shape and ramp up their energy, and after extensive reviews of the literature over the years it's clear the best possible prescription for exercise is 90 minutes a week of movement that raises your heart rate to 70 percent of its maximum capacity (60 percent if you're unfit). Here's how you calculate your target and hit your exercise bulls-eye:

---

220 – Your Age = Your Maximum Heart Rate

Now *to find your target heart rate*, you simply go back to middle school mathematics and calculate 70% of your maximum.

(220 – Your Age) x .70 = *Target Heart Rate*

For example, if you are 40 years old:

220 – 40 = 180 (that's the max)
180 x .70 = 126 (that's the *target*)

A 40-year-old's *Target Heart Rate* is 126 beats per minute. Finally, in order to know you're hitting your target, you need to monitor your pulse during exercise. You can buy a heart rate monitor, or you can simply monitor yourself by pausing briefly to measure your pulse for 15 seconds (sorry, this requires one final math problem).

Target Heart Rate ÷ 4 = 32 (your 15-second *Target Pulse Rate*)

To find your pulse, pause your exercise, place your index and middle fingers lightly on the thumping artery in your neck or inner wrist.

Cultivating Forgiveness

Yesterday I talked about releasing grudges from your thought processes. Try taking the next step—forgiving the person who wronged you. Not paying lip service to forgiving, but really letting go of the wrong, and forgiving the offender. It is amazing how many people in the world do things—unintentionally or purposefully—that harm others. But holding an inner resentment creates a negative energy cycle within you; it reduces your energy. Forgiving does not mean that you have to seek to spend time with the person, though you may have to spend time with him or her at work or socially. Feel compassion toward the other. The act of forgiving, either silently or openly with a direct communication, is incredibly liberating and energizing. If you have been harboring painful feelings for many years, you may have difficulty resetting them on your own. If you have a hard time with this exercise or feel you're thinking negatively all the time, you may benefit from working with a therapist to get past this draining emotional merry-go-round.

10-Minute Meditative Breath Work

Throughout the 21 days I am offering a variety of tips for falling asleep; what works for you will be highly individual. But one thing that is nearly universal to people who have trouble falling asleep is the inability to deal properly with stress (although sometimes it's simply that too much stress overwhelms normally adequate coping skills). To help turn off the thought processes at bedtime, try invoking the morning relaxation exercise, only take it further—try it for 10 minutes. Let your thoughts dissipate and stay focused only on your breathing or your mantra for 10 minutes. You can work on your problems tomorrow. Do this sitting up, then get into bed and try to stay focused in the same neutral mental place. Incorporating this 10-minute meditative breath work into your bedtime routine—and consciously banishing worrying thoughts—can make it much easier to drift off to sleep.

Day Six

- ❑ Power Mind: *Lounge in Bed on Awakening, Daydream*
- ❑ Early Morning Wake-Up Call
- ❑ *Putter in the Morning*
- ❑ Get a Massage
- ❑ *Read Your Stress Log: Identify Triggers of Negative Emotion*
- ❑ *Start Making an Action Plan*

- ❑ Power Food: Organic Menus
- ❑ *The Perils of Red Meat*
- ❑ *Cooking with Spices*

- ❑ Power Exercise: Power Up Workout

- ❑ *Power of Connection: The Communal Meal*

- ❑ Power Rest: *Power Nap*
- ❑ Nighttime: Eight Hours
- ❑ Practice the Sleep Tips That Work for You
- ❑ *Sleep Cycles, What Are They?*

Lounge in Bed on Awakening, Daydream

Take time for yourself today; you've earned it. Instead of jumping out of bed (or crawling if your energy is not yet optimal), lounge and relax before getting up. Let your mind drift to pleasant thoughts or back to your dreams. Reflect back on all you accomplished in the first phase of this plan; and the fresh energy you can look forward to having as you enter the *Cleanse* phase of the plan. Society makes us too goal-oriented so this will be a day to relax and connect with a sense of inner peace. When you get up, practice your early morning wake-up call to allow peacefulness to fill you.

Putter in the Morning

Let there be no hurry—that's today's mantra. If you have chores, stay mindful as you go about them; don't allow yourself to feel dragged down by the weight of all that is expected of you. Know that you will get to what needs to be done.

Read Your Stress Log: Identify Triggers of Negative Emotion Start Making an Action Plan

Up to this point I've had you focus on what causes stress during your day: home, work, relationships, tasks, past issues, anticipation of difficult times ahead . . . you name it. I also encouraged you to let go some of your more destructive thoughts—to release grudges, to feel more compassionate, and to be forgiving. Think about the week to come. Are there easy or practical ways to eliminate stresses? Can you adjust your schedule so you are not so pressed for time during your commute? What may give you similar—or new—stress, which you can minimize with prior planning? With whom can you make peace? How can you better generate the positive energy that you feel within, and give it out to others? Are there any coping strategies that you can adopt for next time? Perhaps you can take a breath break before you encounter a difficult co-worker to help you maintain control. Make reducing stress a priority; you'll be amazed at how much you gain.

The Perils of Red Meat

Here I am telling you to relax, and then I bring up the somewhat troubling concept of eliminating a food you may love to eat. But you need to hear this if you are like the majority of my patients who really don't understand why I want them to eliminate, or at least cut back on, eating red meat. Most people who don't have a cholesterol problem think they're fine eating meat. Cholesterol and saturated fat are particularly dangerous for people with cardiovascular disease, but they are not the only problem with red meat. Animal fat, particularly from red meat (beef, pork, lamb, and veal), can cause overproduction of inflammation-promoting molecules called cytokines, which are implicated in numerous health problems including cancer, heart disease, and arthritis. Some people are more susceptible than others to developing inflammation. (See Chapter 2, for more on inflammation.) In addition, conventional, nonorganic meat can carry antibiotics and pesticide residues, all of which I want you to avoid. Let's see how you feel after three weeks off red meat. Some people feel so wonderful, they never go back to eating meat. Others find they crave it, or actually get energy from it, and in that case there are healthier meats you can eat (see Day 14); but after your 21 days of not eating meat, consume all meat in moderation.

Cooking with Spices

Classic Euro-American cooking imparts flavor by incorporating salt and saturated fat (cream and butter). These two standards both hold and enhance flavors, but are substances I am encouraging you to leave behind for three weeks—and I want you to use dramatically less of them forever. With the 21 days of menus you will replace salt and fats with spices, herbs, and oils that not only impart fantastic flavor, they are some of the most powerful healing substances on the planet. Tonight you will have curry roasted chicken for dinner. Curry contains turmeric among many beneficial spices. Studies have shown that turmeric works on every mechanism involved in reducing inflammation in the body; there is extensive literature about its use as a therapy for inflammatory diseases including cardiovascular disease and some cancers. How wonderful to eat your chicken with a substance that has the potential to prevent a heart attack and cancer! Rosemary, oregano, cinnamon, garlic all have copious research studies attesting to their ability to help the body detoxify, resist infection, regulate blood sugar, and reduce inflammation. Leave the salt and fat behind—switch to healthy herbs and spices to energize your food, and import it with exotic new flavors that will satisfy your palate.

The Communal Meal

Today, consider hosting a meal with friends or family. There is little that is as effective for feeling connected to others as a shared meal—with people you enjoy. I'm not suggesting inviting all the folks who grate on your nerves at obligatory holiday meals. The curry roasted chicken is a perfect, exotic dish to serve as a conversation piece. And you'll note the menu includes a non-alcoholic cocktail to kick off the meal. Invite a group you meet with regularly—surprising them by hosting an event at your place. Or do one of my favorite things—bring people together from different walks of life who will stimulate and be stimulated by each other. Rotate the places at the table throughout the meal so everyone gets to talk with everyone else. Put your positive energy into making others feel part of a greater collective energy.

Sleep Cycles, What Are They?

You should move between the two types of sleep—non-rapid eye movement and REM—about every 90 minutes throughout the night, with the first four stages being more dominant in the first half of your sleep and the fifth vivid dreaming stage being more dominant in the wee hours of the morning. Today, just keep in mind that getting eight hours of uninterrupted sleep allows adequate time to cycle through all of the stages of sleep. For a full understanding of sleep cycles check out Chapter 5.

Day Seven

❑ Power Mind: Early Morning Wake-Up Call
❑ Take the Energy Quiz

❑ Power Food: Organic Menus
❑ *Dr. Merrell's Morning Shake*
❑ *Indulge in a Treat: Dark Chocolate*

❑ Power Exercise: Take a Day Off

❑ Power of Connection: *Establish Your Local Spot to Connect with Nature.*

❑ Power Rest: *Power Nap*
❑ Eight Hours

Dr. Merrell's Morning Shake

Tomorrow you will enter the *Cleanse* phase of this plan, during which you will begin each day with my breakfast shake (see recipe 298). This shake gives a marvelous head start on nutrition for the day. It supplies enough calories to be in line with weight maintenance: a great balance of lean protein, health-promoting fats, complex carbohydrates and fiber, and powerful healing nutrients. This shake incorporates in your breakfast many of the key Power Foods discussed in Chapter 2. It is antioxidant, antiinflammatory, nutritious, and energy-generating. This is a whole meal—you can use it for the rest of your life as breakfast, or a meal replacement, or an energy snack during the day. It is very satisfying—the good fats, protein, complex carbohydrates, and fiber leave you feeling satisfied easily into lunch. (Though I recommend a mid-morning snack each of the 21 days just to prevent you from going famished into lunch.)

Indulge in a Treat: Dark Chocolate

Quick quiz: What is one of nature's most powerful antioxidant foods—four times more powerful than green tea? It's chocolate, scientific name Theobroma coca (theobroma translated literally means food of the gods). It has many health-giving nutrients, powerful antioxidants, and chemicals (including phenylethanolamine) that actually improve mood. Recent studies show it lowers blood pressure, and I'm sure more good news is to come. So why is there any controversy about it? Because the chocolate most of us grew up on—and which is still the most widely consumed—is mainly sugar, often with dairy added. Studies that show chocolate's benefits were done on chocolate with at least 80 percent cocoa mass and very little sugar. Regular commercial chocolate is closer to 10 percent cocoa, with most milk chocolate at between 10 and 15 percent. Even many traditional darker chocolates max out at 30 percent cocoa. The caveat here: for chocolate to work best for health and energy, it needs to be at least 75 percent cocoa, though I'll settle for 70 percent. If not, the rest is mostly sugar and dairy products. People accustomed to high sugar and dairy chocolate may gag on 80 percent-plus. I must say, 90 percent and over is even too bitter for me, a cocoa lover. But the sweet spot should be 75 to 85 percent. In this zone, the bitterness of pure cocoa has been softened with some sugar and cocoa butter, and the natural flavonoids that are so healthy are still abundant. You don't need to eat the whole bar: a few squares should do it. Go ahead: indulge and enjoy in moderation one of nature's great energy foods.

Establish Your Local Spot to Connect with Nature

Today I want you to take the time to get out into nature. Remembering you are part of something beautiful and much larger than yourself, and experiencing awe at that beauty is an essential part of connectivity and of tapping the energy of the universe. While it would be wonderful if you could take a walk in the cathedral of a redwood forest or along the edge of the Grand Canyon, today's exercise can be something as simple as sitting under your favorite tree and truly feeling the energy and wisdom of the tree that's been around for a long time . . . perhaps longer than any human. Think of the tree's connectedness to all living things, many of which have come before you. Even inanimate objects like beautiful rock outcroppings can be equally inspiring. My daughters and I like to skip rocks at a local beach. This is a very mindful time when we're just present with each other and with nature. Wherever it is you love to spend time in nature, make it a regular habit.

Power Nap

I am definitely a fan of short naps, and suggest taking them at least once a week during the 21-Day Plan. The ideal nap is 15–20 minutes long, which allows just enough time to catch the first two stages of non-rapid eye movement sleep that leave you feeling refreshed and, studies show, better able to perform tasks that require thinking and memory. A nap that lasts from 20 minutes to an hour may be too long; it's very likely to leave you feeling groggy as it takes you to a deeper stage without completing a full cycle. While a 90-minute daytime nap will likely take you through an entire sleep cycle and give you energy, it is likely to throw off your body clock and make it harder to fall asleep at bedtime. Take a 20-minute power nap today, then get up and do a two-minute energy boost. You'll feel like a new person.

Week Two: Cleanse

"Matter in its subtlest form is prana, a vital energy which is inseparable from consciousness."

His Holiness the Dalai Lama

From *The Universe in a Single Atom*

Day Eight

- ☐ **Power Mind:** Early Morning Wake-Up Call
- ☐ **Daytime:** Breath Breaks
- ☐ Two-Minute Energy Boost
- ☐ *Book a Massage for Today*
- ☐ *Evening Laugh Log*

- ☐ **Power Food:** Organic Menus
- ☐ *Essential Nutrients: Probiotics*

- ☐ **Power Detox:** *Foods That Detox*

- ☐ **Power Exercise:** Power Up! Workout
- ☐ *Investigate Local Yoga Classes*

- ☐ **Power Sleep:** Asleep by 10
- ☐ *Sleep Tip: Squeezing Lemons*
- ☐ *Evaluate Mattress, Pillow*

Book a Massage

I've told you why I want you to have a massage, but the question is, where to get one? As is the case with all health care providers, word of mouth trumps most all other recommendations. That said, many states and several provinces regulate massage with licensing programs, so that you at least know there is a certain minimum standard of knowledge and experience with any licensed masseur/masseuse. If you don't know where to go, local spas are usually a good bet. Some gyms have good masseurs or masseuses, but spas, which usually cater to a different crowd, often are able to attract more experienced masseurs. Many masseuses with private massage practices or who make home visits are more experienced—they have enough referrals to support a private practice. On the other hand, private masseuses are more likely to have developed their own eclectic style, so make sure to find out exactly what the massage technique is before booking. Local massage schools can give referrals to less expensive massages from students or recent grads.

Evening Laugh Log

Last week I had you keep track of things that added stress to your life, and some things you could do to lessen the burdens. This week, I want you to keep track of those things that make you feel good. I call it a laugh log—but the log is not limited to things you find hilarious. Note what makes you smile, feel warmhearted, fulfilled, and hopeful. Accentuate the positives in your life—in preparation for cultivating them more each day.

Essential Nutrients: Probiotics

I've asked you to add probiotic (helpful bacteria) powder to your shake every morning as part of the cleanse in order to repair and restore your gut, which also strengthens your immune system. There is no supplement class as powerful as probiotics to help digestive function, which is the foundation of a healthy internal detox system (see Chapter 3). In fact, I think of probiotics (including acidophilus and bifidophilus) as the Mr. Fix-Its of digestive health. When the many different types of bacteria get out of balance, however, they can throw your digestion and immune system out of whack. Recent research even suggests that obesity is partly due to improper bacterial colonization of the gut—a person can have too much of certain types of bacteria that extract calories from food! You will improve your health and energy when you set your gut on the right track with probiotics.

It's good if you regularly eat yogurt, which is milk fermented with acidophilus. But you'd have to eat about 10 yogurts to get the amount of probiotics contained in a good supplement. Try to find a higher potency (one billion or greater organisms per capsule) in a refrigerated liquid form or powder concentrate. (There is evidence that the "GG" or "VSL" strains are most effective.) Use quality freeze-dried capsules when you travel. Unlike some of our natural intestinal bacteria, probiotics do not colonize (set up house and multiply) in the intestines—they are mostly eliminated within five days after you ingest them—so to maintain their presence you have to consume probiotics regularly. Buy the powder or liquid, put it in your shake, and let Mr. Fix-It take care of things.

Investigate Local Yoga Classes

The key to starting a yoga practice is going slow and finding a small class. Such classes are tough to find today with so many people getting into yoga, and getting competitive about it! Before you put yourself in someone's hands, check out his or her credentials. Your best bet is to go to a well-known, long-standing yoga studio, preferably one that employs instructors with certification from recognized schools (such as Iyengar, Integral, Sivananda, Kripalu, or the International Yoga Therapy Association). Working one on one with an instructor produces dramatically better results than group work, but many people choose the more economical option of classes where the group dynamics can also help provide a real energy lift. In my experience, classes tend to move quickly, but beginners need to go slowly. Hurrying through postures you're just learning can render them useless and also cause injury. If you can't procure a private session, invest in a video series from one of the nation's top yogis such as beginner DVDs from Jivamukti or Rodney Yee. For most people learning yoga is extremely visual, so the ideal would be to slowly go through a beginner video with a mirror close at hand to match your movements to those of the yogis on the video. For more on getting started with a yoga practice, see Chapter 4.

Sleep Tip: Squeezing Lemons

This short form of muscle relaxation utilizes the image of squeezing lemons. As you lie in bed, pick up two imaginary lemons, hold them straight out in front of you, making a fist. Inhale deeply as you squeeze as hard as you can until all of the "juice" is out of the lemons. Now toss them away as you exhale completely and let your hands go limp. Try this three times.

Evaluate Mattress, Pillow

Is your pillow making you tired? A pillow is supposed to support your head so that your neck, airways, and spine remain in a natural position with good alignment throughout the night. Bottom line: A pillow should support your head and take pressure off your neck.

Pillows frequently contribute to allergies, which prevent a good night's sleep. If you are chronically congested try a nonallergenic foam pillow and place it inside a dust-mite blocking pillow protector that goes under the pillow case (www.greenguide.com is a great source for information on pillow allergies). (Mattress quality is also critical for proper sleep: for details on this, refer to Chapter 5.)

Day Nine

❑ **Power Mind:** Early Morning Wake-Up Call
❑ Two-Minute Energy Break
❑ Breath Breaks
❑ Evening: Laugh Log

❑ **Power Food:** Organic Menus
❑ *Preparing for the Juice Cleanse*

❑ **Power Exercise:** Power Up Workout
❑ *Heart Monitor vs Pedometer*

❑ **Power of Connection**
❑ *Contemplative Time*

❑ **Power Rest:** Asleep by 10
❑ *Light and Your Sleep Hormones*

Preparing for the Juice Cleanse

One of the most powerful tools I have to help jump-start my patients' health is a juice cleanse. Tomorrow, it's your turn; you will ingest only fresh vegetable and fruit juices every three to four hours, maintaining your nutrient and calorie intake while giving your digestive track and natural detox system a rest (see Chapter 3 for more on this). In order to prepare for the cleanse, please read the juice recipes in the recipe section and collect all of the ingredients today. It's essential that you drink fresh juice that you make yourself at home or that is made for you, to your specifications, at a reliable local health food store. Fresh juice lasts for up to three to four hours before enzymes begin to degrade, so you can only make or buy what you will consume within three to four hours. If you are going to purchase a juicer, look for one that includes the fruit or vegetable fiber in the juice. At lunch and dinner you can have a cup of shiitake-miso broth (leftover from tonight's soup). On the cleanse day *especially* you should not drink caffeine or alcohol. A note on store-bought bottled juices: they can be used as a stop-gap when you can't get fresh juice. Make sure to buy organics (Swiss Biotta and American Lakewood are a couple of my favorites). Also make sure there is less than 100 mg of sodium per serving: many conventional vegetable juices contain high levels of sodium. (For more on the health benefits of the cleanse, please see Chapter 3.) The other essential element of tomorrow's cleanse is drinking plenty of fresh water.

Heart Monitor vs. Pedometer

Several years ago the American Heart Association announced that taking 10,000 steps a day reduces the risk of heart disease, which caused a mini-bubble in the market for pedometers that count your steps. But if you want to more effectively increase your energy you have to take a *brisk* walk that raises your heart rate to 70 percent of its maximum capacity, which makes a heart rate monitor the key gadget to employ. A heart rate monitor takes your pulse with a sensor strapped around your chest and transmits the data to a digital readout on a special wristwatch so that you can make sure your heart rate increases gradually to 60 or 70 percent of its maximum for your age. Keep your heart revved for a total of 90 minutes a week and your energy will also rise.

Light and Your Sleep Hormones

Light has a significant effect on your sleep. The primary sleep hormone, melatonin, is produced in darkness, with the peak time being the early hours of the morning. Keep your room very dark when you sleep. Darken your bedroom at night, and throw open the curtains and start moving outside in the morning. (For more on light therapy and sleep hormones see Chapter 5.)

Day Ten

❑ Power Mind: Early Morning Wake-Up Call
❑ Two-Minute Breath Work
❑ Evening: Laugh Log

❑ Power Food: Organic Menu
❑ Juice Cleanse (see menus and recipes)

❑ Power Exercise: Gentle Yoga or 20-Minute Walk or Both

❑ Power Rest: Eight Hours

The Juice Cleanse

This is an exciting day, one you've been preparing for. A juice cleanse is one of the most effective means to repair and rejuvenate, it protects your DNA and improves your ability to create energy. The Juice Cleanse is laid out in detail in Part III, Menus and Recipes. It's critically important that you carefully follow the menu for the day and drink all of the liquids as recommended so that you can maximally repair and restore. The key to this cleanse is that it provides essential nutrients to support your body's detox abilities, and drinking copious amounts of water helps flush out toxins as well as prevent dehydration.

I want you to consider this as a tranquil day. Gentle yoga or a twenty-minute walk is fine, but no exertion. Continue your breath breaks. This sort of cleanse is known to help cultivate mindfulness. With less energy spent on digestion, you are likely to feel more alert throughout the day. Have a quiet evening and take time to reflect on the positives in your life. Finishing with a good eight hours sleep is essential.

Day Eleven

- ❑ Power Mind: Early Morning Wake-Up Call
- ❑ Daytime: Two-Minute Energy Break
- ❑ Breath Breaks
- ❑ Evening: Laugh Log

- ❑ Power Food: Organic Menus

- ❑ Power Detox: *Foods That Detox*

- ❑ Power Exercise: Power Walk 30 Minutes

- ❑ Power of Connection: *Positive Emotional Action*
- ❑ *Get Inspired! Buy Tickets to an Upcoming Show or Event*

- ❑ Power Rest: Asleep by 10

Foods That Detox

In this phase of the plan, you focus on cleaning out your body in order to free up energy. Many of the foods you will eat this week and throughout the plan help boost your body's detox capacity. Here is a quick list of some of the best foods to help your body detoxify; for more complete information about these foods' amazing properties see Chapter 3.

The Brassica family (cruciferous vegetables): broccoli, cauli flower, kale, and Brussel sprouts
The Allium family (sulfurous vegetables): onions, leeks, chives, garlic, and shallots
The Thistle Family: artichokes, dandelions, and burdock
Green tea

Nuts/seeds
Seaweed: arame, hijiki, kombu, wakame
Spices: turmeric, ginger
Red berries

Walking Clubs

If you find it difficult to take up walking on your own, try to do it with a
friend. Equally satisfying is finding a walking club in your local area, and
doing it with a group. The community that comes from this shared desire
to be healthier can be wonderful. The American Volkssport Association
sponsors European-style walking clubs, and their website, www.ava.org
has links to clubs in every state. (The Canadian Volkssport Federation's
website is www.walks.ca.) This is one more creative way to make exercise
a pleasure you look forward to. Your local Road Runners Club (www.rrca
.org) may also have walking clubs as part of their organized activities.

Get Inspired! Buy Tickets to an Upcoming Show or Event

The power of art and entertainment can sweep you out of your everyday
rut. Today, plan to treat yourself to an uplifting event. If you're like me,
you have been looking at the newspaper, saying, I wish I could see this or
go to that. Take yourself up on that challenge. A musical, concert, or play,
not only transports you away from daily concerns, it also plugs you into
the energy of others. Try to maintain the good feelings generated during
the event.

Day Twelve

❑ Power Mind: Early Morning Wake-Up Call
❑ Daytime: Two-Minute Breath Work
❑ Evening: Laugh Log

❑ Power Food: Organic Menu
❑ *Healthy Fats*

❏ **Power Exercise: Power Up Workout**
❏ *Power of the Playground*

❏ **Power of Connection:** *Say You're Sorry*

❏ **Power Rest: Eight Hours**
❏ *Have a TV-free Night*

Healthy Fats

If you've been following the menus—and I sincerely hope that you have—then you know I am not the sort of doctor who is completely against having fat in your diet. The 21-Day food plan has a healthy balance of monounsaturated and omega-3 fats from olive oil; nuts, seeds and nut butters; avocados and fish. The key is that my menus have no trans fats and almost no saturated fat from animal foods. Shifting from saturated to healthy fats changes the way your body responds to inflammation: producing antiinflammatory rather than proinflammatory immune messengers. Your body also needs sufficient healthy plant and fish oil fats to dissolve the fat-soluble vitamins. Your body also utilizes essential fatty acids from healthy oils to build beautiful cell walls that have integrity and can protect your DNA and the many other structures, including the energy-generating mitochondria, that reside inside every one of your cells. A moderate amount of fat in the diet promotes satiety; you may have noticed that, as public health policy shifted toward nonfat foods, the national waistline expanded. You will also find your skin is more supple with eating healthy fats. Bottom line: you will have more energy and, yes, feel and look younger, as you replace bad fats with good.

Power of the Playground

OK, kids, weather's great, it's time to get out and play. After 12 days on the plan you should begin to feel the urge to get outside and move after you've been cooped up inside all day. This is part of the process of reenergizing your body. Today, as you get ready to work out I want you to try to remember the days of your youth when you couldn't wait to get out and run around. When you go outside, embrace the day, breathe deeply as you warm up and feel your body coming alive. You might even hop on your bike today instead of walking, or grab a jump rope and try to get all the way through Miss Mary Mack. Reflect on the joy of going out to play, and then have at it!

Say You're Sorry

I've talked about the energetic lift of letting go of grudges and forgiving others. Today, I want to turn that 180 degrees and have *you* ask someone for forgiveness. This is hard. Asking for forgiveness means swallowing your pride and saying you're sorry; it means admitting you were wrong and that you've hurt someone else. You cannot be sure of the reaction that your apology will bring, but you will have to let go of expectations. If you feel it's appropriate, ask this person what you can do to make it right—or just express that the apology comes from your heart. It is the energy you project that will significantly affect the result. Think about it carefully and rehearse the script if necessary. In my experience, saying "I'm sorry if I hurt you" is less effective than saying, "I'm sorry for what I did." This exercise will help reduce a lot of stress-filled negative emotional energy in your life. It will not necessarily bring back a relationship. But it is part of moving on and cleaning up your emotional baggage. Even if the object of your apology doesn't express open appreciation and forgiveness, your act of giving of yourself will cause a positive energetic shift that will reverberate for quite some time.

Have a TV-free Night

Breaking a bad habit can be incredibly energizing. Nighttime television watching is a habit that's been clearly linked in studies to getting less sleep. Tonight, turn off the TV, and pursue other, more relaxing activities. Take a walk after dinner, listen to your favorite CDs (remember the days when you could just sit and go through the liner notes), read a book, meditate, take a long hot bath. Get out of your habitual, evening couch-potato mode, and you will find that you have better sleep and perhaps even more interesting dreams.

Day Thirteen

- ☐ Power Mind: Lounge in Bed
- ☐ Early Morning Wake-Up Call
- ☐ Putter in the Morning
- ☐ *Review What Made You Laugh This Week*

- ☐ Power Food: Organic Menus
- ☐ *Big 12 Trouble Makers*

- ☐ Power Detox: *Supplements for Detox*

- ☐ Power Exercise: *40 Minutes of Movement*

- ☐ Power of Connection: Concert or Event

- ☐ Power Rest: Eight Hours or Asleep by 10
- ☐ *Sleep Tips—Apnea, Snoring, and Other Impediments*

Review what made you laugh this week

Last week you kept your stress log, and at the end of the week, reviewed it for patterns. I'd like you to review it again this week, but with the goal of getting more of the joy and laughter into your life. My feeling is that as you fill your life with more joy, you'll have less room for stress. When you keep track, you may see that things aren't as bad as they seem. Take the time as you're relaxing and puttering today to reflect on what you love about your life.

The Big 12 Trouble-Makers

As you get ready for your final week of the plan and begin to think of life after the plan I want you to consider your relationship to the 12 most highly reactive foods. Ask yourself, "Might I have a food sensitivity or allergy?" Over the past 13 days, if you've been following the plan, you haven't had most of these foods. Do you feel better? As you add them back, do you notice any reaction? If you think you may have a food allergy, a trip to an allergist for testing can be well worth the time and effort. Identifying chronic energy-draining food sensitivities and allergies—and eliminating those foods for good—is one of the easiest ways to increase energy. (For more on allergies, see Chapter 2.)

Wheat	Coffee
Milk	Alcohol
Corn	Yeast (fermented) foods
Sugar	Citrus
Soy	Shellfish
Peanuts	Eggs

Supplements for Detox

You are at the end of a week of cleansing your system. You should be feeling more energetic at this point, but if you're still not as full of vigor as you want to be, it may be you have a history of being exposed to many toxins. Maybe you were a smoker once, or ate a diet loaded with preservatives or poor quality meats and produce. Maybe you worked in a factory, on in a "sick building." Take a look at the supplements for increasing your detox capacity in Chapter 3.

40 Minutes of Movement

OK, I know I've been telling you that 30 minutes of exercise is sufficient, and it is. But I don't want you to think that's a maximum amount. On the weekend, when you have more time, consider adding more exercise to your regimen. Adding more movement to your day (gentle movement so that you're not sore on Monday like a weekend warrior) is one of the most energizing, life-affirming things you can do with your time.

Apnea, Snoring, and Other Impediments to Sleep

Nothing interferes with restorative sleep more than an abnormal breathing pattern—caused by apnea, heavy snoring, or even chronic sinus congestion—that reduces the oxygen supply to your bloodstream and to the rest of your body. What used to be considered just plain old sawing wood has been increasingly identified by researchers as a cause of significant health problems. For example, sleep apnea (when breathing is frequently obstructed for at least ten seconds throughout the night) has been associated with numerous health problems including hypertension, heart disease, and heart attack. And only recently the American Academy of Otorhinolaryngologists (ear, nose, and throat docs) has recognized chronic sinus congestion as a factor in poor sleep. Amazingly, Breathe Right Nasal Strips that hold open your nostrils to allow in more air can be a quick fix for minor problems. In Chapter 5 I cover a number of possible solutions to sleep-breathing problems. Furthermore, if you or your spouse or partner suspects you might have altered breathing or severe snoring (and if you constantly wake up exhausted), self-help measures may not be enough: please make an appointment to be evaluated at a sleep lab.

Day Fourteen

- ❏ Power Mind: Early Morning Wake-Up Call, Congratulate Yourself!
- ❏ Take the Energy Quiz
- ❏ *Get Ready to Maximize*

- ❏ Power Food: Organic Menus
- ❏ *Life After the Plan: Healthier Meats*

- ❏ Power Exercise: Take a Day Off

- ❏ Power of Connection: An *E-Mail Free Day*, Write a Letter to *Someone Who's Always on Your Mind*

- ❏ Power Rest: Eight Hours
- ❏ *Bedroom Feng Shui*

Get Ready to Maximize

By now you should have made major changes in your energy on many fronts. Congratulations for staying with the plan! You are about to move into week three when the changes will be consolidated and made part of your ongoing lifestyle. Remember there's absolutely no reason that you can't increase your energy throughout your life. Whether you continue to find more vitality and energy through a more varied and plant-based diet, more regular exercise, a cleaner environment, more restorative sleep, or by extending your connections with others or deepening your spiritual or contemplative practice . . . never say never!

Life after the Plan: Healthier Meats

I have had you eliminating red meat during the plan, and limiting poultry. You will most likely feel better energy as a result. If you have no medical conditions that warrant avoiding meat (heart disease, history of colon cancer, autoimmune disorders) and want to resume meat consumption after the plan, limit how often you do so and consider healthier options. Commercially raised red meats and poultry have much higher saturated fat content than wild animals and game. Instead of commercial meat, try venison, bison, or buffalo, which have about the same saturated fat as chicken—much less than beef. The lowest fat in a land animal is ostrich, which may sound weird, but there are commercial ostrich farms and many butchers now carry ostrich meat (which tastes like a cross between chicken and veal, and can be used in chicken and beef recipes). Also consider wild poultry—heritage species, or birds such as quail and partridge, which have less fat than chicken. At the very least, try to find organic (or natural and chemical-free), free-range-raised meats that will contain minimal additives and chemicals.

How you cook your meat and what you eat it with also makes a difference in how healthy it is. Charred meat is high in carcinogens called heterocyclic amines. Brown your meat as you cook it through: don't burn it. Research published in the journal *Carcinogenesis* demonstrated that eating broccoli along with meat increases the liver enzyme systems' removal of heterocyclic amines. Further, eating a diet rich in essential fatty acids (from olive oil, nuts, and fish) counteracts the buildup of cholesterol from saturated fat. In one study conducted by nutrition scientists in

Spain, volunteers who ate a mixture of ground beef and ground walnuts had more antioxidants in their bloodstreams that helped to counteract the harmful inflammatory effects of red meats. Next time you make a hamburger, mix it with some ground walnuts, don't burn the meat, and have a large helping of broccoli on the side. But you'll be even healthier if you eat a veggie burger.

An E-Mail-Free Day, Write a Letter to Someone Who's Always on Your Mind

As you know by now I'm a true believer in reaching out to the energy of others, and making amends with those who have left negative energetic footprints in your life. Along with that comes the need for reflection on how you are communicating with people on a daily basis. I am a fan of e-mail as a work tool, and as a way of keeping in touch with far-flung relatives, but I find that it gets in the way of keeping real connections with the people in your daily life and even interferes with the need to make deeper connections with your inner life. Today, leave the e-mail alone. Sit down, and revisit the art of letter writing. You might even want to get some new stationery to energize your writing further.

Bedroom Feng Shui

Feng shui is a Chinese art of aligning energy within a space to create harmony and health. The physical placement of objects is important, as is color, the orientation of objects, and the relation of the space to nature. Naturally, in the bedroom the goal is to create a harmonious, calm, peaceful, and healthy environment. The placement of your bed is of the utmost importance; feng shui principles in general require the head of the bed to be against a solid wall with no windows, your head should not be in line with the exit door, nor should you be able to see yourself in a mirror from the bed. Equally important is minimizing clutter in the bedroom—absolutely no chotchkes or piles of paper collecting dust. Your belongings, from the contents of your pockets to your shoes and ties to your magazines and perfume bottles, are best kept behind doors in the bedroom to keep the energy flowing and not caught up in a bunch of material objects. Matching bedside tables are thought to promote harmony for couples. And it's considered a good idea to have a comfortable, relaxing chair in the bedroom (placed so the back does not face the door) to promote the tranquil feelings you want to engender at bedtime. Feng shui is as much science as art. I'm certainly no feng shui expert, but I have seen remarkable transformations in peoples' lives as a result of working with feng shui practitioners. If you're interested in pursuing more on the topic, you can consult good books on feng shui or a feng shui school that can provide references to practitioners (www.alexstark.com is a good web resource from a master practitioner).

Week Three: Maximize

"If you miss the present moment, you miss your appointment with life."
Thich Nhat Hanh
From *The Art of Power*

Day Fifteen

☐ **Power Mind: Early Morning Wake-Up Call**
☐ *Start Planning Your Vacation*
☐ *10-Minute Evening Unwind*

☐ **Power Food: Organic Menus**
☐ *Essential Fatty Acids*

☐ **Power Exercise: Power Up! Workout**

☐ **Power Rest: Asleep by 10**
☐ *Life After the Plan: Consistency Is Key for Restorative Rest*

Start Planning Your Vacation

Over the years I have become emphatic about people taking vacations. I don't mean extravagant vacations that cost an arm and a leg. I mean getting away from your everyday existence, preferably communing with nature, and taking the time to unwind. I recently came across a sad study that found that fewer Americans are taking vacations for fear of reprisals at their jobs. I cannot imagine a worse scenario for creating stress than one in which you can't take time off from work for fear of losing your job. Everyone needs time off at least twice a year (Christmas and New Year's don't count because those can actually be stressful or exhausting holidays). Ideally one of these should be for two weeks. The real vacation, when you begin to feel unplugged and recharged, usually starts in the second week. Start planning now, and keep in mind that a good vacation leaves you energized, not needing a vacation from the vacation!

10-Minute Evening Unwind

During the first two weeks of the plan, I had you keep stress and laugh logs, the purpose of which was to review your day in the context of your coping skills. Rather than worrying about how your day went, you identified the important emotional moments from your day; took a step back and reviewed how you managed to cope with them. Then you put any ruminations on your day behind you. If keeping a log particularly resonated with you, please continue to keep it up for 10 minutes in the evening. If writing is not your thing, I'd like you to set aside 10 minutes a day to mentally review and detach from the events of your day. I call this the 10-Minute Unwind—the key is to keep the events of the day in the context of your coping skills. If you could have done better, make a note of that and strategize how to get it right the next time. If you had a wonderfully joyous moment, lock that into the treasury and feed off it when the going gets rough. Then let it go, and move onto the tranquility of your evening routine.

Essential Fatty Acids

I've talked about the healthy plant and fish fats you're eating in the menu plan, but I want to zero in briefly on the important component of those fats, essential fatty acids (EFAs). Your body can't make EFAs, they have to come from the diet, and most people don't get enough. When your diet is low in EFAs (as is the average American diet), your body's ability to fight hundreds of energy-draining inflammatory processes is reduced. You need some source of EFAs every day. If after the 21-Day Plan you find yourself slipping back to old eating habits, take an omega-3 supplement.

Life After the Plan: Consistency Is Key to Restorative Rest

If I can have you remember one tip on maximizing your sleep, it would be for you to go to bed at approximately the same time every night. Maintaining a consistent bedtime and bedtime routine has been shown to be a crucial part of maintaining healthy sleep cycles.

Day Sixteen

- ❏ Power Mind: Early Morning Wake-Up Call
- ❏ Two-Minute Energy Boost
- ❏ 10-Minute Evening Unwind

- ❏ Power Food: Organic Menus
- ❏ *What's the Best Multivitamin?*

- ❏ Power Exercise: Power Walk 30 Minutes

- ❏ Power of Connection: *Investigate Energy Practitioners in Your Area*

- ❏ Power Sleep: 8 Hours
- ❏ *Gentle Sleep Aids*

What's the Best Multivitamin?

By following the 21-Day Menu Plan with its highly diverse foods and wealth of nutrients most people won't need a multivitamin. When you eat a rainbow diet, packed with vegetables, fruits, and lean protein, food alone does have all the nutrients you need. But eating a well-rounded diet is most people's Achilles heel, so, during times of high stress or travel, when eating becomes erratic, or if you have a medical condition, you may need to take a daily multivitamin. In that case, look for a food-based (as opposed to synthetic) multivitamin, which will come as close as scientifically possible to mimicking the nutrient value of food, which has numerous beneficial compounds we have yet to even identify. Vitamin E is a good example. Most supplements only contain one form of E, alpha tocopherol. But in nature (for example, in wheat germ)—and in more sophisticated multivitamins—the whole family of vitamin E is used, including alpha and gamma tocopherols and tocotrieniols. Vitamin C is another good example. A good multivitamin should include the bioflavonoids that always accompany vitamin C in nature. Same for the A vitamins, the caratenoids; beta carotene should come with its whole family (including lycopene, lutein, and zeaxanthin). For a more complete discussion of multiple vitamins see Chapter 2.

Gentle Sleep Aids

If you now have a better diet, increased exercise, you've curtailed alcohol and coffee, and are practicing relaxation exercises, but you are still having trouble falling asleep or staying asleep, there are some gentle sleep aids you can take at bedtime. I reviewed these in detail in Chapter 5, but please reserve these for use on an occasional basis. Using them chronically means you may need to do more work with your sleep habits or seek the help of a sleep specialist to solve your sleep problems.

Investigate Energy Practitioners in Your Area

I can't imagine a more appropriate topic for the week of maximizing energy than locating and having a session with an energy practitioner trained in the art of working with energy fields. I say art because Reiki, therapeutic touch, healing touch, energy healing, Johrei, or any of the dozens of other energy medicine practices are not fully—or even partially—understood by science. However, a number of excellent nursing journals have demonstrated very positive results with energy healing, particularly with the use of Reiki and therapeutic touch in health care settings. Finding a good practitioner requires some perseverance and luck. The interaction is highly personal, and each practitioner brings his or her own background, energy, and training to the experience. Some specific courses confer a certificate; Reiki, for instance, offers standardized mastery levels from 1 thru 5. There is no state licensing for these practices, however, so finding the right person to work with you and your energy is usually best done by getting a referral from someone you trust who has had a positive experience. I have witnessed some remarkable results with my patients so I know it's worth your giving it a try. For more detail on energy medicine see Chapter 6.

Day Seventeen

- ❏ Power Mind: Early Morning Wake-Up Call
- ❏ Five-Minute Breath Work
- ❏ Book a Massage for Day 20
- ❏ 10-Minute Evening Unwind

- ❏ Power Food: Organic Menus
- ❏ *Do You Need an Energy Supplement?*

- ❏ Power Exercise: Power Up! Workout
- ❏ *Maximizing the Routine: Innovative Movement*

- ❏ *Power of Connection: Random Acts of Kindness*

- ❏ Power Sleep: Asleep by 10

Do You Need an Energy Supplement?

If you feel your energy is still substandard, now may be the time to try supplements that have been used to help increase energy, mood, and vitality. These are described in detail in Chapter 2 and include Russian rhodiola, Ayurvedic ashawaganda, Chinese cordyceps, and Chinese and American ginseng. Specific energy-supporting and energy-generating vitamins, minerals, and other nutrients can also be helpful. There is an abundance of energy formulas for sale from supplement manufacturers, but you should exercise extreme caution, as some of these formulas can have unpredictable effects and side-effects. Choosing the right supplement is very important: This almost always requires the input of a knowledgeable health care provider working with you, especially if you have medical problems or are using medications.

Maximizing the Routine: Innovative Movement

At this point in the plan you are advancing your fitness level to a point where you can begin to branch out. I highly recommend exploring the world of martial arts (such as tai chi, karate, and aikido) and martial arts hybrids (like tae bo or capoeira)—exercise systems designed to work specifically with your energy. Start with a local martial arts school. Many gyms, especially in urban settings, are beginning to offer classes that are strictly martial arts or that incorporate aspects of martial arts. Make sure to ask if beginners are welcome.

Random Acts of Kindness

One of the most powerful ways you can generate energy is to give of yourself to others. From random acts of kindness to working with a community group, by giving to others you connect with a larger energy source that enhances your own. As discussed in Chapter 6, community service and helping others is one of the most rewarding, energy-producing activities you can do, and it's been shown to reduce depression. You receive back many-fold times more energy than you give when you give selflessly, out of love and compassion for humankind—both giver and recipient are enveloped in a more healing energy environment. Today, do something that helps. I'm not asking you to sign on for hundreds of hours of obligations to a charitable organization if you don't have the time or inclination. Try some random acts of kindness. All too often ambitious intentions fall by the wayside, but it's the little things—like brightening someone else's day with a positive comment—that most frequently add up to big changes.

Day Eighteen

☐ Power Mind: Early Morning Wake-Up Call
☐ Breath Breaks
☐ 10-Minute Evening Unwind

☐ Power Food: Organic Menus
☐ *A Note on Bitters*

❏ Power Detox: *Antioxidants, To Have or Have Not*
❏ Power Exercise: 30-Minute Power Walk

❏ Power Sleep: Eight Hours

A Note on Bitters

Quaffing a teaspoon of bitters is a great way to assist digestion occasionally and stop the energy drain of slow or poor digestion. Made from bitter herbs such as gentian and thistle, many digestive bitters were originally manufactured as patent medicines. All bitters—whether alcohol-based Angostura, or alcohol-free Swedish Bitters, or bitter aperitifs (Peychaud, Monin, Campari, Cinzano, Fernet Branca)—stimulate the flow of all of your body's natural digestive chemicals. Only a teaspoonful is needed, and only on occasion. (Enzymes sold in health food stores as digestive aids can work sometimes, but then only supply one part of the digestive picture, the pancreas's enzymes.)

Antioxidants: To Have or Have Not

The majority of people who come to me taking more than one vitamin supplement per day use some form of antioxidant. For most, the old-fashioned vitamins E-C-beta carotene has given way to newer antioxidant pills containing more exotic ingredients such as quercetin, pycnogenol, grapeseed, and resveratrol. Do you need these? Rarely. With the menus in the 21-Day Plan, you are eating many foods that are anti-inflammatory and antioxidant. And your lifestyle these three weeks produces dramatically fewer free radicals in the first place. Food can be your medicine here. Fruits, vegetables, herbs, and spices should be doing most of the work for you, so that you don't need supplements. Pill forms should be reserved for the handful of people whose lifestyle and health risk factors predispose them to heavier free radical burdens (such as heart disease, chronic arthritis, inflammatory bowel disease, and recent smokers). In these instances, taking a pill may be useful: the caveat is that you should take one that has ingredients containing as much of the whole food as possible, rather than only one extracted molecule from a food. This is best done in consultation with a knowledgeable integrative health care professional (naturopath, physician, pharmacist, osteopath, nurse practitioner, physician assistant, or nutritionist).

Day Nineteen

☐ **Power Mind:** Early Morning Wake-Up Call
☐ *Mindfulness Meditation*
☐ **Breath Breaks**
☐ 10-Minute Unwind

☐ **Power Food:** Organic Menus
☐ *Other Supplement Options*

☐ **Power Detox:** *How Green Is Your Grass?*

☐ **Power Exercise:** Power Up Workout or Class

☐ **Power Rest:** Eight Hours

Mindfulness Meditation

I want you to begin to cultivate what the great healer/philosphers Jon Kabat-Zinn and Thich Nhat Hanh teach us—be mindful all day. In his book *True Love*, Nhat Hanh explains mindfulness as: "Mindfulness is like a light, enabling concentration to really be there, and that also makes it possible for us to look deeply into the heart of things." Mindfulness is the opposite of multitasking. It's about being in the moment—not thinking of twenty other things you want to do—especially the things that worry you most; and in that moment absolutely feeling love and compassion toward yourself, the task you are engaged in, or the person you are with. Whether you are washing dishes, driving the car, practicing breath breaks or sitting in a meeting, be mindful.

Mindfulness meditation is rather like filling your cup of consciousness with positive energy. Again, I like Thich Nhat Hanh's explanation in *True Love*: "Our immediate awareness is something like our living room. The task of the meditator is not to chase away or suppress the energy of anger that is there but rather to invite another energy that will be able to care for the anger." It's quite extraordinary that it's possible to effect such a transformation with your thoughts.

I recommend you explore the books and tapes published by Kabat-Zinn and Thich Nhat Hanh. For today you can try one of the mindfulness meditations in Chapter 1 or as you do your breath work today try the following healing meditation from Thich Nhat Hanh, *The Energy of Prayer*:

Breathing in, I see myself as a five-year-old child.
Breathing out, I smile to the five-year-old child.
Breathing in, I see the five-year-old child, who is myself, as very fragile and vulnerable.
Breathing out, I smile to the five-year-old child in myself, with understanding and compassion.

There are infinite varieties of mindfulness meditations you can use to transform your energy. Try a few. Occasionally, I encounter patients who simply can't get the hang of it on their own, but there are excellent meditation teachers and coaches who can help. Your stress will be less, you will make more meaningful connections with those around you, and you will feel an energy surge as you begin to banish the many negative thoughts that interfere all day in coping with life's challenges.

How Green Is Your Grass?

Yes, I'm talking about your lawn. The suburbs may be blanketed with grass as green as the hills of Ireland, but they are also awash in chemicals that achieve the green. Over 100 million pounds of herbicides and pesticides are applied around American residences each year. Most of us know to stay off the lawn after a treatment until the grass has had a good soaking. But few people think to have their well water checked for the presence of chemicals like atrazine, a weed killer that keeps the crab grass at bay. The nation's lakes and streams are contaminated with atrazine enough to affect as many as 3,600 drinking water systems throughout the United States according to the Natural Resource Defense Council. Think about the chemicals you're putting on your grass. Investigate integrative pest management lawn services that use organic methods to control the lawn, and in this case, perhaps try to think *less* green. The good news for your own drinking water is that a simple activated carbon-based water filter like the ones commonly available in grocery stores can filter out atrazine and other chemicals. Reduce and remove . . . that's your mantra.

Day Twenty

- ❏ Power Mind: Lounge in Bed
- ❏ Putter in the Morning
- ❏ Get a Massage
- ❏ *Crisis Management*

- ❏ Power Food: Organic Menus

- ❏ Power Exercise: *Get a Game*

- ❏ Power of Connection: Positive Emotional Action
- ❏ Reach Out—Make Plans with Friends for the Weekend

- ❏ Power Rest: Afternoon Nap
- ❏ Eight hours

Crisis Management

Unfortunately, many people use food as crisis management medicine. Comfort foods—rich in refined carbohydrates and fats—provide instant emotional rewards: they raise blood sugar, giving an immediate energy boost, and briefly elevate neurotransmitters, counteracting the effects of stress hormones. But this short-lived fix causes all manner of destructive inflammation, glycation, and oxidation. An abrupt elevation of your happy molecules—blood sugar and neurotransmitters—is always followed by a crash in the same, leaving you much worse off than when you began—suffering from low blood levels and the roller coaster ride down. Don't triage yourself with junk food; support yourself with nature and natural nurture.

My Crisis Management First Aid Kit

Lean protein and whole grains (for sustained energy).
A cup of green tea contains L-Theanine for a gentle lift.
Licorice (sweetened with molasses) or licorice root to
   support the adrenals (chew every couple of hours).
Protein shake made with fruit and veggie juices (once a day).
A square of 70 percent or greater dark chocolate
   (1–2 times per day).
Tonic herbal tea, such as chamomile (as often as needed).
Antianxiety tincture, Bach Flower "Rescue Remedy."
Calming essential oils like lavender (dab on the wrist daily).
Adaptogenic herbs, ashwaganda or cordyceps (twice daily).
Multivitamin to support increased energy demands (daily).
Relaxation exercises, morning meditation, yoga stretches,
   and frequent breath breaks (daily).

Get a Game

Game playing is a bit of a lost art, and I'd encourage you to consider reviving it. I grew up watching my parents play bridge monthly and my father play his weekly golf game (even through the frigid days of November). I came to appreciate the value these games had in keeping them connected with friends and in truly energizing their lives even at times when the going was rough for my father at work or my mother was besieged by having four teenage boys in the house. One of my patients who was going through a very rough time in her life joined a volleyball league in New York (a game she'd not played since high school), which became a real anchor for her during turbulent times. She'd go out and forget about her troubles during the practices and games and get a bit of a workout to boot. Computer games don't count in my book—they cause you to lose sleep and can be addictive. Keep the level of competition healthy. One of my patients felt little stress at home or work, but became highly anxious in his ultracompetitive weekly golf outings. If you're consumed by winning, then game playing may have moved out of the health-promoting category for you. In that case, perhaps taking up a new sport would be a better idea.

Day Twenty-one

☐ Power Mind: Early Morning Wake-Up Call, Congratulate Yourself
☐ Take the Energy Quiz—You're Graduating Today

☐ Power Food: Organic Menus

☐ Power Exercise: A Day Off *or* Your Favorite New Workout

☐ Power of Connection: *Connecting to a Greater Energy*

☐ Power Rest: Eight Hours

Connecting to a Greater Energy

You've been through a transformative journey these past 21 days. You've fixed a lot of mechanical energy problems and healed emotional energy drains. I'd like you to finish this journey with the intention to connect to a greater energy beyond yourself—through family, community, religion, nature, or spirituality. Your vital spirit touches others; it energizes them and is magnified back to you in a reverberating circuit. Beyond your ability to see or even comprehend fully, the universe exists as a limitless energy field that you can tap for greater personal energy. Today, take some contemplative time to commune with this energy of the cosmos, with a higher power, that which is, the absolute. You are a vital part of it. You can sense it within you and around you. Breathe, relax, and feel joy.

PART THREE

Menus and Recipes

with Stefanie Bryn Sacks, M.S.

Culinary Nutritionist Stefanie Bryn Sacks contributed the menus and recipes for the 21-Day Plan. Stefanie has helped many of my patients transform their eating lives, and I think you will find that her menus and recipes presented here will do the same for you.

Pantry Notes

A food processor is required for some of the recipes. You don't need to get a huge expensive piece of equipment; a three-cup model from a reputable manufacturer will suffice and can be found for under $50.

Agave syrup (nectar) is a sweetener, derived from the leaves of a plant native to Mexico, and is a good alternative to table sugar as it has a low glycemic index.

Amazon.com—yes, formerly the bookseller—is a great place to purchase many of the staple items in our recipes.

Canola mayo is rich in heart healthy monounsaturated fats giving it a healthier fat profile than traditional mayonnaise. Canola mayonnaise can be found at most markets.

Certified organic is the best choice when choosing animal foods such as eggs, dairy, or meats, meaning the animal has been raised without hormones or antibiotics, given organic feed, and treated humanely. If not organic, next best option is hormone and antibiotic free.

Curry powder can be found at markets with good international food sections. Make sure the one you choose does not contain monosodium glutamate (MSG) or artificial ingredients. You can also order it online (an excellent source for spices is www.penzeys.com).

Gomasio is an Asian seasoning made from sea salt, sesame seeds, and seaweed. One teaspoon has 80 mg of sodium while one teaspoon of table salt has 2,360 mg sodium.

Juices, which are naturally sweet, are typically high in natural fruit sugar (fructose). Many juices on the market today contain added sugar whether in the form of high fructose corn syrup, cane sugar, or even other juices and juice extracts. When buying juices, try to choose those that are 100 percent juice (preferably 100 percent single fruit juice).

Mirin is a seasoned, rice-based wine often used in Japanese cuisine. It is similar to sake but has a lower alcohol content. Mirin can be found in markets where soy sauce and tamari are displayed. Make sure to buy real mirin versus those products that call themselves mirin but are only corn syrup, water, and flavorings.

Quinoa (pronounced keen-wah) is a whole grain native to South America. It can be substituted for rice in most recipes. It has one of the highest protein contents of any grain.

Red curry paste is made with red chilies and is commonly found in the condiment or international foods sections of grocery stores.

White miso is a Japanese seasoning paste made from soy that can be found refrigerated in the produce or dairy sections of many markets. Don't substitute *sweet* white miso, which can change the taste of the recipe.

Whole cardamon pods encase the tiny brown seeds that are ground to make the powdered spice. Cardamom has a peppery floral essence. The pods can be found in most spice departments. Look for unbleached, green varieties.

—**Stefanie Bryn Sacks, M.S.**

A note for vegetarians and vegans: This plan is designed to help everyone transition toward a plant-based diet. If you are already there, you can substitute the poultry or fish dishes with any one of the many vegetarian dishes in the menus and recipes.

DAY ONE

Breakfast
Plain low-fat Greek yogurt topped with honey,
wheat germ, and walnuts
Blueberries
12 ounces filtered water
Green tea (decaf or regular) or herbal tea

Snack
Burst of Energy Trail Mix (page 350)
12 ounces filtered water

Lunch
Lemon Parsley Hummus Wrap (page 344)
12 ounces filtered water or noncaffeinated, unsweetened drink
Herbal tea

Snack
Rice cake with almond butter (1 tablespoon)
8 ounces filtered water or noncaffeinated unsweetened drink

Dinner
Garlic Roasted Asparagus (page 325)
Walnut-Pesto Wild Salmon (page 340)
Harvest Wild Rice (page 336)
Citrus Mint Mixed Berries (page 353)
8 ounces filtered water

DAY TWO

Breakfast
Almond butter (1 tablespoon) and strawberries on wheat-free toast
12 ounces filtered water
Green tea (decaf or regular) or herbal tea

Snack
Rice crackers with Lemon Parsley Hummus (leftover)
12 ounces filtered water or noncaffeinated, unsweetened drink

Lunch
Watercress Arugula Salad (page 321)
Rye crisp bread
12 ounces filtered water
Herbal tea

Snack
2 dark (65%+) chocolate squares
8 ounces filtered water or noncaffeinated, unsweetened drink

Dinner
Papaya Fizz (page 361)
Mesclun greens with balsamic vinaigrette (page 315)
Vegetarian Chili (page 348)
Brown rice (follow directions on package)
8 ounces filtered water

DAY THREE

Breakfast
Vegetable Goat Cheese Egg-White Omelet (page 302)
12 ounces filtered water
Green tea (decaf or regular) or herbal tea

Snack
Red grapes
12 ounces filtered water or noncaffeinated, unsweetened drink

Lunch
Vegetarian Chili (leftover)
12 ounces filtered water
Herbal tea

Snack
Rice crackers with Walnut Pesto (leftover)
8 ounces filtered water or noncaffeinated, unsweetened drink

Dinner
Juicy, Sweet Roasted Broccoli (no kidding!) (page 326)
Tofu Vegetable Stir-Fry (page 346)
Rice noodles or 100% buckwheat soba noodles (follow directions
on package)
Coco-nutty Banana (page 354)
8 ounces filtered water

DAY FOUR

Breakfast
Power Up Granola (page 300) with soy or rice milk and mixed berries
12 ounces filtered water
Green tea (decaf or regular) or herbal tea

Snack
Rice cake with hard boiled egg
12 ounces filtered water or noncaffeinated, unsweetened drink

Lunch
Mediterranean Tuna Salad on Crispy Greens (page 314)
12 ounces filtered water
Herbal tea

Snack
Fresh cut veggies with Guacamole (page 351)
8 ounces filtered water or noncaffeinated, unsweetened drink

Dinner
Cool Mint Lemonade (page 358)
Arugula Salad with Crushed Walnuts and Goat Cheese (page 310)
Warm French Lentils (page 335)
Savory Herb Marinated Chicken (page 342)
8 ounces filtered water

DAY FIVE

Breakfast
Wheat-free toast topped with goat cheese and chopped watercress
12 ounces filtered water
Green tea (decaf or regular) or herbal tea

Snack
Small apple
12 ounces filtered water or noncaffeinated, unsweetened drink

Lunch
Savory Herb Chicken Salad Wrap (page 317)
12 ounces filtered water
Herbal tea

Snack
Celery with almond butter (1 tablespoon)
8 ounces filtered water or noncaffeinated, unsweetened drink

Dinner
Sweet Spinach Salad (page 318)
Quinoa with Scallions and Toasted Sesame Oil (page 327)
Miso Baked Cod (page 338)
Dark Chocolate Dairy-Free Mousse (page 356)
8 ounces filtered water

DAY SIX

Breakfast
Plain low-fat Greek yogurt topped with honey,
wheat germ, and walnuts
12 ounces filtered water
Green tea (decaf or regular) or herbal tea

Snack
Antioxidant Fruit Salad (page 309)
12 ounces filtered water or noncaffeinated, unsweetened drink

Lunch
Nitrate-free sliced turkey with avocado in a wheat-free wrap
12 ounces filtered water
Herbal tea

Snack
2 dark (65%+) chocolate squares
8 ounces filtered water or noncaffeinated, unsweetened drink

Dinner
Cranberry Tea Infusion (page 359)
Sauteed Kale with Garlic (page 330)
Cinnamon Roasted Acorn Squash (page 323)
Curry Roasted Chicken (page 341)
8 ounces filtered water

DAY SEVEN

Breakfast
Scrambled Tofu with Vegetables (page 301)
Wheat-free toast
Blueberries
12 ounces filtered water

Snack
Half grapefruit
12 ounces filtered water or noncaffeinated, unsweetened drink

Lunch
Vegetarian Cobb (page 319)
12 ounces filtered water
Herbal tea

Snack
Burst of Energy Trail Mix (page 350)
8 ounces filtered water or noncaffeinated, unsweetened drink

Dinner
Mango-Peach Freeze (page 361)
Watercress Arugula Salad (page 321)
Red Lentil Soup (page 305)
8 ounces filtered water

DAY EIGHT

Breakfast
Dr. Merrell's Morning Shake (page 298)
12 ounces filtered water
Green tea (decaf or regular) or herbal tea

Snack
Burst-of-Energy Trail Mix (page 350)
12 ounces filtered water or noncaffeinated, unsweetened drink

Lunch
Red Lentil Soup (leftover)
Rye Crisp Bread
12 ounces filtered water
Herbal tea

Snack
Fresh Cut Veggies with Guacamole (page 351)
8 ounces filtered water or noncaffeinated, unsweetened drink

Dinner
Warm Hijiki Salad (page 320)
Tofu Vegetable Stir-Fry (page 346)
Brown rice (follow directions on package)
Fresh berries
8 ounces filtered water

DAY NINE

Breakfast
Dr. Merrell's Morning Shake (page 298)
12 ounces filtered water
Green tea (decaf or regular) or herbal tea

Snack
Rice Crackers with Lemon Parsley Hummus (page 352)
12 ounces filtered water or noncaffeinated, unsweetened drink

Lunch
Leafy Greens and Chickpea Salad (page 313)
12 ounces filtered water
Herbal tea

Snack
Apple half with almond butter (1 tablespoon)
8 ounces filtered water or noncaffeinated, unsweetened drink

Dinner
Shitake Miso Soup (page 307)
Quinoa with Sliced Avocado (page 328)
Fresh berries
8 ounces filtered water

WEEK TWO ■ CLEANSE ■ MENUS

DAY TEN—JUICE CLEANSE

7:30 a.m.
Dr. Merrell's Morning Shake (page 298)
Green tea (decaf or regular) or herbal tea

9:00 a.m.
8 ounces filtered water or noncaffeinated, unsweetened drink

10:30 a.m.
8 ounces Dr. Merrell's Veggie Juice (page 360)

12:00 p.m.
1 cup Shitake Miso Broth (leftover)
8 ounces filtered water
1 cup noncaffeinated, unsweetened herbal tea

1:30 p.m.
8 ounces Dr. Merrell's Veggie Juice

3:00 p.m.
1 cup herbal noncaffeinated, unsweetened drink
8 ounces filtered water

4:30 p.m.
12 ounces Dr. Merrell's Fruit Juice (page 360)

6:00 p.m.
8 ounces Dr. Merrell's Veggie Juice
1 cup Shitake Miso Broth (leftover)
8 ounces filtered water

7:30 p.m.
8 ounces noncaffeinated, unsweetened beverage

9:00 p.m.
8 ounces Dr. Merrell's Veggie Juice

10:30 p.m.
1 cup noncaffeinated, unsweetened herbal tea

DAY ELEVEN

Breakfast
Dr. Merrell's Morning Shake (page 298)
12 ounces filtered water
Green tea (decaf or regular) or herbal tea

Snack
1 small apple
12 ounces filtered water or noncaffeinated, unsweetened drink

Lunch
Leafy Greens and Chickpea Salad (page 313)
12 ounces filtered water
Herbal tea

Snack
Fresh veggies with Guacamole (page 351)
8 ounces filtered water or noncaffeinated, unsweetened drink

Dinner
Cucumber Wakame Salad (page 312)
White Bean Kale Soup (page 308)
Brown rice (follow directions on package)
Fresh berries
8 ounces filtered water

DAY TWELVE

Breakfast
Dr. Merrell's Morning Shake (page 298)
12 ounces filtered water
Green tea (decaf or regular) or herbal tea

Snack
Celery sticks with almond butter (1 tablespoon)
12 ounces filtered water or noncaffeinated, unsweetened drink

Lunch
Power Protein Mixed Green Salad (page 316)
Half grapefruit
12 ounces filtered water
Herbal tea

Snack
Power Up Granola (page 300)
8 ounces filtered water or noncaffeinated, unsweetened drink

Dinner
Sweet and Spicy Collard Greens (page 334)
Red Curry Tofu with Basil (page 345)
Quinoa (follow directions on package)
Fresh berries
8 ounces filtered water

DAY THIRTEEN

Breakfast
Dr. Merrell's Morning Shake (page 298)
12 ounces filtered water
Green tea (decaf or regular) or herbal tea

Snack
Burst of Energy Trail Mix (page 350)
12 ounces filtered water or noncaffeinated, unsweetened drink

Lunch
Immune-Boost Soup (page 303)
Wheat-free bread drizzled with extra virgin olive oil
12 ounces filtered water
Herbal tea

Snack
Orange wedges
8 ounces filtered water or noncaffeinated, unsweetened drink

Dinner
Tangerine Spritzer with Papaya Ice (page 363)
Braised Chard (page 322)
Vegetable Biryani (page 347)
8 ounces filtered water

DAY FOURTEEN

Breakfast
Dr. Merrell's Morning Shake (page 298)
12 ounces filtered water
Green tea (decaf or regular) or herbal tea

Snack
Power Up Granola (page 300)
12 ounces filtered water or noncaffeinated, unsweetened drink

Lunch
Rosemary Butternut Squash Soup (page 306)
Black Bean Salad (page 311)
12 ounces filtered water
Herbal tea

Snack
Half grapefruit
8 ounces filtered water or noncaffeinated, unsweetened drink

Dinner
Scrumptious Brussels Sprouts (page 331)
Trout with Lemon and Herbs in Parchment (page 339)
Brown rice (follow directions on package)
Berry Parfait (page 353)
8 ounces filtered water

DAY FIFTEEN

Breakfast
Plain low-fat Greek yogurt topped with honey, wheat germ, and
walnuts
12 ounces filtered water
Green tea (decaf or regular) or herbal tea

Snack
Burst of Energy Trail Mix (page 350)
12 ounces filtered water or noncaffeinated, unsweetened drink

Lunch
Rosemary Butternut Squash Soup (page 306)
Watercress Arugula Salad (page 321)
12 ounces filtered water
Herbal tea

Snack
Rice cake with hard boiled egg
8 ounces filtered water or noncaffeinated, unsweetened drink

Dinner
Mango Peach-Freeze (page 361)
Sweet and Spicy Collard Greens (page 334)
Vegetarian Chili Burritos (page 349)
8 ounces filtered water

DAY SIXTEEN

Breakfast
Dr. Merrell's Morning Shake (page 298)
Wheat-free toast drizzled with extra virgin olive oil
12 ounces filtered water
Green tea (decaf or regular) or herbal tea

Snack
Antioxidant Fruit Salad (page 309)
12 ounces filtered water or noncaffeinated, unsweetened drink

Lunch
White Bean Kale Soup (page 308)
Rye crisp bread with goat cheese
12 ounces filtered water
Herbal tea

Snack
Power Up Granola (page 300)
8 ounces filtered water or noncaffeinated, unsweetened drink

Dinner
Juicy Sweet Roasted Broccoli (no kidding!) (page 326)
Halibut Puttanesca (page 337)
Brown rice (follow directions on package)
Dark Chocolate Dairy-Free Mousse (page 356)
8 ounces filtered water

DAY SEVENTEEN

Breakfast
Vegetable Goat Cheese Egg-White Omelet (page 302)
12 ounces filtered water
Green tea (decaf or regular) or herbal tea

Snack
Red grapes
12 ounces filtered water or noncaffeinated, unsweetened drink

Lunch
Nitrate-free sliced turkey with avocado in a wheat-free wrap
12 ounces filtered water
Herbal tea

Snack
Half apple with almond butter (1 tablespoon)
8 ounces filtered water or noncaffeinated, unsweetened drink

Dinner
Peach Spritzer with Cranberry Ice (page 362)
Crunchy Bok Choy with Tangy Chili Vinaigrette (page 324)
Red Curry Tofu with Basil (page 345)
Quinoa with Scallions and Toasted Sesame Oil (page 327)
8 ounces filtered water

DAY EIGHTEEN

Breakfast
Power Up Granola (page 300) with soy or rice milk and mixed berries
12 ounces filtered water
Green tea (decaf or regular) or herbal tea

Snack
Grapefruit wedges
12 ounces filtered water or noncaffeinated, unsweetened drink

Lunch
Vegetarian Cobb (page 319)
12 ounces filtered water
Herbal tea

Snack
Celery and jicama (or carrot) with Lemon Parsley Hummus (page 352)
8 ounces filtered water or noncaffeinated, unsweetened drink

Dinner
Arugula Salad with Crushed Walnuts and Goat Cheese (page 310)
Turkey Bolognese over Spaghetti Squash (page 343)
Berry Parfait (page 353)
8 ounces filtered water

DAY NINETEEN

Breakfast
Plain low-fat Greek yogurt topped with honey,
wheat germ, and walnuts
12 ounces filtered water
Green tea (decaf or regular) or herbal tea

Snack
Fresh cut veggies with Guacamole (page 351)
12 ounces filtered water or noncaffeinated, unsweetened drink

Lunch
Power Protein Mixed Green Salad (page 316)
12 ounces filtered water
Herbal tea

Snack
Power Up Granola (page 300)
8 ounces filtered water or noncaffeinated, unsweetened drink

Dinner
Cranberry Tea Infusion (page 359)
Quick Italian Vegetable Soup (page 304)
Warm French Lentils (page 335)
Brown rice (follow directions on package)
8 ounces filtered water

DAY TWENTY

Breakfast
Wheat-free toast drizzled with extra virgin olive oil and sliced hard-boiled egg
12 ounces filtered water
Green tea (decaf or regular) or herbal tea

Snack
Rice crackers with Walnut Pesto (page 340)
12 ounces filtered water or noncaffeinated, unsweetened drink

Lunch
Quick Italian Vegetable Soup (leftovers)
Black Bean Salad (page 311)
12 ounces filtered water
Herbal tea

Snack
Fresh berries
8 ounces filtered water or noncaffeinated, unsweetened drink

Dinner
Spiced Coconut Cauliflower (page 332)
Curry Roasted Chicken (page 341)
Harvest Wild Rice (page 336)
Dark Chocolate Chunk Almond Cookies (page 355)
8 ounces filtered water

DAY TWENTY-ONE

Breakfast
French Toast (page 299)
Blueberries
12 ounces filtered water
Green Tea (decaf or regular) or herbal tea

Snack
Burst of Energy Trail Mix (page 350)
12 ounces filtered water or noncaffeinated, unsweetened drink

Lunch
Mesclun Greens with Balsamic Vinaigrette (page 315)
Red Lentil Soup (page 305)
Wheat-free bread drizzled with extra virgin olive oil
12 ounces filtered water
Herbal tea

Snack
Half grapefruit
8 ounces filtered water or noncaffeinated, unsweetened drink

Dinner
Steamed Artichokes with Lemon Aioli (page 333)
Walnut-Pesto Wild Salmon (page 340)
Quinoa Tabouli (page 329)
Spiced Apples with Pecan Crumble (page 357)
8 ounces filtered water

Dr. Merrell's Morning Shake

Serves two

      1½ cups mixed frozen berries (or fresh cut pineapple or papaya*)
      1 cup pineapple juice (or pomegranate or cherry juice)
      ½ cup water
      ¾ cup unsweetened soy milk or rice milk (for soy allergies use whey
         or organic brown rice protein powder**)
      1½ teaspoons fresh ginger root, peeled and minced
         (or ½ teaspoon ground cinnamon or turmeric)
      1 heaping tablespoon flax meal
      1 teaspoon flax oil
      1 tablespoon probiotic powder or liquid***

Combine all ingredients in a blender and puree until smooth.

   *   Can cut pineapple or papaya ahead of time and store in airtight
      container or bag in fridge for up to three days.
  ** Combine 2 heaping tablespoons of powder with ½ cup water (use
      instead of soy milk).
*** Make sure contains, at least, acidophilus and bifidophilus. Available
      in refrigerator section of most health food stores.

NUTRITION PER SERVING

Calories: 193; *Total fat (g)*: 5.2; *Saturated fat (g)*: 0.6; *Cholesterol (mg)*: 0.0; *Monounsaturated fat (g)*: 1.1; *Polyunsaturated fat (g)*: 3.5; *Total carbohydrate (g)*: 33.3; *Sugars (g)*: 21.3; *Dietary fiber (g)*: 4.1; *Protein (g)*: 4.6; *Sodium (mg)*: 51.0

French Toast

Serves two

2 medium eggs
¼ cup soy milk, plain, unsweetened
1½ teaspoons pure vanilla extract
¼ teaspoon cinnamon
½ tablespoon canola oil*
½ tablespoon butter, unsalted
4 slices bread, wheat-free
2 tablespoons maple syrup or agave syrup

1. In a medium bowl, combine eggs, soy milk, vanilla and cinnamon; mix well with fork.
2. Heat oil and butter in large saute pan on medium.
3. Soak bread in egg mixture. Then gently place bread in pan and cook until browned on each side (about 3 minutes per side). Repeat with remaining bread slices.
4. Serve with maple syrup or agave syrup.

* If using a nonstick pan, use 1 tablespoon oil instead of oil and butter.

NUTRITION PER SERVING

Calories: 325; *Total fat (g):* 11.6; *Saturated fat (g):* 3.9; *Cholesterol (mg):* 193; *Monounsaturated fat (g):* 5.1; *Polyunsaturated fat (g):* 2.6; *Total carbohydrate (g):* 41.2; *Sugars (g):* 15.9; *Dietary fiber (g):* 1.4; *Protein (g):* 10.2; *Sodium (mg):* 417.0

Power Up Granola*

Serves eight

½ cup whole raw almonds, coarsely chopped
½ cup pecans, coarsely chopped
½ cup walnuts, coarsely chopped
½ cup rolled oats
¼ cup wheat germ
¼ cup unsweetened coconut
¼ teaspoon ground cinnamon
1 tablespoon maple syrup
¼ cup brown rice syrup or honey
½ tablespoon canola oil

1. Preheat oven to 350°F.
2. Cover cookie sheet with parchment paper; set aside.
3. Place chopped nuts in a bowl with remaining ingredients and mix well.
4. Spread mixture onto cookie sheet; bake for 10 minutes.
5. Remove from oven (it will look like a big cookie) and allow granola to cool for 10 minutes before breaking into chunks.
6. Once thoroughly cooled, store in airtight container in cool dry place for up to three weeks. Can measure ¼ cup serving into small plastic bags for on-the-go eating.

* Make once for entire 21 Day Plan.

NUTRITION PER SERVING

Calories: 330; *Total fat (g)*: 23.2; *Saturated fat (g)*: 5.8; *Cholesterol (mg)*: 0.0; *Monounsaturated fat (g)*: 10.0; *Polyunsaturated fat (g)*: 7.4; *Total carbohydrate (g)*: 24.6; *Sugars (g)*: 11.6; *Dietary fiber (g)*: 5.4; *Protein (g)*: 7.7; *Sodium (mg)*: 3.0

Scrambled Tofu and Vegetables

Serves two

½ block extra firm tofu, crumbled

1 tablespoon canola oil
1 small yellow onion, diced (about ½ cup)
1 small zucchini, diced (about 1 cup)
2 teaspoons tamari soy sauce, low sodium
½ teaspoon curry powder
⅛ teaspoon salt

1. In a medium sauté pan, heat oil on medium and sauté onions until translucent. Add zucchini and sauté for another 3 minutes.
2. Drain tofu well. Crumble tofu into pan and mix well. Add tamari, curry, and salt, mix well and cook for another 3 minutes.

NUTRITION PER SERVING

Calories: 256; Total fat (g): 16.3; Saturated fat (g): 2.8; Cholesterol (mg): 0.0; Monounsaturated fat (g): 3.5; Polyunsaturated fat (g): 10.0; Total carbohydrate (g): 11.3; Sugars (g): 2.6; Dietary fiber (g): 2.2; Protein (g): 16.9; Sodium (mg): 330.0

Vegetable Goat Cheese Egg-White Omelet

Serves two

6 egg whites, separated from yolks
½ tablespoon extra virgin olive oil*
½ tablespoon butter, unsalted
¼ cup scallions, thinly sliced
¼ cup broccoli florets, finely chopped**
¼ cup (2 ounces) goat cheese
fresh ground pepper, to taste

1. Using two bowls, separate whites from yolks (discard yolks). Add scallions and broccoli to whites and mix well.
2. In a medium sauté pan, heat olive oil and butter on medium.
3. When pan is hot, pour in egg. As edges start to set, gently lift edges, tilting pan slightly to allow uncooked egg to flow underneath cooked edges.
4. When most of the egg is set, spread goat cheese over top of the omelet. Cook for another minute, until cooked entirely through.
5. Fold omelet in half over itself, and slide onto plate.

*   If using a nonstick pan, use 1 tablespoon oil instead of oil and butter.
** Fresh or frozen. If frozen, run package under hot water for 30 seconds to defrost before chopping.

NUTRITION PER SERVING

Calories: 211; *Total fat (g):* 14; *Saturated Fat (g):* 8.2; *Cholesterol (mg):* 29.0; *Monounsaturated fat (g):* 5.1; *Polyunsaturated fat (g):* 0.7; *Total carbohydrate (g):* 2.8; *Sugars (g):* 1.7; *Dietary fiber (g):* 0.3; *Protein (g):* 17.4; *Sodium (mg):* 313.0

Immune-Boost Soup

*Serves four (includes leftovers)**

> 1 tablespoon extra virgin olive oil
> 1 clove garlic, coarsely chopped
> ½ small onion, diced (about ¼ cup)
> 1 small carrot, cut into rounds
> ½ teaspoon paprika**
> ¼ teaspoon ground coriander
> 1 small head broccoli, trimmed and coarsely chopped
>   (about 5–6 cups)
> 4 cups water
> pinch of salt
> fresh ground pepper, to taste

1. In a medium pot, heat oil on medium. Sauté garlic, onion, carrot, and spices for 3–5 minutes, until soft.
2. Trim and coarsely chop broccoli. Add broccoli and water to pot and simmer, covered, on low for 15 minutes (until broccoli is soft).
3. Uncover and cool for 5–10 minutes. Place in blender and puree until creamy.***
4. Season with salt and pepper.

*   Store leftovers in airtight container in fridge for up to three days, or immediately freeze for up to three months.
** Preferably smoked Spanish paprika, but regular will do.
*** Be cautious when pureeing warm/hot items in blender. Hold top down firmly with hand. Otherwise, top could easily pop off while pureeing thus creating a mess.

NUTRITION PER SERVING

Calories: 117; *Total fat (g)*: 3.6; *Saturated fat (g)*: 0.6; *Cholesterol (mg)*: 0.0; *Monounsaturated fat (g)*: 2.5; *Polyunsaturated fat (g)*: 0.5; *Total carbohydrate (g)*: 17.6; *Sugars (g)*: 4.9; *Dietary fiber (g)*: 6.6; *Protein (g)*: 6.7; *Sodium (mg)*: 83.

Quick Italian Vegetable Soup

Serves four (includes leftovers)*

    2 tablespoons extra virgin olive oil
    1 clove garlic, minced
    1 small yellow onion, thinly sliced (about ½ cup)
    2 teaspoons dried oregano
    1 teaspoon dried thyme
    1 medium yellow squash, sliced lengthwise, and cut into half moons
        (about 1 cup)
    1 medium zucchini, sliced lengthwise, and cut into half moons
        (about 1 cup)
    ½ cup red bell pepper, thinly sliced
    10 oz bag mixed frozen vegetables (whichever are your favorites)
    2 tablespoons balsamic vinegar
    4 cups water
    1 handful parsley, stems tied with string
    ½ teaspoon salt
    fresh ground pepper, to taste
    4 teaspoons Parmesan cheese

1. In a large pot heat oil on medium. Add garlic, onion, and dried herbs and sauté until onion is translucent (about 3 minutes).
2. Add remaining vegetables (including frozen), balsamic vinegar, water, and parsley. Cover, bring to a boil, then reduce heat and simmer for 20 minutes.
3. Discard parsley and season with salt and pepper. Serve with a sprinkling of Parmesan.

* Store leftovers in airtight container in fridge for up to three days, or immediately freeze for up to three months.

NUTRITION PER SERVING
Calories: 152; *Total fat (g)*: 7.6; *Saturated fat (g)*: 1.5; *Cholesterol (mg)*: 1.0; *Monounsaturated fat (g)*: 5.2; *Polyunsaturated fat (g)*: 1.0; *Total carbohydrate (g)*: 17.8; *Sugars (g)*: 4.7; *Dietary fiber (g)*: 4.9; *Protein (g)*: 5.0; *Sodium (mg)*: 333.0

Red Lentil Soup

Serves four (includes leftovers)*

1 tablespoon extra virgin olive oil
1 small yellow onion, thinly sliced (about ½ cup)
1 cup celery, diced, about 2 stalks
1 cup red lentils
3 cups water
2 cups vegetable broth, low sodium
pinch of salt
fresh ground pepper, to taste

In medium pot, heat olive oil on medium, add vegetables and sauté until soft (about 3 minutes). Add lentils, water, and broth. Simmer, uncovered, for about 30 minutes. Season with salt and pepper.

*   Store leftovers in airtight container in fridge for up to three days, or immediately freeze for up to three months.

NUTRITION PER SERVING
Calories: 225; *Total fat (g)*: 5.0; *Saturated fat (g)*: 0.9; *Cholesterol (mg)*: 0.0; *Monounsaturated fat (g)*: 3.0; *Polyunsaturated fat (g)*: 1.1; *Total carbohydrate (g)*: 32.2; *Sugars (g)*: 1.4; *Dietary fiber (g)*: 5.9; *Protein (g)*: 14.7; *Sodium (mg)*: 59

S
O
U
P

■

R
E
C
I
P
E
S

Rosemary Butternut Squash Soup

*Serves four (includes leftovers)**

    1 medium (2 lbs) butternut squash (about 4 cups cubed)
    3 cups water
    1 large sprig fresh rosemary
    pinch of salt

1. Peel squash, cut lengthwise, and remove seeds; cut into large cubes.
2. Combine squash, water, and rosemary in medium pot. Cover and cook on medium to low until squash is soft (about 20 minutes).
3. Cool for 5–10 minutes. Remove sprig of rosemary and discard. Add squash to blender with ½ the cooking liquid and puree. Add more cooking liquid as needed to achieve thick, creamy consistency.**
4. Season with salt.

* Store leftovers in airtight container in fridge for up to three days, or immediately freeze for up to three months.
** Be cautious when pureeing warm/hot items in blender. Hold top down firmly with hand. Otherwise, top could easily pop off while pureeing thus creating a mess.

NUTRITION PER SERVING

Calories: 63; *Total fat (g)*: 0.1; *Saturated fat (g)*: 0.0; *Cholesterol (mg)*: 0.0; *Monounsaturated fat (g)*: 0.0; *Polyunsaturated fat (g)*: 0.1; *Total carbohydrate (g)*: 16.4; *Sugars (g)*: 3.1; *Dietary fiber (g)*: 2.9; *Protein (g)*: 1.4; *Sodium (mg)*: 5.0

Shitake-Miso Soup

*Serves four (includes leftover broth for cleanse)**

6 medium dry shitake mushrooms
1 cup warm water (to soak mushrooms)
7 cups water
1 small yellow onion, thinly sliced (about ½ cup)
1 large carrot, thinly sliced into rounds
10 medium fresh shitake mushrooms, destemmed and thinly sliced
2 slices fresh ginger, unpeeled, ¼ inch thick
1½ tablespoons white miso
3 stalks bok choy, thinly sliced
Tamari soy sauce, low sodium, wheat-free, to taste
Gomasio, to taste

1. In bowl, soak dry mushrooms in 1 cup warm water.
2. Prep vegetables.
3. In a large pot, place water plus all vegetables (including ginger) except for bok choy. Cover and bring to boil. Turn down heat and simmer, covered for 20–40 minutes.
4. Meanwhile, when soaking mushrooms are soft, remove from water, slice thin (may need to remove tough stems) and add to simmering soup with soaking liquid.
5. When soup is finished, turn off heat, remove and discard ginger. Add miso, mixing thoroughly. Add bok choy.
6. Season with tamari and gomasio.

* With whatever is leftover, strain the broth, discard vegetables and save in the fridge for the cleanse day.

NUTRITION PER SERVING

Calories: 69; *Total fat (g):* 0.5; *Saturated fat (g):* 0.1; *Cholesterol (mg):* 0.0; *Monounsaturated fat (g):* 0.1; *Polyunsaturated fat (g):* 0.3; *Total carbohydrate (g):* 16.0; *Sugars (g):* 3.9; *Dietary fiber (g):* 2.8; *Protein (g):* 2.5; *Sodium (mg):* 262

White Bean Kale Soup

*Serves four (includes leftovers)**

1 can (15 ounces) white beans, drained and rinsed
1 tablespoon extra virgin olive oil
1 small yellow onion, thinly sliced (about ½ cup)
1 clove garlic, minced
2 vine ripe tomatoes, diced
3 cups water
3 cups low sodium vegetable broth
1 sprig fresh thyme
1 sprig fresh oregano
1 small bunch kale, ripped from stem or cut into small pieces
pinch of salt
fresh ground pepper, to taste

1. In a large pot, heat olive oil on medium. Sauté onion and garlic until lightly golden. Add beans, tomatoes, water, broth, and herbs. Simmer, covered for 15 minutes.
2. Remove and discard herb stems. Add kale and continue to simmer, covered, for 20 minutes more.
3. Season to taste.

* Store leftovers in airtight container in fridge for up to three days, or immediately freeze for up to three months.

NUTRITION PER SERVING

Calories: 217; *Total Fat (g)*: 5.0; *Saturated fat (g)*: 1.0; *Cholesterol (mg)*: 0.0; *Monounsaturated fat (g)*: 3.0; *Polyunsaturated fat (g)*: 1.0; *Total carbohydrate (g)*: 32.0; *Sugars (g)*: 2.2; *Dietary fiber (g)*: 9.1; *Protein (g)*: 14.2; *Sodium (mg)*: 73

Antioxidant Fruit Salad*

Serves two

1 cup papaya, peeled, halved, seeds removed, and cubed
½ cup kiwi, peeled and sliced into rounds
½ cup blueberries
1 tablespoon fresh mint leaves, coarsely chopped

In a bowl combine all ingredients and mix gently.

* Can be made the night before if desired. Can also buy fresh fruit salad at local market if easier (make sure it is fresh fruit and not a fruit cocktail with added sugar).

NUTRITION PER SERVING

Calories: 75; *Total Fat (g):* 0.3; *Saturated fat (g):* 0.1; *Cholesterol (mg):* 0.0; *Monounsaturated fat (g):* 0.1; *Polyunsaturated fat (g):* 0.2; *Total carbohydrate (g):* 19.0; *Sugars (g):* 11.8; *Dietary fiber (g):* 3.7; *Protein (g):* 1.3; *Sodium (mg):* 3.0

Arugula Salad with Crushed Walnuts and Goat Cheese

Serves two

2 cups arugula, packed
½ head radicchio, shredded
1 small pear, peeled and thinly sliced
¼ cup (2 ounces) goat cheese, crumbled
2 tablespoons walnuts, coarsely chopped
1 tablespoon extra virgin olive oil
1 tablespoon balsamic vinegar
fresh ground pepper, to taste

1. Thoroughly wash and dry arugula and radicchio (pat with paper towel or use salad spinner) and place in medium salad bowl.
2. Add pear, goat cheese, and walnuts, and gently toss.
3. Add oil, vinegar and pepper. Toss gently.

NUTRITION PER SERVING

Calories: 267; Total fat (g): 18.9; Saturated fat (g): 7.1; Cholesterol (mg): 22.0; Monounsaturated fat (g): 8.1; Polyunsaturated fat (g): 3.7; Total carbohydrate (g): 15.5; Sugars (g): 9.7; Dietary fiber (g): 3.2; Protein (g): 9.0; Sodium (mg): 154.0

Black Bean Salad

Serves two

1 can (15 ounces) black beans, drained and rinsed
½ cup grape tomatoes, halved
½ avocado, diced
1 small red onion, diced (about ½ cup)
¼ cup cilantro, stems and leaves coarsely chopped
1 tablespoon extra virgin olive oil
1 lime, juiced
¼ teaspoon salt

1. Drain and rinse black beans in a fine mesh strainer; add to medium salad bowl.
2. Add remaining ingredients and mix well.

NUTRITION PER SERVING

Calories: 422; *Total fat (g):* 12.2; *Saturated fat (g):* 2.0; *Cholesterol (mg):* 0.0; *Monounsaturated fat (g):* 8.4; *Polyunsaturated fat (g):* 1.2; *Total carbohydrate (g):* 60.0; *Sugars (g):* 3.0; *Dietary fiber (g):* 22.0; *Protein (g):* 20.4; *Sodium (mg):* 298.0

Cucumber Wakame Salad

Serves two

1 large cucumber, peeled, deseeded, and thinly sliced
1 tablespoon brown rice vinegar
½ lemon, juiced
2 teaspoons gomasio
½ cup dry wakame seaweed, cut into ½ inch strips with scissors,
    soaked in ½ cup cold water until soft (about 5 minutes),
    and drained

1. In medium bowl combine cucumber slices, vinegar, lemon juice, and gomasio.
2. Drain wakame, add to bowl, and toss.

NUTRITION PER SERVING

Calories: 30; *Total fat (g)*: 0.1; *Saturated fat (g)*: 0.0; *Cholesterol (mg)*: 0.0; *Monounsaturated fat (g)*: 0.0; *Polyunsaturated fat (g)*: 0.0; *Total carbohydrate (g)*: 7.9; *Sugars (g)*: 1.9; *Dietary fiber (g)*: 2.2; *Protein (g)*: 1.2; *Sodium (mg)*: 257.0

Leafy Greens and Chickpea Salad

Serves two

1 cup Swiss chard, packed
1 cup baby spinach, packed
¼ cup flat leaf parsley leaves
1 cup garbanzo beans (chickpeas), drained and rinsed
2 tablespoons unsalted almonds, chopped
½ cup red grapes, halved

DRESSING
1 tablespoon extra virgin olive oil
½ tablespoon mirin
2 tablespoons brown rice vinegar
⅛ teaspoon salt

1. Thoroughly wash and dry chard, spinach, and parsley (pat with paper towel or use salad spinner).
2. In a large bowl, combine all salad ingredients and toss well.
3. In a small bowl, whisk together dressing ingredients.
4. Dress the salad and toss.

NUTRITION PER SERVING
Calories: 285; *Total fat (g):* 12.7; *Saturated fat (g):* 1.5; *Cholesterol (mg):* 0.0; *Monounsaturated fat (g):* 8.3; *Polyunsaturated fat (g):* 2.8; *Total carbohydrate (g):* 34.1; *Sugars (g):* 11.4; *Dietary fiber (g):* 7.9; *Protein (g):* 10.2; *Sodium (mg):* 257.0

SALAD ■ RECIPES

Mediterranean Tuna Salad

Serves two

1 can low sodium chunk light tuna in water
1 tablespoon fresh dill, chopped
2 tablespoons scallions, thinly sliced
1 tablespoon extra virgin olive oil
1 tablespoon red wine vinegar
1 tablespoon lime juice
pinch of salt
fresh ground pepper, to taste

CRISPY GREENS
2 cups mesclun greens, packed
1 tablespoon lime juice

1. Drain tuna and place in medium bowl. Add remaining ingredients and mix well.
2. Thoroughly wash and dry greens (pat with paper towel or use salad spinner). In another bowl, toss with lime juice.
3. Serve tuna over crispy greens.

NUTRITION PER SERVING

Calories: 164; *Total fat (g)*: 7.2; *Saturated fat (g)*: 1.1; *Cholesterol (mg)*: 24.0; *Monounsaturated fat (g)*: 5.1; *Polyunsaturated fat (g)*: 1.0; *Total carbohydrate (g)*: 2.4; *Sugars (g)*: 0.5; *Dietary fiber (g)*: 0.5; *Protein (g)*: 21.6; *Sodium (mg)*: 49.0

Mesclun Greens with Balsamic Vinaigrette

Serves two

> 2 cups mesclun greens, packed
> ½ cup flat leaf parsley, leaves and stems, coarsely chopped
> 1 tablespoon extra virgin olive oil
> 2 teaspoons balsamic vinegar (or more to taste)
> ½ lemon, juiced
> fresh ground pepper, to taste

1. Thoroughly wash and dry mesclun greens and parlsey (pat with paper towel or use salad spinner). Place in salad bowl.
2. Add remaining ingredients and toss.

NUTRITION PER SERVING

Calories: 78; *Total fat (g):* 6.7; *Saturated fat (g):* 1.0; *Cholesterol (mg):* 0.0; *Monounsaturated fat (g):* 5.0; *Polyunsaturated fat (g):* 0.8; *Total carbohydrate (g):* 5.4; *Sugars (g):* 1.0; *Dietary fiber (g):* 2.0; *Protein (g):* 1.2; *Sodium (mg):* 16.0

SALAD ■ RECIPES

Power Protein Mixed Green Salad

Serves two

1 can (15 ounces) white (cannelloni or great northern) beans,
    drained and rinsed
½ red bell pepper, diced
¼ small red onion, diced (about 2 tablespoons)
1 heaping tablespoon fresh dill, chopped

DRESSING
1 tablespoon extra virgin olive oil
1½ tablespoons brown rice vinegar
1½ tablespoons red wine vinegar
pinch of salt
fresh ground pepper, to taste

BED OF GREENS
2 cups mesclun greens, packed

1. In a medium bowl combine beans, pepper, onion, and dill.
2. In a small bowl whisk together dressing ingredients, and add to
    bean mixture, tossing well.
3. Thoroughly wash and dry mesclun greens (pat with paper towel or
    use salad spinner).
4. Serve bean mixture over bed of greens.

NUTRITION PER SERVING

Calories: 333; *Total fat (g)*: 7.4; *Saturated fat (g)*: 1.2; *Cholesterol (mg)*: 0.0; *Monounsaturated fat (g)*: 5.0; *Polyunsaturated fat (g)*: 1.1; *Total carbohydrate (g)*: 48.7; *Sugars (g)*: 2.1; *Dietary fiber (g)*: 16.1; *Protein (g)*: 18.6; *Sodium (mg)*: 12.0

Savory Herb Chicken Salad

Serves two

¾ lb Savory Herb Marinated Chicken, chopped (page 342)
1 teaspoon canola oil mayonnaise
1 teaspoon Dijon mustard
1 tablespoon capers
1 teaspoon caper juice
1 tablespoon red onion, diced
2 thin slices avocado
2 wheat-free tortilla wraps, 7–8 inches in diameter

1. Chop chicken into bit size pieces.
2. In a small bowl combine all ingredients (except for avocado and wrap) and mix well.
3. Serve in a wheat-free wrap with avocado slices.

NUTRITION PER SERVING

Calories: 393; *Total fat (g)*: 20.7; *Saturated fat (g)*: 3.7; *Cholesterol (mg)*: 127; *Monounsaturated fat (g)*: 13.3; *Polyunsaturated fat (g)*: 3.7; *Total carbohydrate (g)*: 5.6; *Sugars (g)*: 0.3; *Dietary fiber (g)*: 0.9; *Protein (g)*: 46.7; *Sodium (mg)*: 402.0

SALAD ■ RECIPES

Sweet Spinach Salad

Serves two

4 cups baby spinach, packed
½ small red onion, thinly sliced (about ¼ cup)
½ avocado, cubed
2 tablespoons pine nuts, toasted

DRESSING
1 tablespoons extra virgin olive oil
1 lemon, juiced
½ teaspoon maple syrup
pinch of salt
fresh ground pepper, to taste

1. Thoroughly wash and dry spinach (pat with paper towel or use salad spinner). Place in large salad bowl with onion and avocado.
2. To toast pine nuts, toss constantly in small sauté pan over low flame until golden (about 3 minutes). Add to salad.
3. In a small bowl, whisk together olive oil, lemon juice, and maple syrup.
4. Dress salad and toss. Season with salt and pepper.

NUTRITION PER SERVING

Calories: 209; Total fat (g): 16.3; Saturated fat (g): 2.1; Cholesterol (mg): 0.0; Monounsaturated fat (g): 9.9; Polyunsaturated fat (g): 4.3; Total carbohydrate (g): 15.4; Sugars (g): 2.1; Dietary fiber (g): 5.5; Protein (g): 4.3; Sodium (mg): 150.0

Vegetarian Cobb

Serves two

2 eggs, hard boiled, yolks discarded, chopped
1 head romaine lettuce, coarsely chopped
1 bunch watercress, ends trimmed and coarsely chopped
½ avocado, cubed
½ cup grape tomatoes, halved
2 tablespoons pitted Kalamata olives, chopped
¼ cup (2 ounces) goat cheese, crumbled
1 tablespoon flax meal

DRESSING
1 tablespoon extra virgin olive oil
1½ tablespoons white balsamic vinegar (or regular balsamic)
1 teaspoon Dijon mustard
½ tablespoon fresh thyme

1. Place two eggs in small pot with cold water. Bring to a low boil for 10 minutes. Remove and cool.
2. In a small bowl, combine dressing ingredients and mix well.
3. Thoroughly wash and dry greens (pat with paper towel or use salad spinner). Place in large salad bowl, and toss with ½ of dressing. Add remaining ingredients (including chopped egg whites), and drizzle with remaining dressing.

NUTRITION PER SERVING

Calories: 395; *Total fat (g)*: 27.2; *Saturated fat (g)*: 9.4; *Cholesterol (mg)*: 208.0; *Monounsaturated fat (g)*: 13.8; *Polyunsaturated fat (g)*: 3.9; *Total carbohydrate (g)*: 20.0; *Sugars (g)*: 7.9; *Dietary fiber (g)*: 11.0; *Protein (g)*: 18.1; *Sodium (mg)*: 498.0

SALAD ■ RECIPES

Warm Hijiki Salad

Serves two

½ cup dry hijiki seaweed, soaked
2 teaspoons sesame oil
½ small yellow onion, thinly sliced (about ¼ cup)
1 small carrot, cut into half moons
½ tablespoon mirin
1 teaspoon low sodium tamari
1 tablespoon sesame seeds

1. Soak seaweed according to instructions on package.
2. In a large pan heat oil on medium. Sauté onion and carrot until lightly browned (about 5 minutes). Drain hijiki and add to pan with mirin, tamari, and sesame seeds; mix well.

NUTRITION PER SERVING

Calories: 133; *Total fat (g)*: 7.6; *Saturated fat (g)*: 1.1; *Cholesterol (mg)*: 0.0; *Monounsaturated fat (g)*: 3.1; *Polyunsaturated fat (g)*: 3.4; *Total carbohydrate (g)*: 19.8; *Sugars (g)*: 3.0; *Dietary fiber (g)*: 2.0; *Protein (g)*: 3.8; *Sodium (mg)*: 418.0

Watercress Arugula Salad

Serves two

1 cup arugula, coarsely chopped and packed
1 cup watercress, coarsely chopped and packed
2 cups romaine lettuce, coarsely chopped and packed
½ cup grape tomatoes, halved
½ small red onion, thinly sliced (about ¼ cup)
2 tablespoons pitted Kalamata olives, chopped
¼ cup (2 ounces) goat's milk feta cheese, crumbled

DRESSING
1 tablespoon extra virgin olive oil
1 tablespoon red wine vinegar
1 teaspoon dried oregano
fresh ground pepper, to taste

1. Thoroughly wash and dry greens (pat with paper towel or use salad spinner). Place in medium bowl.
2. Add remaining vegetables, olives, and goat cheese. Gently toss.
3. In a small bowl, combine dressing ingredients and whisk with fork. Add to salad and toss.

NUTRITION PER SERVING

Calories: 182; *Total fat (g)*: 14.6; *Saturated fat (g)*: 5.5; *Cholesterol (mg)*: 25.0; *Monounsaturated fat (g)*: 7.9; *Polyunsaturated fat (g)*: 1.2; *Total carbohydrate (g)*: 7.3; *Sugars (g)*: 3.8; *Dietary fiber (g)*: 2.7; *Protein (g)*: 6.0; *Sodium (mg)*: 552.0

SALAD ■ RECIPES

Braised Chard

Serves two

1 small bunch Swiss chard, leaves coarsely chopped
1 teaspoon extra virgin olive oil
2 teaspoons water or low sodium vegetable broth
2 teaspoons gomasio

1. Thoroughly wash and dry chard (pat with paper towel or use salad spinner).
2. In a large sauté pan, heat oil on medium.
3. Sauté chard for 3–5 minutes, tossing while cooking
4. Finish with gomasio.

NUTRITION PER SERVING

Calories: 26; *Total fat (g)*: 2.2; *Saturated fat (g)*: 0.3; *Cholesterol (mg)*: 0.0; *Monounsaturated fat (g)*: 1.7; *Polyunsaturated fat (g)*: 0.3; *Total carbohydrate (g)*: 1.4; *Sugars (g)*: 0.4; *Dietary fiber (g)*: 0.6; *Protein (g)*: 0.6; *Sodium (mg)*: 156.0

Cinnamon Roasted Acorn Squash

Serves two

1 acorn squash, halved and de-seeded
2 teaspoons extra virgin olive oil
1 teaspoon cinnamon

1. Preheat oven to 350°F.
2. Cut squash in half (cut off ends, place vertically on cutting board, guide knife down middle of squash, and split open). Scoop out seeds and pulp.
3. Brush entire squash with olive oil and sprinkle with cinnamon.
4. Place squash flesh side down onto baking dish.
5. Bake for 30 minutes or until you can easily poke fork through the skin.

NUTRITION PER SERVING

Calories: 128; *Total fat (g)*: 4.5; *Saturated fat (g)*: 0.7; *Cholesterol (mg)*: 0.0; *Monounsaturated fat (g)*: 3.3; *Polyunsaturated fat (g)*: 0.6; *Total carbohydrate (g)*: 23.5; *Sugars (g)*: 0.0; *Dietary fiber (g)*: 3.9; *Protein (g)*: 1.8; *Sodium (mg)*: 6.0

SIDE ■ RECIPES

Crunchy Bok Choy with
Tangy Chili Vinaigrette

Serves two

1 small head bok choy, trimmed and shredded
1 small carrot, shredded or julienned
½ small red onion, thinly sliced (about ¼ cup)

DRESSING
1 tablespoon extra virgin olive oil
1 tablespoon brown rice vinegar
1 teaspoon Dijon mustard
1 lime, juiced
⅛ teaspoon chili powder
pinch of salt
fresh ground pepper, to taste

1. Trim top and bottom of bok choy. Holding bunch together, thinly slice. Place in large bowl. Add carrot and onion and toss.
2. In a small bowl, combine dressing ingredients.
3. Toss dressing with vegetables. Season with salt and pepper.

NUTRITION PER SERVING

Calories: 139; Total fat (g): 7.3; Saturated fat (g): 1.1; Cholesterol (mg): 0.0; Monounsaturated fat (g): 5.1; Polyunsaturated fat (g): 1.2; Total carbohydrate (g): 15.3; Sugars (g): 7.3; Dietary fiber (g): 5.4; Protein (g): 7.0; Sodium (mg): 320.0

Garlic Roasted Asparagus

Serves two

1 bunch asparagus, trimmed
½ tablespoon extra virgin olive oil
1 lemon, juiced
2 cloves garlic, coarsely chopped

1. Preheat oven to 350°F.
2. Cut bottom ends off asparagus (about 1 inch). Place asparagus in small baking dish.
3. Add to baking dish olive oil, lemon juice, and garlic, and toss, gently coating asparagus.
4. Bake, uncovered, for 15–20 minutes.

NUTRITION PER SERVING

Calories: 64; *Total fat (g)*: 3.5; *Saturated fat (g)*: 0.5; *Cholesterol (mg)*: 0.0; *Monounsaturated fat (g)*: 2.5; *Polyunsaturated fat (g)*: 0.5; *Total carbohydrate (g)*: 10.7; *Sugars (g)*: 1.9; *Dietary fiber (g)*: 4.7; *Protein (g)*: 3.0; *Sodium (mg)*: 4.0

SIDE ■ RECIPES

Harvest Wild Rice

Serves two

½ cup wild rice (100% wild rice)
1½ cups water
1 vegetable bouillon cube, low sodium
½ tablespoon extra virgin olive oil
2 tablespoons flat leaf parsley, coarsely chopped
3 tablespoons currants, optional
2 tablespoons pecans, coarsely chopped
pinch of salt
fresh ground pepper, to taste

1. In a small pot, combine rice, water, and bouillon. Cover pot and bring to a boil on medium to high. Turn to low and simmer for 40 to 50 minutes (or until all water is absorbed).
2. Chop parsley and pecans.
3. When rice is finished, add olive oil, parsley, currants, and pecans and mix well. Season with salt and pepper.

NUTRITION PER SERVING

Calories: 286; *Total fat (g)*: 14.0; *Saturated fat (g)*: 1.5; *Cholesterol (mg)*: 0.0; *Monounsaturated fat (g)*: 8.8; *Polyunsaturated fat (g)*: 3.6; *Total carbohydrate (g)*: 34.7; *Sugars (g)*: 2.6; *Dietary fiber (g)*: 4.4; *Protein (g)*: 7.8; *Sodium (mg)*: 23.0

Juicy Sweet Roasted Broccoli (no kidding)

Serves two

½ head broccoli, cut into small pieces (about 3 cups)
1 tablespoon extra virgin olive oil
pinch of salt or 1 tablespoon of gomasio

1. Preheat oven to 350°F.
2. Trim 1 inch from bottom of broccoli stem. Cut broccoli in half (save other half for another day). Cut half into small pieces using stem and florets. Place in small baking dish and drizzle with olive oil and salt or gomasio. Toss to coat.
3. Cover dish with foil. Bake in oven, tossing occasionally, until brown for about 15 minutes (or less for crunchier broccoli).

NUTRITION PER SERVING
Calories: 137; *Total fat (g)*: 6.8; *Saturated fat (g)*: 1.0; *Cholesterol (mg)*: 0.0; *Monounsaturated fat (g)*: 5.0; *Polyunsaturated fat (g)*: 0.8; *Total carbohydrate (g)*: 15.1; *Sugars (g)*: 3.9; *Dietary fiber (g)*: 5.9; *Protein (g)*: 6.4; *Sodium (mg)*: 75.0

SIDE ■ RECIPES

Quinoa with Scallions and Toasted Sesame Oil

Serves two

½ cup quinoa
¾ cup water
½ tablespoon sesame oil
1 teaspoon toasted sesame oil
2 tablespoons scallions, thinly sliced
1 tablespoon gomasio or ⅛ teaspoon salt

1. Place quinoa in fine mesh strainer and rinse with water. In a small pot combine water and quinoa. Place covered pot on medium/high and bring to a boil. Then simmer, covered, until grain is light and fluffy (about 10 minutes).
2. Clean and slice scallions.
3. When quinoa is finished cooking, add sesame oils and gomasio or salt and mix well.

NUTRITION PER SERVING

Calories: 207; *Total fat (g):* 7.8; *Saturated fat (g):* 1.1; *Cholesterol (mg):* 0.0; *Monounsaturated fat (g):* 2.9; *Polyunsaturated fat (g):* 3.8; *Total carbohydrate (g):* 27.7; *Sugars (g):* 0.1; *Dietary fiber (g):* 3.1; *Protein (g):* 6.1; *Sodium (mg):* 121.0

Quinoa with Sliced Avocado

Serves two

½ cup quinoa
¾ cup water
½ avocado, thinly sliced
2 teaspoons extra virgin olive oil
pinch of salt

1. Place quinoa in fine mesh strainer and rinse with water. In a small pot combine water and quinoa. Place covered pot on medium/high and bring to a boil. Then simmer, covered, until grain is light and fluffy (about 10 minutes).
2. Slice avocado.
3. When quinoa is finished, add olive oil and season with salt.
4. Serve topped with avocado slices.

NUTRITION PER SERVING

Calories: 252; Total fat (g): 11.4; Saturated fat (g): 1.6; Cholesterol (mg): 0.0; Monounsaturated fat (g): 7.3; Polyunsaturated fat (g): 2.5; Total carbohydrate (g): 30.2; Sugars (g): 0.1; Dietary fiber (g): 5.3; Protein (g): 6.7; Sodium (mg): 4.0

Quinoa Tabouli

Serves two

½ cup quinoa
¾ cups water
½ small cucumber, peeled, deseeded, and diced
2 tablespoons scallions, thinly sliced
2 tablespoons mint leaves, coarsely chopped
½ orange, juiced
½ lime, juiced
1 tablespoon extra virgin olive oil
pinch of salt
fresh ground pepper, to taste

1. Place quinoa in fine mesh strainer and rinse with water. In a small pot, combine water and quinoa. Place covered pot on medium/high and bring to boil. Then simmer, covered, until grain is light and fluffy (about 10 minutes).
2. Prepare vegetables and mint and place in small bowl with olive oil and citrus juices.
3. When quinoa is finished, add to bowl and gently toss. Season with salt and pepper.

NUTRITION PER SERVING

Calories: 242; *Total fat (g):* 9.0; *Saturated fat (g):* 1.2 *Cholesterol (mg):* 0.0; *Monounsaturated fat (g):* 5.6; *Polyunsaturated fat (g):* 2.1; *Total carbohydrate (g):* 34.1; *Sugars (g):* 3.9; *Dietary fiber (g):* 4.4; *Protein (g):* 6.8; *Sodium (mg):* 3.0

Sauteed Kale with Garlic

Serves two

1 tablespoon extra virgin olive oil
1 clove garlic, minced
1 bunch leafy green kale*, pulled from stems and coarsely chopped
½ lemon, juiced
1 tablespoon water
pinch of salt

1. Heat oil on medium to low in a large sauté pan. Add garlic and sauté until lightly browned.
2. Thoroughly wash and dry kale (pat with paper towel or use salad spinner).
3. Chop kale and add to pan with lemon juice and water and sauté for 3–5 minutes, tossing regularly to braise evenly without burning.
4. Finish with a pinch of salt.

* You can also use lacinato kale (sometimes called dinosaur kale); it's the sweetest variety.

NUTRITION PER SERVING

Calories: 91; *Total fat (g)*: 6.9; *Saturated fat (g)*: 1.0; *Cholesterol (mg)*: 0.0; *Monounsaturated fat (g)*: 5.0; *Polyunsaturated fat (g)*: 0.9; *Total carbohydrate (g)*: 8.4; *Sugars (g)*: 0.0; *Dietary fiber (g)*: 2.1; *Protein (g)*: 2.1; *Sodium (mg)*: 22.0

Scrumptious Brussels Sprouts

Serves two

1 small container Brussels sprouts (about 2 cups uncut), quartered
½ tablespoon extra virgin olive oil
pinch of salt
fresh ground pepper, to taste

1. Preheat oven to 350°F.
2. Slice off bottom of sprouts and peel off outer leaves. Slice into quarters (or shave thin) and place in roasting pan with olive oil, salt, and pepper. Toss and spread sprouts evenly across pan.
3. Bake for 20–30 minutes, turning occasionally, until soft and crispy.

NUTRITION PER SERVING

Calories: 67; *Total fat (g):* 3.5; *Saturated fat (g):* 0.5; *Cholesterol (mg):* 0.0; *Monounsaturated fat (g):* 2.5; *Polyunsaturated fat (g):* 0.5; *Total carbohydrate (g):* 7.9; *Sugars (g):* 1.9; *Dietary fiber (g):* 3.3; *Protein (g):* 3.0; *Sodium (mg):* 22.0

Spiced Coconut Cauliflower

Serves two

½ head cauliflower, cut into bite-sized pieces (about 4 cups)
½ tablespoon canola oil
1½ teaspoons brown mustard seeds
1½ teaspoons cumin seeds
½ cinnamon stick
3 whole cloves
2 cardamom pods
⅛ teaspoon red pepper flakes
1 cup light coconut milk
⅛ teaspoon salt

1. In a large sauté pan, heat oil on medium to low and add all spices. Cook for about 3 minutes mixing frequently to avoid burning.
2. Add cauliflower to pan with coconut milk and mix thoroughly.
3. Cover pan and simmer for 15 minutes.
4. Season with salt.

NUTRITION PER SERVING

Calories: 318; *Total fat (g):* 26.7; *Saturated fat (g):* 22.2; *Cholesterol (mg):* 0.0; *Monounsaturated fat (g):* 2.2; *Polyunsaturated fat (g):* 2.3; *Total carbohydrate (g):* 16.2; *Sugars (g):* 3.8; *Dietary fiber (g):* 6.1; *Protein (g):* 6.5; *Sodium (mg):* 212.

Steamed Artichokes with Lemon Aioli

Serves two

2 medium artichokes
water

AIOLI
½ cup plain low-fat Greek yogurt
1 lemon, juiced
1 small clove garlic, minced
½ tablespoon extra virgin olive oil
¼ teaspoon salt
fresh ground pepper, to taste

1. Slice off ½ inch at bottom of artichoke stem and discard. Pull off and discard smaller leaves at the base.
2. In large pot, place 3 inches of water. Add artichokes so that they stand (preferably in a steaming basket). Cover and bring to a boil, then reduce heat and simmer for 30 minutes.
3. In a small bowl combine aioli ingredients. Place in refrigerator.
4. When artichokes are finished (you should be able to pull out the leaves easily) serve with aioli dip.

NUTRITION PER SERVING

Calories: 140; *Total fat (g)*: 4.4; *Saturated fat (g)*: 1.2; *Cholesterol (mg)*: 3.0; *Monounsaturated fat (g)*: 2.7; *Polyunsaturated fat (g)*: 0.5; *Total carbohydrate (g)*: 24.0; *Sugars (g)*: 5.6; *Dietary fiber (g)*: 9.5; *Protein (g)*: 8.4; *Sodium (mg)*: 454.0

Sweet and Spicy Collard Greens

Serves two

1 bunch collard greens. chiffonade
4 cloves garlic, minced
¼ teaspoon red pepper flakes
1 tablespoon extra virgin olive oil
2 tablespoons apple juice
pinch of salt

1. In a large sauté pan heat oil on medium. Add garlic, red pepper flakes and sauté until garlic is lightly browned.
2. Rinse collards and pat dry with paper towel.
3. Slice collard leaves off stems. Place leaves on top of one another, fold in half lengthwise and roll tightly going from top of leaf to bottom. Firmly holding rolled collards, thinly slice (will look like spaghetti strands).
4. Add collards to pan with apple juice and simmer, covered, on low for 15 minutes, tossing occasionally.
5. Season with salt.

NUTRITION PER SERVING
Calories: 83; *Total fat (g)*: 6.7; *Saturated fat (g)*: 1.0; *Cholesterol (mg)*: 0.0; *Monounsaturated fat (g)*: 5.0; *Polyunsaturated fat (g)*: 0.8; *Total carbohydrate (g)*: 5.5; *Sugars (g)*: 1.9; *Dietary fiber (g)*: 1.2; *Protein (g)*: 1.1; *Sodium (mg)*: 6.0

SIDE ■ RECIPES

Warm French Lentils

Serves two

½ cup French lentils
1½ cups water
¾ cup grape tomatoes, quartered (about 10–15 tomatoes)
½ cup scallion, thinly sliced
1 tablespoon red onion, finely chopped
1 small clove garlic, minced
¼ cup flat leaf parsley, coarsely chopped
¼ cup lemon juice (about 1 large lemon)
1 tablespoon extra virgin olive oil
pinch of salt
fresh ground pepper, to taste

1. Place lentils and water in a small pot. Cover and bring to a boil on medium heat. Reduce to simmer and cook, covered, for about 15 minutes.
2. In a small bowl, combine remaining ingredients and mix well.
3. When lentils are finished (chewy but not hard) drain using a fine mesh strainer, rinse with warm water, and add to bowl. Mix well, and season with salt and pepper.

NUTRITION PER SERVING

Calories: 260; *Total fat (g):* 7.1; *Saturated fat (g):* 1.0; *Cholesterol (mg):* 0.0; *Monounsaturated fat (g):* 5.1; *Polyunsaturated fat (g):* 1.0; *Total carbohydrate (g):* 37.0; *Sugars (g):* 4.0; *Dietary fiber (g):* 16.4; *Protein (g):* 13.8; *Sodium (mg):* 13.0

Halibut Puttanesca

Serves two

¾ lb. halibut fillet (also works well with cod or other white fish)
½ lemon, juiced
1 teaspoon salt

1 tablespoon extra virgin olive oil
1 clove garlic, minced
1 small yellow onion, thinly sliced (about ½ cup)
1 pint grape tomatoes
2 tablespoons pitted Kalamata olives, chopped
2 tablespoons capers
1 tablespoon caper liquid
2 tablespoons flat leaf parsley, coarsely chopped

1. Preheat oven to 350°F.
2. In a small sauté pan heat olive oil on medium. Sauté garlic and onion until golden brown.
3. Add tomatoes, olives, capers and caper liquid and simmer, covered, stirring occasionally for 15 minutes or until tomatoes have softened.
4. While puttanesca simmers, wash fish with salt and lemon juice, rinse under cold water and pat dry with a paper towel. Place in baking dish.
5. Add parsley to finished puttanesca sauce. Pour over fish and bake in oven for 20 minutes.

NUTRITION PER SERVING

Calories: 306; Total fat (g): 10.9; Saturated fat (g): 1.7; Cholesterol (mg): 54.0; Monounsaturated fat (g): 6.9; Polyunsaturated fat (g): 2.2; Total carbohydrate (g): 13.7; Sugars (g): 5.5; Dietary fiber (g): 4.4; Protein (g): 37.9; Sodium (mg): 429.0

ENTREE, FISH ■ RECIPES

Miso Baked Cod

Serves two

¾ lb. cod (also works well with salmon or black sea bass)
½ lemon, juiced
1 teaspoon salt

1 tablespoon white miso (not sweet variety)
1 tablespoon honey
1 teaspoon low sodium tamari
2 teaspoons fresh ginger, peeled and minced

1. Preheat oven to 375°F.
2. Wash fish with salt and lemon juice, rinse under cold water and pat dry with a paper towel. Place in baking dish.
3. In a small bowl, mix miso, honey, tamari, and ginger so that it becomes a paste. Spread evenly over fish.
4. Bake uncovered for 15–20 minutes, then finish under broiler for 5–7 minutes.

NUTRITION PER SERVING

Calories: 195; *Total fat (g):* 1.3; *Saturated fat (g):* 0.3; *Cholesterol (mg):* 73.0; *Monounsaturated fat (g):* 0.3; *Polyunsaturated fat (g):* 0.7; *Total carbohydrate (g):* 14.4; *Sugars (g):* 9.2; *Dietary fiber (g):* 1.8; *Protein (g):* 31.8; *Sodium (mg):* 500.0

Trout with Lemon and Herbs in Parchment

Serves two

¾ lb. rainbow trout (also works well with flounder or sole)
½ lemon, juiced
1 teaspoon salt

2 teaspoons extra virgin olive oil
1 lemon, juiced
2 sprigs fresh thyme
2 sprigs fresh oregano
¼ teaspoon salt
fresh ground pepper to taste

1. Preheat oven to 350°F.
2. Cut two rectangles of parchment, approximately 13 inches by 15 inches.
3. Wash fish with salt and lemon juice, rinse under cold water and pat dry with a paper towel. Split fish into two equal servings.
4. Place fish on parchment. Drizzle each piece with olive oil, lemon juice, and place a sprig each of thyme and oregano on top of fish. Season with salt and pepper.
5. Seal parchment by bringing together the two lengthwise ends and folding them down like you'd fold a brown paper bag to close; then twist the ends of the packet like a candy wrapper. Place on baking dish and bake for 20 minutes.
6. Remove fish from parchment to serve.

NUTRITION PER SERVING

Calories: 310; *Total fat (g)*: 14.6; *Saturated fat (g)*: 2.6; *Cholesterol (mg)*: 98.0; *Monounsaturated fat (g)*: 8.8; *Polyunsaturated fat (g)*: 3.2; *Total carbohydrate (g)*: 9.5; *Sugars (g)*: 0.0; *Dietary fiber (g)*: 4.4; *Protein* (g): 36.5; *Sodium (mg)*: 295.0

Walnut-Pesto Wild Salmon

Serves two

¾ lb. wild Alaskan salmon fillet (also works well with any fish)
1 lemon, juiced
1 teaspoon salt

PESTO*
2 cups basil leaves, rinsed and packed tightly in the cup
4 cloves garlic, whole, peeled
½ cup walnuts, no shell
6 tablespoons extra virgin olive oil

1. Preheat oven to 350°F.
2. Combine all pesto ingredients in food processor and purée.
3. Wash fish with salt and lemon juice, rinse under cold water and pat dry with a paper towel. Place fish in baking dish.
4. Use ½ of the pesto to generously coat the top of each fillet.
5. Cover baking dish with tightly fitting top or aluminum foil and bake for 20–25 minutes (15 minutes for rare).

*   Save half walnut-pesto for snack another day. Can be stored in airtight container in fridge for up to one week, or immediately freeze for up to three months.

NUTRITION PER SERVING

Calories: 529; *Total fat (g)*: 37.7; *Saturated fat (g)*: 5.0; *Cholesterol (mg)*: 93.0; *Monounsaturated fat (g)*: 20.7; *Polyunsaturated fat (g)*: 12.0; *Total carbohydrate (g)*: 4.9; *Sugars (g)*: 0.8; *Dietary fiber (g)*: 1.4; *Protein (g)*: 38.2; *Sodium (mg)*: 75.0

Curry Roasted Chicken

Serves four

Small whole roaster chicken (about 3 pounds)
1 lemon, juiced
2 teaspoons salt

1 large yellow onion, quartered

CURRY RUB
½ cup extra virgin olive oil
2 teaspoons salt
3 tablespoons curry powder
1 bunch cilantro, coarsely chopped

1. Preheat oven to 375°F; place rack in the center of the oven.
2. Discard any spare parts inside of chicken. Wash chicken with salt and lemon juice, rinse under cold water and pat dry with a paper towel. Place chicken in large baking dish, breast-side up.
3. Quarter unpeeled onion and place inside cavity.
4. In a small bowl, combine olive oil, 2 teaspoons salt, curry powder and cilantro; mix well.
5. Rub the curry mixture all over the chicken, placing some under the breast skin by creating a pocket between skin and flesh with your fingers.
6. Bake for 1 hour and 30 minutes. Baste regularly during baking (about every 20–30 minutes). When done, remove chicken from oven, cover with foil, and let sit for 15 minutes.

NUTRITION PER SERVING

Calories: 533; *Total fat (g)*: 21.1; *Saturated fat (g)*: 4.3; *Cholesterol (mg)*: 221.0; *Monounsaturated fat (g)*: 13.0; *Polyunsaturated fat (g)*: 3.9; *Total carbohydrate (g)*: 9.4; *Sugars (g)*: 1.8; *Dietary fiber (g)*: 3.6; *Protein (g)*: 70.6; *Sodium (mg)*: 262.0

ENTREE, POULTRY ■ RECIPES

Savory Herb Marinated Chicken

Serves four (includes leftovers)

1½ pounds skinless, boneless chicken breast, cubed
1 teaspoon salt
½ lemon, juiced

MARINADE
2 tablespoons extra virgin olive oil
1 clove garlic, minced
1 lemon, juiced
1 tablespoon fresh thyme, remove from stem
1 tablespoon fresh oregano, chopped
1 tablespoon fresh basil, chopped
¼ teaspoon salt

1 tablespoon extra virgin olive oil, for cooking

1. Wash chicken with salt and lemon juice; rinse under cold water and pat dry with a paper towel.
2. Combine marinade ingredients in a large bowl; mix well.
3. Place chicken into the marinade and coat completely. (Can refrigerate at this point for up to a day.)
4. Heat tablespoon of olive oil in a large sauté pan on medium. Sauté herb-marinated chicken until browned on all sides and cooked through (about 10–12 minutes).

NUTRITION PER SERVING

Calories: 285; *Total fat (g):* 12.1; *Saturated fat (g):* 2.1; *Cholesterol (mg):* 96.0; *Monounsaturated fat (g):* 8.2; *Polyunsaturated fat (g):* 1.8; *Total carbohydrate (g):* 4.4; *Sugars (g):* 0.2; *Dietary fiber (g):* 1.8; *Protein* (g): 38.3; *Sodium (mg):* 87.0

Turkey Bolognese over Spaghetti Squash

Serves two

½ lb. ground turkey
1 teaspoon extra virgin olive oil
1 clove garlic, minced
1 small yellow onion, thinly sliced (about ½ cup)
1 teaspoon dried thyme, or fresh picked
1 teaspoon dried oregano, or fresh picked
1 teaspoon dried rosemary, or fresh minced
2 cups (16 ounces) canned crushed tomatoes
2 tablespoons tomato paste
Pinch of salt
2 teaspoons Parmesan cheese, grated (optional)
1 small spaghetti squash, halved and de-seeded
1 teaspoon extra virgin olive oil

1. Preheat oven to 350°F for spaghetti squash.
2. Split spaghetti squash in half (cut off ends, place vertically on cutting board, guide knife down middle of squash and split open). De-seed, rub with olive oil, and place facedown on a baking sheet. Bake for 30 minutes until fork easily pierces skin. (For microwave, pierce skin with fork and cook on high for 15 minutes turning once; allow to cool before opening.)
3. While spaghetti squash is cooking, heat olive oil in a large sauté pan on medium. Sauté garlic and onions until lightly browned. Add dried herbs and sauté for another 2 minutes (if using fresh herbs, add with crushed tomatoes). Add ground turkey, breaking apart with fork as you continue to sauté for 5 minutes, until lightly browned. Add crushed tomatoes, tomato paste, salt (and fresh herbs if using) and simmer, uncovered, for 20 minutes.
4. Scoop "spaghetti" out of squash; top with Bolognese and a sprinkle of Parmesan if desired.

NUTRITION PER SERVING

Calories: 370; *Total fat (g):* 7.7; *Saturated fat (g):* 2.0; *Cholesterol (mg):* 67.0; *Monounsaturated fat (g):* 4.0; *Polyunsaturated fat (g):* 1.7; *Total carbohydrate (g):* 44.7; *Sugars (g):* 11.4; *Dietary fiber (g):* 10.6; *Protein (g):* 34.8; *Sodium (mg):* 440.0

ENTREE, POULTRY ■ RECIPES

Lemon Parsley Hummus Wrap

Serves two

½ cup Lemon Parsley Hummus (page 352)*
½ avocado, pitted, removed from skin, thinly sliced
1 small vine ripe tomato, thinly sliced
½ cup bean sprouts, rinsed and patted dry with paper towel**
2 wheat-free tortilla wraps, 7–8 inches diameter

1. Spread ¼ cup hummus on one side of tortilla.
2. Top with ¼ avocado, ½ tomato, and ¼ cup sprouts. Roll or fold.

*   Store-bought hummus with all-natural ingredients is fine. Watch out for those brands with preservatives such as potassium sorbate or potassium benzoate.
** Make sure sprouts are fresh, meaning that there are no browned or spoiled areas; they can carry harmful bacteria.

NUTRITION PER SERVING

Calories: 174; *Total fat (g)*: 9.8; *Saturated fat (g)*: 1.4; *Cholesterol (mg)*: 0.0; *Monounsaturated fat (g)*: 6.3; *Polyunsaturated fat (g)*: 2.0; *Total carbohydrate (g)*: 17.3; *Sugars (g)*: 1.5; *Dietary fiber (g)*: 5.5; *Protein (g)*: 4.4; *Sodium (mg)*: 153.0

Red Curry Tofu with Basil

Serves two

½ block extra firm tofu, cut into slabs*

½ tablespoon sesame oil
1 clove garlic, minced
½ tablespoon fresh ginger, minced
½ cup scallions, thinly sliced

1 cup light coconut milk
1 teaspoon red curry paste
½ lime, juiced
⅛ teaspoon salt
½ cup basil leaves, coarsely chopped

1. In a small pan, add sesame oil, garlic, and ginger. Sauté garlic and ginger on medium flame until golden.
2. Add remaining ingredients (except basil and tofu) and mix well until curry paste dissolves. Add basil and simmer, uncovered, for 10 minutes.
3. Drain tofu well. Cut into ¼-inch slabs, and cut each slab in half.
4. Place tofu in pan, making sure to cover with sauce. Continue simmering, covered for 10 more minutes, gently stirring.

* Leftover tofu can be stored in an airtight container with fresh water; change water every 2 days.

NUTRITION PER SERVING

Calories: 448; *Total fat (g)*: 37.4; *Saturated fat (g)*: 23.7; *Cholesterol (mg)*: 0.0; *Monounsaturated fat (g)*: 5.1; *Polyunsaturated fat (g)*: 8.6; *Total carbohydrate (g)*: 12.8; *Sugars (g)*: 0.8; *Dietary fiber (g)*: 1.9; *Protein (g)*: 18.7; *Sodium (mg)*: 166.0

Tofu Vegetable Stir-Fry

Serves two

½ block extra firm tofu*, cubed

1 tablespoon sesame oil
1 small yellow onion, thinly sliced (about ½ cup)
1 small carrot, cut into ½ moons, about ⅛" thick
1 small zucchini, cut into ½ moons, about ⅛" thick
1 cup broccoli florets, cut into small pieces
2 teaspoons tamari, wheat-free, low sodium
2 teaspoons mirin
2 tablespoons water
½ teaspoon toasted sesame oil
½ tablespoon gomasio

1. In a large sauté pan or wok, heat sesame oil on medium and sauté onions until translucent.
2. Add remaining vegetables, tamari, mirin, and water, mix well and cook for another 3 minutes.
3. Drain tofu well and cut into ½" cubes. Add tofu and water to pan. Gently mix, cover pan, and simmer for 5 more minutes.
4. Turn off heat and season with toasted sesame oil and gomasio.

*   Leftover tofu can be stored in an airtight container with fresh water; change water every 2 days.

NUTRITION PER SERVING

Calories: 288; *Total fat (g)*: 18.4; *Saturated fat (g)*: 2.8; *Cholesterol (mg)*: 0.0; *Monounsaturated fat (g)*: 5.7; *Polyunsaturated fat (g)*: 9.8; *Total carbohydrate (g)*: 17.3; *Sugars (g)*: 5.1; *Dietary fiber (g)*: 2.7; *Protein* (g): 17.0; *Sodium (mg)*: 254.0

Vegetable Biryani

Serves two

½ cup brown basmati rice
1 cup water
½ can (about 7 ounces) garbanzo
    beans, drained and rinsed

1 tablespoon sesame oil
1 clove garlic, minced
1 small yellow onion, sliced thin

SPICES
1½ teaspoons brown or yellow
    mustard seeds
1½ teaspoons whole cumin seeds
3 whole cardamom pods
3 whole cloves
½ cinnamon stick
1½ teaspoons curry powder

VEGETABLES (OR 2 CUPS MIXED
    FROZEN VEGETABLES)
1 small carrot, sliced lengthwise,
    and cut into half moons
½ cup cauliflower, cut into small
    pieces
½ cup snow peas, trimmed
½ cup yellow squash, sliced
    lengthwise, and cut into
    half moons

¼ cup vegetable broth or water
¼ cup light coconut milk
pinch of salt

1. In a small pot, combine water and rice, cover and bring to boil; reduce to simmer and cook, covered, for 40–50 minutes.
2. In a large sauté pan, heat oil on medium to low; add garlic, onion, and spices and sauté for 3–5 minutes stirring regularly to avoid burning. Turn off heat.
3. Prep all other vegetables and add to pan with garbanzo beans, broth (or water), and coconut milk; mix well. Turn heat back on and simmer, uncovered, for 20 minutes.
4. Discard cinnamon stick, cardamom pods, and cloves. Add rice to the pan. Cook, gently stirring for another 2 minutes.

NUTRITION PER SERVING
Calories: 534; *Total fat (g)*: 17.2; *Saturated fat (g)*: 7.2; *Cholesterol (mg)*: 0.0; *Monounsaturated fat (g)*: 4.9; *Polyunsaturated fat (g)*: 5.1; *Total carbohydrate (g)*: 80.1; *Sugars (g)*: 10.0; *Dietary fiber (g)*: 15.1; *Protein (g)*; 16.6; *Sodium (mg)*: 50.0

ENTREE, VEGETARIAN ■ RECIPES

Vegetarian Chili

Serves four (includes leftovers)*

1 can (15 ounces) red kidney beans, drained and rinsed
1 can (15 ounces) black beans, drained and rinsed

1 tablespoon extra virgin olive oil
2 cloves garlic, chopped
1 small yellow onion, thinly sliced (about ½ cup)
1 teaspoon ground cumin
1 teaspoon chili powder
¼ teaspoon ground cinnamon
½ cup red bell pepper, diced
1 small zucchini, sliced lengthwise, and cut into half moons (about 1 cup)
1 small yellow squash, sliced lengthwise, and cut into half moons (about 1 cup)
1 can (15 ounces) diced tomatoes
1 can (5 ounces) tomato paste
½ cup cilantro, chopped
pinch of salt
1 cup plain low-fat Greek yogurt (optional)

1. In a large pot, heat oil on medium. Add garlic and onion and sauté until soft and slightly golden. Add spices, pepper, zucchini, and squash and continue to sauté for 3–5 minutes.
2. Add beans to pot with diced tomatoes and tomato paste and stir well. Cover and simmer for 10 minutes. Remove cover and simmer for another 10 minutes.
3. Stir in cilantro to finish. Season with salt.
4. Serve with dollop of plain Greek yogurt.

*   Store leftovers in airtight container in fridge for up to three days, or immediately freeze for up to three months.

NUTRITION PER SERVING

Calories: 437; Total fat (g): 5.6; Saturated fat (g): 1.4; Cholesterol (mg): 3.0; Monounsaturated fat (g): 3.0; Polyunsaturated fat (g): 1.2; Total carbohydrate (g): 75.2; Sugars (g): 16.4; Dietary fiber (g): 20.7; Protein (g): 26.0; Sodium (mg): 327.0

Vegetarian Chili Burritos

Serves two

2 cups Vegetarian Chili (page 348)
4 tablespoons Guacamole* (page 351)
4 tablespoons plain low-fat Greek yogurt (optional)
2 wheat free or corn tortillas

1. In small pot, heat chili on medium.
2. Warm tortillas in oven.
3. Place 1 cup chili, 2 tablespoons guacamole, and 2 tablespoons of yogurt in center of tortillas. Tightly wrap and enjoy.

* Can use store bought guacamole.

NUTRITION PER SERVING

Calories: 516; *Total fat (g):* 10.6; *Saturated fat (g):* 1.7; *Cholesterol (mg):* 1.0; *Monounsaturated fat (g):* 6.1; *Polyunsaturated fat (g):* 2.2; *Total carbohydrate (g):* 80.1; *Sugars (g):* 19.6; *Dietary fiber (g):* 22.7; *Protein (g);* 29.6; *Sodium (mg):* 518.0

ENTREE, VEGETARIAN ■ RECIPES

Burst of Energy Trail Mix

Serves eight (includes leftovers)

½ cup walnuts
½ cup raw almonds
¼ cup raw pumpkin seeds (also known as pepitas)
¼ cup unsalted sunflower seeds, shelled
¼ cup dried cranberries
¼ cup dried papaya, coarsely chopped

1. Place all ingredients in a bowl and toss.
2. Measure ¼ cup serving into small plastic bags and store in cool dry place. Great for on the go eating.

*   Make once for entire 21-Day Plan

NUTRITION PER SERVING

Calories: 189; *Total fat (g):* 14.6; *Saturated fat (g):* 1.7; *Cholesterol (mg):* 0.0; *Monounsaturated fat (g):* 6.3; *Polyunsaturated fat (g):* 6.7; *Total carbohydrate (g):* 8.8; *Sugars (g):* 3.3; *Dietary fiber (g):* 3.1; *Protein (g):* 7.4; *Sodium (mg):* 2.0

Guacamole

Serves two

2 ripe avocados
1 lime, juiced (about 2 tablespoons)
½ small red onion, diced (about ¼ cup)
¼ cup cilantro, with stems, coarsely chopped
pinch of salt
fresh ground pepper, to taste

1. Peel and halve avocados. Remove pit and use spoon to scoop flesh.
2. In large bowl, mash avocado with fork. Add all other ingredients and mix well. Season with salt and pepper.
3. Serve with vegetables, rice crackers, or in vegetarian chili burrito.

NUTRITION PER SERVING
Calories: 240; *Total fat (g)*: 18.7; *Saturated fat (g)*: 2.9; *Cholesterol (mg)*: 0.0; *Monounsaturated fat (g)*: 13.3; *Polyunsaturated fat (g)*: 2.5; *Total carbohydrate (g)*: 15.5; *Sugars (g)*: 1.6; *Dietary fiber (g)*: 9.7; *Protein (g)*: 3.0; *Sodium (mg)*: 11.0

SNACK ■ RECIPES

Lemon Parsley Hummus

Serves four (includes leftovers)*

1 can (15 ounces) garbanzo beans, drained and rinsed
2 lemons, juiced, about 4 tablespoons
⅓ cup extra virgin olive oil
1 small clove garlic
2 tablespoon parsley leaves
½ teaspoon salt

Place drained and rinsed beans in food processor with remaining
ingredients and puree until smooth and creamy.

*   Store leftovers in airtight container in fridge for up to three days.

NUTRITION PER SERVING

Calories: 345; *Total fat (g)*: 19.7; *Saturated fat (g)*: 2.8; *Cholesterol (mg)*: 0.0; *Monounsaturated fat (g)*: 13.8; *Polyunsaturated fat (g)*: 3.2; *Total carbohydrate (g)*: 35.3; *Sugars (g)*: 5.1; *Dietary fiber (g)*: 10.7; *Protein (g)*: 10.2; *Sodium (mg)*: 300.0

Berry Parfait

Serves two

1 cup plain low-fat Greek yogurt
2 tablespoons honey
1 cup raspberries
1 cup blackberries
4 tablespoons Power Up Granola (page 300)

1. Using a stemmed champagne or parfait glass, layer first yogurt, then honey and finally berries.
2. Top with Power Up Granola.

NUTRITION PER SERVING

Calories: 277; Total fat (g): 5.8; Saturated fat (g): 1.8; Cholesterol (mg): 7.0; Monounsaturated fat (g): 2.0; Polyunsaturated fat (g): 1.9; Total carbohydrate (g): 48.3; Sugars (g): 35.2; Dietary fiber (g): 9.2; Protein (g): 10.5; Sodium (mg): 90.0

Citrus Mint Mixed Berries

Serves two

½ cup blackberries
½ cup blueberries
½ cup strawberries, quartered
½ cup raspberries
¼ cup orange juice, fresh squeezed
2 teaspoons fresh mint leaves, coarsely chopped

In a medium bowl, gently combine berries with orange juice and mint.

NUTRITION PER SERVING

Calories: 77; Total fat (g): 0.5; Saturated fat (g): 0.0; Cholesterol (mg): 0.0; Monounsaturated fat (g): 0.1; Polyunsaturated fat (g): 0.4; Total carbohydrate (g): 18.8; Sugars (g): 11.2; Dietary fiber (g): 5.8; Protein (g): 1.7; Sodium (mg): 0.0

Coco-nutty Banana

Serves two

1 large banana, sliced into rounds and quartered (about 1 cup)
2 tablespoons shredded unsweetened coconut
1 cup blueberries
½ lemon, juiced

1. Slice banana and place in medium bowl with lemon juice. Mix gently. Add coconut and mix again to coat bananas.
2. Divide between two small bowls and top with blueberries.

NUTRITION PER SERVING

Calories: 201; *Total fat (g):* 9.0; *Saturated fat (g):* 8.2; *Cholesterol (mg):* 0.0; *Monounsaturated fat (g):* 0.4; *Polyunsaturated fat (g):* 0.3; *Total carbohydrate (g):* 32.5; *Sugars (g):* 17.8; *Dietary fiber (g):* 7.1; *Protein (g);* 2.6; *Sodium (mg):* 6.0

Dark Chocolate Chunk Almond Cookies

*One dozen**

1 cup smooth almond butter
⅓ cup canola oil
½ cup maple syrup
1 teaspoon vanilla
1½ cups spelt flour
½ cup dark chocolate coarsely chopped (2 ounces, about ½ large bar)

1. Cover cookie sheet with parchment (or brush lightly with canola oil).
2. Preheat oven to 350°F.
3. In a large bowl mix almond butter, oil, maple syrup, and vanilla. Add spelt flour to form dough. Stir in dark chocolate pieces.
4. Drop small balls of dough (about 1 inch diameter) onto cookie sheet. Press with spoon to form ¼ inch thick cookie.
5. Bake for 15–20 minutes until cookies are lightly browned on edges.
6. Cool before removing from sheet.

* Store in airtight container in cool dry place for up to one week or freeze for up to three months.

NUTRITION PER SERVING

Calories: 292; *Total fat (g):* 19.0; *Saturated fat (g):* 3.9; *Cholesterol (mg):* 0.0; *Monounsaturated fat (g):* 9.6; *Polyunsaturated fat (g):* 5.5; *Total carbohydrate (g):* 26.0; *Sugars (g):* 8.1; *Dietary fiber (g):* 3.5; *Protein (g):* 5.9; *Sodium (mg):* 5.0

Dark Chocolate Dairy-Free Mousse

Serves two

1 box (12 ounces) silken tofu
5 tablespoons cocoa powder*
1½ teaspoons pure vanilla extract
⅓ cup plus 2 tablespoons maple syrup
⅛ teaspoon cinnamon, optional

1. Place all ingredients into a food processor or blender and puree until smooth and creamy.
2. Chill for 1 hour or overnight.

* Preferably Nestlé's Unsweetened Cocoa (non-dutched).

NUTRITION PER SERVING

Calories: 273; Total fat (g): 6.0; Saturated fat (g): 1.7; Cholesterol (mg): 0.0; Monounsaturated fat (g): 1.5; Polyunsaturated fat (g): 2.8; Total carbohydrate (g): 48.8; Sugars (g): 34.8; Dietary fiber (g): 4.7; Protein (g); 10.8; Sodium (mg): 15.0

Spiced Apples with Pecan Crumble

Serves two

2 small Gala apples (or Fuji), cored
2 cups apple juice
4 whole cloves
⅛ inch slice fresh ginger root, unpeeled

PECAN CRUMBLE
¼ cup pecans, coarsely chopped
¼ teaspoon ground cinnamon
1½ teaspoons dark brown sugar

1. Rinse and core apples, do not peel. Place apples in a medium pot with apple juice, cloves, and ginger. Bring to a boil, then simmer, covered, for 10 minutes (apples should be fork tender).
2. In a small bowl combine pecans, cinnamon, and brown sugar.
3. Remove apples from pot and serve warm, topped with crumble.

NUTRITION PER SERVING

Calories: 407; *Total fat (g)*: 20.9; *Saturated fat (g)*: 2.1; *Cholesterol (mg)*: 0.0; *Monounsaturated fat (g)*: 12.5; *Polyunsaturated fat (g)*: 6.2; *Total carbohydrate (g)*: 55.9; *Sugars (g)*: 45.0; *Dietary fiber (g)*: 6.2; *Protein (g)*: 3.5; *Sodium (mg)*: 17.0

DESSERT ■ RECIPES

Cool Mint Lemonade

Serves two

2½ lemons, juiced (about ½ cup)
2½ cups cold water
½ cup warm water
2 tablespoons honey
2 sprigs fresh mint

1. In a pitcher, dissolve honey in ½ cup warm water by stirring vigorously.
2. Add remaining water and lemon juice and mix well.
3. Add mint. Refrigerate for at least an hour for mint to impart full flavor.
4. Serve on the rocks.

NUTRITION PER SERVING

Calories: 93; *Total fat (g)*: 0.2; *Saturated fat (g)*: 0.1; *Cholesterol (mg)*: 0.0; *Monounsaturated fat (g)*: 0.0; *Polyunsaturated fat (g)*: 0.1; *Total carbohydrate (g)*: 32.2; *Sugars (g)*: 17.2; *Dietary fiber (g)*: 6.8; *Protein (g)*: 1.9; *Sodium (mg)*: 6.0

Cranberry Tea Infusion

Serves two

4 bags cranberry tea
2½ cups water
½ cup apple juice
2 sprigs fresh mint
½ orange, sliced into wedges (optional)

1. Heat water to warm.
2. In a pitcher, add tea bags, warm water, apple juice, and mint.
3. Refrigerate until cool.
4. Serve in stem glass on the rocks with an orange wedge.

NUTRITION PER SERVING
Calories: 49; *Total fat (g)*: 0.1; *Saturated fat (g)*: 0.0; *Cholesterol (mg)*: 0.0; *Monounsaturated fat (g)*: 0.0; *Polyunsaturated fat (g)*: 0.1; *Total carbohydrate (g)*: 12.2; *Sugars (g)*: 9.7; *Dietary fiber (g)*: 1.2; *Protein (g)*: 0.5; *Sodium (mg)*: 3.0

Dr. Merrell's Fruit Juice

Serves two

1½ cups fresh pineapple, peeled, cored, and cut into large cubes (or
     fresh papaya)
1 cup mixed frozen berries
½ cup pineapple juice (or pomegranate or cherry juice)
½ cup water (optional)

Combine all ingredients in a blender and puree until smooth. May
add water (small amounts at a time) to reach desired consistency.

NUTRITION PER SERVING

Calories: 184; *Total fat (g)*: 0.2; *Saturated fat (g)*: 0.0; *Cholesterol (mg)*: 0.0; *Monounsaturated fat (g)*: 0.0; *Polyunsaturated fat (g)*: 0.1; *Total carbohydrate (g)*: 47.0; *Sugars (g)*: 39.1; *Dietary fiber (g)*: 3.7; *Protein (g)*: 1.7; *Sodium (mg)*: 3.0

Dr. Merrell's Veggie Juice

Serves two

2 medium cucumbers, peeled
2 stalks celery
2 large carrots (or 2 small apples)
½ cup flat leaf parsley, packed
fresh ginger root, nickel size piece
3 cups kale, packed
1 lemon, juiced

1. Juice all vegetables in a vegetable juicer.
2. Finish with lemon juice.

NUTRITION PER SERVING

Calories: 125; *Total fat (g)*: 0.8; *Saturated fat (g)*: 0.2; *Cholesterol (mg)*: 0.0; *Monounsaturated fat (g)*: 0.1; *Polyunsaturated fat (g)*: 0.5; *Total carbohydrate (g)*: 29.2; *Sugars (g)*: 7.0; *Dietary fiber (g)*: 9.1; *Protein (g)*: 6.5; *Sodium (mg)*: 138.0

Mango-Peach Freeze

Serves two

2 cups frozen peaches
2 cups mango nectar
½ lime, cut in half

1. Combine peaches and nectar in blender and puree until smooth.
2. Serve in stemmed glass with a spritz of lime.

NUTRITION PER SERVING

Calories: 193; *Total fat (g)*: 0.4; *Saturated fat (g)*: 0.0; *Cholesterol (mg)*: 0.0; *Monounsaturated fat (g)*: 0.2; *Polyunsaturated fat (g)*: 0.2; *Total carbohydrate (g)*: 49.5; *Sugars (g)*: 44.5; *Dietary fiber (g)*: 3.2; *Protein (g)*: 1.8; *Sodium (mg)*: 12.0

Papaya Fizz

Serves two

1½ cups papaya nectar
1½ cups seltzer
1 lime, quartered

1. In a pitcher, combine nectar and seltzer.
2. Serve on the rocks with a spritz of lime (½ lime per serving).

NUTRITION PER SERVING

Calories: 112; *Total fat (g)*: 0.3; *Saturated fat (g)*: 0.1; *Cholesterol (mg)*: 0.0; *Monounsaturated fat (g)*: 0.1; *Polyunsaturated fat (g)*: 0.1; *Total carbohydrate (g)*: 29.1; *Sugars (g)*: 26.4; *Dietary fiber (g)*: 1.2; *Protein (g)*: 0.4; *Sodium (mg)*: 46.0

Peach Spritzer with Cranberry Ice

Serves two

    2 cups peach nectar
    1 cup seltzer

    CRANBERRY ICE CUBES
    ¼ cup cranberry concentrate
    ¼ cup water

1. To make ice cubes, mix cranberry concentrate with water in a large measuring cup, then pour into ice cube tray and freeze overnight (makes 4 cubes).
2. In pitcher combine nectar and seltzer.
3. Serve over cranberry ice cubes.

NUTRITION PER SERVING

Calories: 148; *Total fat (g)*: 0.1; *Saturated fat (g)*: 0.0; *Cholesterol (mg)*: 0.0; *Monounsaturated fat (g)*: 0.0; *Polyunsaturated fat (g)*: 0.0; *Total carbohydrate (g)*: 38.5; *Sugars (g)*: 37.0; *Dietary fiber (g)*: 1.5; *Protein (g)*: 0.8; *Sodium (mg)*: 42.0

Tangerine Spritzer with Papaya Ice

Serves two

1½ cups tangerine juice, fresh squeezed (or can use orange juice)
1½ cups seltzer
½ lime, cut in half

PAPAYA ICE CUBES
½ cup papaya nectar

1. To make ice cubes, pour papaya nectar into ice cube tray and freeze overnight (makes four ice cubes).
2. In pitcher combine tangerine juice (or orange juice) and seltzer.
3. Cut lime and squeeze juice into pitcher.
4. Serve over papaya ice cubes.

NUTRITION PER SERVING
Calories: 117; *Total fat (g)*: 0.3; *Saturated fat (g)*: 0.1; *Cholesterol (mg)*: 0.0; *Monounsaturated fat (g)*: 0.1; *Polyunsaturated fat (g)*: 0.1; *Total carbohydrate (g)*: 28.7; *Sugars (g)*: 27.2; *Dietary fiber (g)*: 0.8; *Protein (g)*: 1.1; *Sodium (mg)*: 41.0

Recipe Index

Breakfast

Dr. Merrell's morning shake   298
French toast   299
Power Up granola   300
Scrambled tofu with
    vegetables   301
Vegetable goat cheese
    Egg-white omelet   302

Soups

Immune-boost soup   303
Quick Italian vegetable soup   304
Red lentil soup   305
Rosemary butternut
    squash soup   306
Shitake-miso soup   307
White bean kale soup   308

Salads

Antioxidant fruit salad   309
Arugula salad with crushed
    walnuts and goat cheese   310
Black bean salad   311
Cucumber wakame salad   312

Leafy greens and chickpea
    salad   313
Mediterranean tuna salad   314
Mesclun greens with
    balsamic vinaigrette   315
Power protein mixed
    green salad   316
Savory herb chicken salad   317
Sweet spinach salad   318
Vegetarian Cobb   319
Warm hijiki salad   320
Watercress arugula salad   321

Sides

Braised chard   322
Cinnamon roasted acorn
    squash   323
Crunchy bok choy with
    tangy chili vinaigrette   324
Garlic roasted asparagus   325
Harvest Wild Rice   326
Juicy sweet roasted broccoli   327
Quinoa with scallions and
    toasted sesame oil   328
Quinoa with sliced avocado   329

Quinoa tabouli 330
Sauteed kale with garlic 331
Scrumptious Brussels
sprouts 332
Spiced coconut
cauliflower 333
Steamed artichokes with
lemon aioli 334
Sweet and spicy collard greens 335
Warm French lentils 336

Entrees

Fish
Halibut puttanesca 337
Miso baked cod 338
Trout with lemon and
herbs in parchment 339
Walnut-pesto wild
salmon 340

Poultry
Curry roasted chicken 341
Savory herb marinated
chicken 342
Turkey bolognese over
spaghetti squash 343

Vegetarian
Lemon parsley
hummus wrap 344
Red curry tofu with basil 345
Tofu vegetable stir-fry 346
Vegetable biryani 347

Vegetarian chili 348
Vegetarian chili burritos 349

Snacks

Burst of energy trail mix 350
Guacamole 351
Lemon parsley hummus 352

Desserts

Berry parfait 353
Citrus mint mixed berries 353
Coco-nutty banana 354
Dark chocolate chunk
almond cookies 355
Dark chocolate dairy-free
mousse 356
Spiced apples with
pecan crumble 357

Beverages

Cool mint lemonade 358
Cranberry tea infusion 359
Dr. Merrell's fruit juice 360
Dr. Merrell's veggie juice 360
Mango peach-freeze 361
Papaya fizz 361
Peach spritzer with
cranberry ice 362
Tangerine spritzer with
papaya ice 363

Acknowledgments

The energetic costs of writing a book are astronomical, and this one was no different. A multitude of thanks goes out to the community that gathered around to make *Power Up* a reality. First, to my soul mate and writing partner, Kathy, you were the cornerstone of this project, and without you it would never have happened. I am grateful for this literary partnership, and thankful that we made it out intact! I am deeply indebted to Kim Witherspoon and Richard Pine for their persistence, patience, and guidance in honing the concept for this book and for knowing that Kathy and I could do this together. Monumental thanks go to Leslie Meredith for being our editorial champion and offering such thoughtful guidance, and to Dominick Anfuso for his unwavering support. I offer much gratitude to Donna Loffredo for her tireless effort and attention to detail throughout the process, and to Carol de Onís for her incredible labors and detailed reading.

Deep gratitude goes out to the many masters who have taught me the value of using lifestyle changes and energetic management as healing modalities. In particular I want to thank Jeff Bland, Larry Dossey, and Dan Goleman for their friendship and visionary leadership in the healing arts. For years, Mehmet Oz and Christiane Northrup have shared ideas and collaborated in bringing integrative medicine to a greater audience. Specifically for this book I received invaluable input from Marion Nestle, Alan Hipkiss, and Harold Koenig, all of whom took time to speak with me about their pioneering work.

I am eternally grateful to my parents, June and Charles Merrell, for their unconditional love and for giving me my earliest lessons in healing energy. Deep thanks go to Kathy's parents, Donald and Colleen Healy, for their thoughtful input on the book, constant cheerleading and loving support throughout. Christian Wright gave her characteristically insightful commentary as well as inspiration for the title and for this we are deeply grateful. Many thanks go to Stefanie Bryn Sacks for offering her culinary magic and precious time.

Last but not least, I am forever grateful to all of my patients, for teaching me in countless ways how to create energy.

Index

Abdominal breathing, 39
Acceptance, stoic, 35
Acetaldehyde, 232
Acetylcholine, 28
Acidophilus, 125, 129, 246
Acorn Squash, Cinnamon Roasted, 323
ACTH, 30
Acupressure, 48, 235
Acupuncture, 4, 20, 23, 37, 45–48, 174, 182
Acupuncture Foundation Institute of Canada, 47
Adaptogens, 86–88, 264
Adenosine, 162, 163, 175
Adenosine triphosphate (ATP), 7–8, 60–61, 84, 93, 135, 138, 153, 154
Adrenal glands, 28, 29, 86, 88
Adrenaline, 20, 28–31, 87
Adriamycin, 99
Aerobic exercise, 137–140, 229
AFM Safecoat paint, 115
Agave syrup (nectar), 275
Aging, sleep and, 169–170
Aging process, 58–59
Agriculture, U.S. Department of, 104, 109, 155
Air pollution, 68, 72, 94, 101, 233
Airplane interiors, 118
Alameda County, California, 196
Albert Einstein College of Medicine, 6
Alcohol use, 26, 73, 79, 91, 96, 160, 166, 171–173, 175, 231–232
Alexander Technique, 142
Alginic acid, 123

Allergies, 15, 24
    food, 55, 70, 76–77, 173–174, 227–228, 256
    pillows, 178
Allicin, 122
Allium family, 122, 251
Allostatic load, 34
Almond Cookies, Dark Chocolate Chunk, 355
Alpha-linolenic acid, 69
Aluminum, 119
Alzheimer's disease, 54, 68, 134
Amazon.com, 275
Ambien, 177
American Academy of Acupuncture and Oriental Medicine, 47
American ginseng (Panax quinquefolium), 87, 264
American Heart Association, 249
Amino acids, 52, 53, 59, 63, 64, 66, 84, 100, 183
Amphetamines, 175–176
Anaphylactic allergic reaction, 77
Anemia, 15
Antacids, 174
Anthocyanins, 71
Anthocyanodins, 73
Antianxiety drugs, 22
Antibacterial soap, 116
Antibiotics, 97, 126, 176
    in food, 78, 79, 107, 108, 275
Antidepressant drugs, 22, 30, 53, 136–137, 176, 177
Antihistamine drugs, 176, 177

Antiinflammatory drugs, 176
Antioxidant Fruit Salad, 309
Antioxidants, 64, 66, 72–73, 84–86, 95, 122, 128, 243, 266–267
Antiseizure drugs, 53, 176
Anxiety, 22, 26. *See also* Depression
Apples, Spiced, with Pecan Crumble, 357
Arachidonic acid, 69, 108
Archives of Internal Medicine, 192, 193
Armstrong, Lance, 152
Arsenic, 108, 109
Art therapy, 201
Arthritis, 6, 15, 57, 68, 174, 241
Artichokes with Lemon Aioli, Steamed, 334
Arugula Salad with Crushed Walnuts and Goat Cheese, 310
Ashtanga yoga, 48
Asian ginseng (Panax), 87, 264
Asparagus, Garlic Roasted, 325
ASPCA (American Society for the Prevention of Cruelty to Animals), 108
Astaxanthin, 155
Asthma, 6, 15, 89–90, 93
ATP. *See* Adenosine triphosphate (ATP)
Atrazine, 215, 268–269
Autoimmune diseases, 93, 174
Autonomic nervous system (ANS), 27, 28, 31, 47, 50, 87, 220–221
Ayurvedic Ashwaganda (Withania somnifera), 86, 264

B complex vitamins, 61, 66, 85
Bacon, 106
Bad vs. good stress, 22, 32–35
Baked goods, 75, 78, 105, 228
Balance boards, 146
Balls, exercise, 145
Bands, exercise, 145
Barbiturates, 177
Beatles, the, 40
Bedrooms, 259–260
Bedtime routine, 177–178, 224–225, 238
Behavioral medicine, 186
Behavioral therapy, 181
Benadryl, 177
Benjamin Moore paints, 114
Benson, Herbert, 25–26, 31, 37, 194, 213
Benzodiazepines, 177
Berry Parfait, 353
Beta blockers, 176
Beta-carotene, 83, 263

Beta-Glucan, 125
Beverage recipes
  Cool Mint Lemonade, 358
  Cranberry Tea Infusion, 359
  Dr. Merrell's Fruit Juice, 360
  Dr. Merrell's Veggie Juice, 360
  Mango-Peach Freeze, 361
  Papaya Fizz, 361
  Peach Spritzer with Cranberry Ice, 362
  Tangerine Spritzer with Papaya Ice, 363
Bifidophilus, 125, 129, 246
Biking, 138
Biofeedback, 31, 32, 43–44
Bioflavonoids, 71, 263
Biomolecular medicine, 7
Biotin, 60
Bisphenol A (BPA), 116–117
Bitters, 125, 266
Black Bean Salad, 311
Blackburn, Elizabeth H., 25
Bladder cancer, 106
Bland, Jeffrey, 57
Blood carbon dioxide levels, 39
Blood pressure, 30, 39, 87–88
Blood pressure drugs, 176
Blue-green algae, 85
Bok Choy with Tangy Chili Vinaigrette, 324
Bomb calorimeter, 65
Botanicals (herbs), 53–54, 83, 123, 183–184
Bowel dysfunction, 15
Brain-derived neurotrophic factor (BDNF), 135
Braised Chard, 322
Brassica family, 121–122, 128, 251
Breakfast recipes
  Dr. Merrell's Morning Shake, 298
  French Toast, 299
  Power Up Granola, 300
  Scrambled Tofu and Vegetables, 301
  Vegetable Goat Cheese Egg-White Omelet, 302
Breast cancer, 41, 94, 104, 166
Breast milk, 94, 118
Breath breaks, 36, 38–39, 220–221
Breath work, 16, 20, 21, 149–150
Breathe Right Nasal Strips, 173, 257
Broccoli, 121–122
  Juicy Sweet Roasted, 327
Brussels Sprouts, Scrumptious, 332
Buddhism, 188, 191, 194

Building materials, 114
Burritos, Vegetarian Chili, 349
Burst of Energy Trail Mix, 350
Byrd, Randolph, 193

Cadmium, 119
Caffeine, 52, 55, 56, 66, 79, 91, 175–176, 228, 232
  metabolizing of, 97–99
Calcium, 60, 136, 143, 153, 154
Calcium disodium EDTA, 106
Calories, 63, 65, 81, 105, 235
CalPacific Medical Center, 193
Camellia sinensis, 228
Canadian Food Inspection Agency, 102
Cancer, 33, 71, 84, 93, 111, 241
  bladder, 106
  breast, 41, 94, 104, 166
  colon, 106
  lung, 83, 115
  prostate, 41, 104
  skin, 83
  stomach, 106
Cane sugar, 276
Canine therapy, 202
Canola mayo, 275
Car interiors, 118
Carbohydrates, 70, 74, 76, 78, 235
  complex, 63–64, 66, 75, 79, 81, 153
  loading, 14
Cardamon, 276
Cardiac conditions. See Heart attack; Heart disease
L-carnitine, 84
Carotenes, 73, 82–83
Carotenoids, 124, 263
Carpets, 89, 90, 114, 115, 222
Cat yoga posture, 49
Catalase, 72
Catechins, 71, 228
Cauliflower, Spiced Coconut, 333
Celiac disease, 228
Center for Mindfulness Medicine, University of Massachusettes Department of Medicine, 41
Center of Spirituality, Theology and Health, Duke University Medical Center, 191
Centers for Disease Control, 10, 91
Certified organic labeling, 107, 275
Chakras, 141, 142
Chamomile, 53, 183

Chaplin, Charlie, 24
Chard, Braised, 322
Chemicals. See Toxins
Chewing, 219–220
Chicago Rush Medical Center Department of Ear, Nose, and Throat Medicine, 174
Chicken, 108–110, 258. See also Poultry recipes
  Curry Roasted, 341
  Savory Herb Marinated, 342
  Savory Herb Salad, 317
Child, Julia, 236
Chili, Vegetarian, 348
Chiropractic, 174
Chlorella, 85
Chlorophyll, 73
Chocolate, dark, 243–244
Cholesterol, 6, 69, 96, 240
Chopra, Deepak, 44
Chromosomes, 25, 26
Chronic fatique, 5, 68
Chronic infection, 15
Chronic pain
  sleep and, 174
  stress and, 21
Cigarette smoking, 21, 26, 68, 73, 96, 97, 99
Cinnamon Roasted Acorn Squash, 323
Cipro, 176
Circadian rhythms, 165, 168, 177, 180–182
Citrate, 154
Citrus fruits, 123
Citrus Mint Mixed Berries, 353
Cleaning products, 115–116, 223
Cleveland Clinic, Department of Rehabilitation Medicine and Biomedical Engineering, 152
Co-enzyme Q10 (Ubiquinone), 84
Co-factors, 59, 64, 75, 84–85
Cobb Salad, Vegetarian, 319
Cobra yoga posture, 49
Coco-nutty Banana, 354
Cod, Miso Baked, 338
Codeine, 177
Coffee, 79, 175–176, 228, 232
Coffee enemas, 130
Collard Greens, Sweet and Spicy, 335
Colon cancer, 106
Colonics, 129–130
Colonoscopy, 15, 130

Columbia University, 136, 187
  College of Physicians and Surgeons, 3,
    6, 23
  Department of Medicine, 167
  Mailman School of Public Health,
    Department of Epidemiology, 167
Commerce, U.S. Department of, 105
Communal meal, 241–242
Community service, 197–199, 265
Complex carbohydrates, 63–64, 66, 75, 79,
    81, 153, 236
Conjugators, 97, 98, 100, 122, 128
Connectedness. *See* Spiritual
    connectedness
Consumer Reports, 179
*Consumer's Dictionary of Food Additives,
    A* (Winters), 103
Continuous positive airway pressure
    device (CPAP), 172, 173
Conversational aerobics, 229
Cool Mint Lemonade, 358
Copernicus, 23
Coping styles, 33, 35–36, 40
Copper, 60, 61, 66, 85, 124
Cordyceps (Cordyceps sinensis), 86, 87,
    264
Core training, 141–142
Corn oil, 69, 105
Corn syrup, 105
Coronary artery disease, 6, 68
Cortisol, 28–30, 39, 41, 86, 87, 141, 162,
    165, 169, 187
Cortisone, 20, 30, 86
Corvallis Psychiatric Clinic, Oregon, 181
Cosmetics, 101, 119, 120, 223
Coumarin paradisin, 99
Cousins Center for
    Psychoneuroimmunology, University
    of California at Los Angeles
    Neuropsychiatric Institute, 51
Cow's milk, 78–79, 107–108
Cranberry Tea Infusion, 359
Creatine, 154
Crisis management, 269–270
Crohn's disease, 68
Cruciferous vegetables, 121–122, 251
Crunches, 142, 144, 158, 229–230
Crunchy Bok Choy with Tangy Chili
    Vinaigrette, 324
Cucumber Wakame Salad, 312
Curry powder, 275
Curry Roasted Chicken, 341

Cytochrome (P450s), 97–99, 232
Cytokines, 41, 68–70, 165, 169, 174, 175,
    188, 241
Cytoplasm, 26

Daily Spiritual Experience Scale, 190
Dairy products, 78–79, 107–108
Dalai Lama, 188, 245
Dalmane, 177
Dance therapy, 201
Dark Chocolate Chunk Almond Cookies,
    355
Dark Chocolate Dairy-Free Mousse, 356
Dark therapy, 180–181
David Geffen School of Medicine,
    University of California at Los
    Angeles, 197–198
DDT, 102, 111
De Qi sensation, 46
Decongestants, 176
Dehydration, 123, 126
Delayed food allergies, 76
Denial, of stress, 35
Depression
    antidepressant drugs, 22, 30, 53,
        136–137, 176, 177
    exercise and, 136–137
    SAMe (S-adenosyl-methionine) and, 53
    seasonal affective disorder (SAD), 180
    spirituality and, 191
    stress leading to, 26
Descartes, René, 23
Dessert recipes
    Berry Parfait, 353
    Citrus Mint Mixed Berries, 353
    Coco-nutty Banana, 354
    Dark Chocolate Chunk Almond
        Cookies, 355
    Dark Chocolate Dairy-Free Mousse,
        356
    Spiced Apples with Pecan Crumble,
        357
Detoxification, 8, 10, 91, 94–101, 121–130
    fasting, 127–128
    food and, 121–123, 251–252
    gut optimization, 121, 128–129
    juice cleanse, 121, 127–128, 249,
        250–251
    saunas, 121, 126
    sleep and, 62, 81, 121–130
    supplements and, 121, 124–125, 256
    in 21-Day Plan, 221–224, 231–232

Diabetes, 6, 15, 68, 71, 93, 117, 155, 161, 166
Diet. *See* Food and nutrition
Diethanolamine (DEA), 120
Digestion. *See also* Food and nutrition
  stress and, 32
Dioxane, 120
Dioxins, 111, 126
Disinfectants, 111
DNA (deoxyribonucleic acid), 7, 8, 25–27, 30, 32, 56–58, 63, 65–66, 71, 93, 126, 132
Dr. Merrell's Fruit Juice, 360
Dr. Merrell's Morning Shake, 243, 298
Dr. Merrell's Veggie Juice, 360
Dopamine, 30, 52, 104, 137
Dossey, Larry, 194, 206
Douglas, William O., 202
Down's syndrome, 53
Downward-Facing Dog yoga posture (Adhomukha Svanasana), 49, 156–157
Dreaming, 160, 163–165, 233–234
Drugs. *See* Medications
Du Pont Corporation, 102
Duke University, 136, 190, 191
Dust, 89, 115
Dyes, 94

Early Morning Wake-Up Call, in 21-Day Plan, 171, 212–213, 218–219, 226, 239
Eating. *See* Food and nutrition
E.coli, 102, 107
Elavil, 177
Electro-encephalograms (EEGs), 194
Elimination diet, 77–79, 173–174
Ellagic acid, 123
Emory University, Rollins School of Public Health, 105
Emotional Intelligence (Goleman), 36
Endorphins, 24, 30, 31, 41, 47, 133, 182, 187
Enemas, coffee, 130
Energy drinks and bars, 5, 66, 75, 76
Energy medicine, 203–204, 263–264
Energy metabolism, 7–8
Energy of Prayer, The (Nhat Hanh), 43
Ensure Complete Balanced Nutrition, 76
Entrees. *See* Fish entrees; Poultry entrees. Vegetarian entrees
Environmental Defense Fund, 112

Environmental Health Perspectives (National Institute of Environmental Health Sciences), 102
Environmental pollution, 62, 68, 72, 94, 101, 233
Environmental Protection Agency (EPA), 92, 102, 110, 114
Environmental Science and Technology, 118
Environmental toxins. *See* Toxins
Environmental Working Group, 94, 101
Enzymes, 63, 64, 95–97, 135, 136, 220, 266
Equine therapy, 202
Erythromycin, 97
Essential fatty acids (EFAs), 70, 71, 258, 261
Estrogen, 104, 122
Exercise, 8, 10, 73, 131–158. *See also* Yoga
  aerobic, 137–140, 229
  benefits of, 132–133
  brain and, 134–135
  case history, 131–132
  core training, 141–142
  crunches, 142, 144, 158, 229–230
  depression and, 136–137
  energy creation and, 133–136
  equipment, 145–146
  food and nutrition and, 153
  heart rate and, 132, 138, 139, 141, 152, 237, 249
  hopping, 157–158
  interval training, 140
  martial arts, 146–149
  music and, 151–152, 158
  overexercising, 137, 140–141
  push-ups, 144, 145, 158, 230
  strength training, 143–145
  supplements and, 153–155
  in 21-Day Plan, 224, 226, 229–230, 237, 247, 253–254, 256
  visualization techniques and, 151, 156
  walking, 138, 139, 156, 224, 229, 237, 249, 252
  warm ups, 152–153
Expiration dates, 117
Expressive writing, 201

FACIT *Spiritual Well Being* scale, 190
Family doctors, 187
Family risk factors, 15
Family structure, 199, 200
Farmed fish, 111, 236

Fatique, 4–5, 19–20, 24, 33, 34
  chronic fatigue, 5, 68
Fats, 63–65, 68–70, 78, 81, 96, 240, 241,
    253, 258
Fatty acids, 59, 84, 155
Feng shui, 259–260
Fenugreek seed, 155
Fetzer Institute, 187
Fiber, 79, 81, 122, 123, 128, 129
Fibrin, 68
Fight-or-flight mechanism, 28
Fighting spirit, 35
Fish, 57, 64, 69, 79, 91, 99
  farmed, 111, 236
  monthly allotment of, 112–113
  shopping for, 236
  toxins in, 110–113
Fish recipes
  Halibut Puttanesca, 337
  Miso Baked Cod, 338
  Trout with Lemon and Herbs in
    Parchment, 339
  Walnut-Pesto Wild Salmon, 340
Fishing industry, 111
Flavonoids, 73, 244
Flavorings and flavor enhancers, 103
Flaxseed oil, 57, 69
Flu vaccine, 167
Flu viruses, 96
Folic acid, 83
Food additives, 96
Food allergies, 55, 70, 76–77, 173–174,
    227–228, 256
Food and Drug Administration (FDA),
    102, 117
Food and nutrition, 8, 10, 55–88. See also
    Supplements
  baked goods, 75, 78, 105, 228
  calories, 63, 65, 81, 105, 235
  carbohydrates, 63, 70, 74, 76, 78, 235
  L-carnitine, 84
  case history, 55–56
  complex carbohydrates, 63–64, 66, 75,
    79, 81, 153, 236
  crisis management and, 269–270
  detoxification and, 121–123, 251–252
  elimination diet, 77–79, 173–174
  energy drinks and bars, 66, 75, 76
  exercise and, 153
  fats, 63–65, 68–70, 78, 81, 96, 240, 241,
    253, 258
  fiber, 79, 81, 122, 123, 128, 129

fish, 57, 64, 69, 79, 91, 99, 110–113, 236
  flavorings and flavor enhancers, 103
  food allergies, 55, 70, 76–77
  food labels, 58
  food sensitivities, 76–77
  foods to avoid, 78–79
  frozen food, 81
  fruit, 59, 73–74, 103–104, 123
  glycation and, 62, 67, 74–75, 78, 269
  green drinks, 85
  green tea, 52, 73, 122, 228–229, 232, 251
  inflammation and, 62, 67–71, 78, 269
  Krebs cycle and, 61, 62
  making energy, 59–65
  meat, 64, 65, 69, 73, 78, 79, 105,
    107–108, 240–241, 258–259
  organic food, 103–108, 219, 275
  oxidation and, 62, 67, 72–74, 78, 269
  pantry notes, 275–276
  power foods, 79–82
  processed foods, 56, 57, 105–107
  proteins, 63, 64, 79, 81, 96
  salt, 101, 106, 241, 276
  sugar, 63, 64, 66, 67, 73–76, 79
  toxins and, 102–113
  in 21-Day Plan, 214, 219, 220, 226–228,
    240–241, 243–244, 246–247,
    258–259
  vegetables, 59, 65, 73–74, 79, 81,
    121–122
  whole grains, 56, 57, 63–64, 123
  yogurt, 123, 128, 129
Food labels, 58, 73
Food processor, 275
Food pyramids, 64
Food sensitivities, 76–77
Forgiveness, 219, 238, 254
Formaldehyde, 115, 120
Free radicals, 58, 61, 66, 72–73, 78, 84, 91,
    93, 96, 100, 122, 136, 140, 162, 266
French fries, 63
French Toast, 299
Frozen food, 81
Fructo-Oligo-Saccharides, 125
Fruit, 59, 73–74, 103–104, 123
Functional medicine, 4, 57
Functional MRIs (fMRI), 194

GABA (gamma-aminobutyric acid)
    receptor, 52, 165
Galen, 137
Game playing, 270–271

Gamma-linolenic acid, 69
Garlic, 122
Garlic Roasted Asparagus, 325
Gastro-Esophageal Reflux Disease
    (GERD), 174
Gastrointestinal disorders, stress and,
    21
Genetic polymorphism, 97
Genetically modified (GMO) crops,
    105–106
German Sleep Medicine Lab, 178
Ghrelin, 167–168
Ginseng, 85, 87, 264
Global warming, 92
Glucose, 59, 84, 96, 155
Glutamate receptors, 52
L-glutamine, 125
Glutathione reductase, 72
Gluten, 227–228
Glycation, 62, 67, 74–75, 78, 269
Glycemic index (GI), 70, 75
Glycemic load (GL), 74, 75
Glycine, 125
Glycogen, 96, 140, 155
GMP (good manufacturing principles),
    83
God, Faith and Healing (Levin), 197
Goleman, Daniel, 36, 198
Gomasio, 276
Gomez-Pinilla, Fernando, 134
Good vs. bad stress, 22, 32–35
Gottschall, L. Douglas, 195, 196
Granola, 66
    recipe, 300
Grapefruit juice, 99
Green drinks, 85
Green Guide, The, 222
Green tea, 52, 73, 122, 228–229, 232, 251
Greenguard.org, 114
Growth hormone, 30, 78, 79, 107, 169
Grudges, letting go of, 219, 230, 254
Guacamole, 351
Guided imagery, 31, 32, 44–45

Halibut Puttanesca, 337
Handwashing, 116
Harvard Medical School, 190
Harvard School of Public Health, 61,
    167
Harvard University, 37, 190, 199
Harvest Wild Rice, 326
Hatha yoga, 48

Headaches, 15, 26
Healing Beyond the Body (Dossey), 194
Healing Foods (Murray and Pizzorno), 74
Heart attack, 59–60, 170, 172
    caffeine and, 97–99
    Type A personalities and, 33–34
Heart disease, 15, 21, 57, 71, 83, 161, 166,
    167, 241
Heart rate
    exercise and, 132, 138, 139, 141, 152,
        237, 249
    responsiveness, 41
Heart rate variability (HRV), 31–32, 52
HeartMath, 43
Heavy metals, 68, 85, 110, 115, 119, 121,
    123
HEPA filters, 90, 115, 233
Herbicides, 102, 111, 219, 268
Herbs, 4, 53–54, 83, 123, 183–184
    adaptogens, 86–88, 264
Heterocyclic amines, 258
High fructose corn syrup, 67, 75, 105, 106,
    276
Hijiki Salad, Warm, 320
Hipkiss, Alan R., 127, 135
Histamine, 77
Hoffman, Hunter, 44
Holotropic breath work, 38
Homeopathy, 4, 54
Hopping, 157–158
Hormonal imbalance, 15
Hormone disruption, 104, 116–118
Hormones
    adrenaline, 20, 28–31, 87
    cortisol, 28–30, 39, 41, 86, 87, 141, 162,
        165, 169, 187
    dopamine, 30, 52, 104, 137
    endorphins, 24, 30, 31, 41, 47, 133, 182,
        187
    estrogen, 104, 122
    melatonin, 24, 165, 168, 180, 182–183,
        250
    serotonin, 24, 30, 31, 41, 52, 53, 87, 133,
        137, 162
    testosterone, 11, 169
Hot dogs, 106
Household products, 114–116
5-HTP (5-hydroxy-tryptophan), 53, 183
Humane Farm Animal Care Program,
    108
Hummus Wrap, Lemon Parsley, 344
Humor, sense of, 24

Hydrocodone, 177
Hydroquinone, 120
Hypertension, 6, 87
Hypothalamic-pituitary-adrenal (HPA)
    axis, 27, 28–31, 47, 188
Hypothalamus, 28, 29
Hypothyroid, 15

IgE and IgG antibodies, 77
Immediate food allergies, 76
Immune-Boost Soup, 303
Immune system, 15, 24, 29, 30, 33, 67–68,
    86, 96, 111, 131, 166, 174, 188
Inderal, 176
Indigestion, 32, 220
Indole-3 carbinol, 122
Infertility, 104
Inflammation, 62, 67–71, 78, 174–175,
    214, 269
Insomnia, 159–160, 166, 170–171,
    175–177, 180, 181
Institute of Noetic Sciences, 204
Insulin, 29, 65, 154, 162, 235
Interleukin 6, 169, 175, 196
Interleukin 12, 162
Interleukins, 30, 174
Internet communities, 199
Interval training, 140
Intestinal tract, 95–96
Intimate relationships, 199–200
Inulin, 125
Iodide, 101–102
Iron, 60, 61, 64, 85
Irritable bowel syndrome, 6, 26
Isolation, feelings of, 197–198
Iyengar, B.K.S., 150, 157
Iyengar yoga, 48

Jet lag, 168, 177, 183
Jivamukti, 247
Jivamukti yoga, 48
Johns Hopkins School of Medicine, 190,
    191
Journal of Holistic Nursing, 204
Journal of the American Medical
    Association (JAMA), 97, 187, 201
Journal of the U.S. National Institute of
    Environmental Health, 99
Journaling, 201
Juice cleanse, 15, 121, 127–128, 249,
    250–251
Juices, 276

Juicy Sweet Roasted Broccoli, 327
Jump ropes, 146, 157

Kabat-Zinn, Jon, 41, 267, 268
Kale with Garlic, Sauteed, 331
Kava kava, 184
Ketchup, 63
Kindness, random acts of, 265
Klonopin, 177
Koenig, Harold, 188, 191
Krebs cycle, 61, 62, 154
Krebs Cycle Nutrient Co-Factors, 84–85
Krieger, Dolores, 204
Kripalu yoga, 48
Kundalini yoga, 38, 48

Lactic acid, 136
Lactobacillus, 123
Lactose intolerance, 77
Laser acupuncture, 48
Lasker Prize, 25
Laugh log, 246, 261
Laughter, 24
Laundry detergent, 116
Lavender oil (Lavandula
    officinalis/angustifolia), 54
Lawns, 268
Laxatives, 130
Lead, 93, 119, 120, 215
Leafy Greens and Chickpea Salad, 313
Lemon balm (Melissa officinalis), 53–54
Lemon Parsley Hummus, 352
Lemon Parsley Hummus Wrap, 344
Lemonade, Cool Mint, 358
Lentils, Warm French, 336
Leptin, 167–168, 235
Letter writing, 259
Levin, Jeffrey, 197
Levitin, Daniel J., 201
Licorice root, 87–88
Life expectancy, 58
Light therapy, 179–180, 183, 250
Linolenic acid, 69
Lipitor, 84
Lipoic acid, 125
Liver detox, 93, 95–100
Liver disease, 15
Locus of control, 34
Loneliness, 197–198
Longevity, 58–59
Lunch meat, 106
Lunesta, 177

Lung cancer, 83, 115
Lutein, 263
Lycopene, 263
Lyme disease, 174
Lymphatic system, 96

Magnesium, 53, 60, 85, 90, 153
Magnesium citrate, 154
Magneto-acupuncture, 48
Mammograms, 15
Mango-Peach Freeze, 361
Mantras, 40–42
Marine algae extract, 155
Martial arts, 146–149, 265
Massachusetts General Hospital, 190, 235
Massage, 234–235, 245–246
Mattresses, 178–179, 222, 248
Meat, 64, 65, 69, 73, 78, 79, 97, 105, 107–108, 240–241, 258–259
Medical problems, screening for, 15
Medications
   antianxiety, 22
   antidepressant, 22, 30, 53, 136–137, 176, 177
   antihistamine, 176, 177
   antiinflammatory, 176
   antiseizure, 53, 176
   blood pressure, 176
   grapefruit juice and, 99
   side effects, 15
   sleep and, 176–177
   sleeping pills, 5, 22, 159–160, 177
   SSRIs (selective serotonin reuptake inhibitors), 30, 53, 176, 177
   statins, 6, 84
   steroids, 6, 173
   triptan, 30
Meditation, 4, 20, 21, 25–26, 31, 32, 36, 40–45, 191
   benefits of, 41
   biofeedback, 31, 32, 43–44
   environment for, 42
   guided imagery, 31, 32, 44–45
   mantras, 40–42
   mindfulness, 40, 42–43, 191, 219, 267–268
   mountain stream, 45
   position for, 41
   single-pointed, 40, 42
Mediterranean Tuna Salad, 314
Melatonin, 24, 165, 168, 180, 182–183, 250

Men's Health magazine, 145
Menstrual cycle, 118
Menuhin, Yehudi, 212
Menus, 11, 277–297
Mercury, 93, 95, 110–112, 119, 120, 121, 126, 215, 236
Mesclun Greens with Balsamic Vinaigrette, 315
Metabolism, 3, 58, 73, 167
Methionine, 52
Migraines, 30
Milk thistle, 122, 125
Mind-body connection, 22, 23–26, 30
Mind/Body Medical Institute, Harvard University, 37
Mindfulness meditation, 40, 42–42, 191, 219, 267–268
Minerals, 59–61, 63, 64, 83, 85, 124
Mirin, 276
Miso Baked Cod, 338
Mitchell, Edgar, 204
Mitochondria, 7, 8, 26, 27, 57, 59–62, 72, 84, 128, 132, 135, 166
Mixed Green Salad, Power Protein, 316
Modern Times (movie), 24
Mold, 89, 90
Monosodium glutamate (MSG), 275
Monounsaturated fats, 64, 66, 70, 253
Monterey Bay Aquarium Seafood Watch, 236
Mormons, 195–196
Mountain stream meditation, 45
Mountain with Bound Arms yoga posture, 49
Mousse, Dark Chocolate Dairy-Free, 356
Moving Toward Balance (Yee), 157
MRI (magnetic resonance imaging), 23
MSM (Methyl-sulf-methane), 125
Multiple sclerosis, 174
Multivitamins, 262–263
Murray, Michael, 74
Muscle fatique and soreness, 136
Musculoskeletal and Human Physiology Lab, Oklahoma State University, 179
Music, exercise and, 151–152, 158
Music therapy, 201

NAC/glutathione, 125
NAC (N-acetyl-cysteine), 124, 154–155
Naparstek, Belleruth, 37–38
Napping, 161, 162, 167, 244
Naproxen, 176

Narcotics, 177
Nasonex, 173
National Institute of Environmental
    Health Sciences, 102, 108
National Institutes of Health, 114
Natural killer cells, 33, 68, 235
Nature, 202–203, 244
Nestle, Marion, 106, 107
Neuropeptide web (NPW), 27, 30, 31,
    204–205
Neuropeptides, 24, 30, 31, 47
Neurotransmitters, 39, 41, 46, 47, 53, 133,
    137, 162, 182, 228
NF-kB (nuclear factor-kappa beta), 71
Nhat Hanh, Thich, 42, 43, 260,
    267–268
Nightmares, 170, 176
Nitrate, 106
Nitrite, 106
NMDA (N-methyl-D-aspartate)
    receptors, 53, 165
Non-rapid eye movement (NREM) sleep,
    164, 165, 169, 178, 181, 242
Nonlocality, 205, 206
Noradrenaline, 137
NSF International, 215, 216
Nurses Health Study, 167
Nursing mothers, 24
Nutrient deficiencies, 15
Nuts/seeds, 122, 252

Obesity, 21, 68, 93, 117, 129, 161,
    166–168, 171, 235
Offgassing, 115
Oklahoma State University
    Musculoskeletal and Human
    Physiology Lab, 179
Omega-3 fatty acids, 64, 69, 70, 90, 110,
    111, 236, 253, 261
Omega-6 fatty acids, 69
One-day juice cleanse, 121, 127–128, 249,
    250–251
Onions, 122, 219
Orexins, 165
Organic food, 103–108, 219, 275
Organophosphate pesticides, 96
Ornish, Dean, 44, 197
Overexercising, 137, 140–141
Oxidation, 62, 67, 72–74, 78, 269
Oxidative stress, 100
Oxygen, 41, 59, 72, 134, 149
Ozone, 118

Pain management, guided imagery and,
    44–45
Paints, 114, 115, 222
Pantry notes, 275–276
Papaya Fizz, 220, 361
Parabens, 120
Parasympathetic nervous system, 28, 31,
    40, 41, 47, 50, 133, 164, 170, 173
Parkinson's disease, 53, 68
Passion flower (Passiflora incarnata), 54,
    184
Paxil, 177
PCBs (polychlorinated biphenyls), 95, 99,
    102, 111, 126
Peach Spritzer with Cranberry Ice, 362
Peale, Norman Vincent, 36
Peanuts, allergy to, 76, 77
Penn State University Division of Allergy,
    173
Perchlorate, 101–102
Perspiration, 126
Pert, Candace, 24
Pesticides, 78, 94–97, 99, 102–105, 111,
    219, 268
PET scans, 194
Phase I and II liver detox system, 97–100,
    122, 128
Phenobarbital, 177
Phenylenediamine, 120
Phenylethanolamine, 243
Phosphocreatine, 154
Phthalates, 118, 120
Physician's Desk References (PDR), 84
Phytochemicals, 121–122, 128
Pilates, 142
Pillows, 178, 248
Pineal gland, 165
Pituitary gland, 29, 30
Pizzorno, Joseph, 74
Plasters, 114
Plastics, 116–118
Platelets, 68
Polyethyelene, 117
Polypharmacy, 177
Polyphenols, 71
Polypropylene, 117
Polyunsaturated fats, 69
Polyvinyl chloride (PVC), 118
Positive thinking, power of, 36
Posture, 142–143
    breath breaks and, 39
Potassium, 154–155

Poultry recipes
   Curry Roasted Chicken, 341
   Savory Herb Marinated Chicken, 342
   Turkey Bolognese over Spaghetti
      Squash, 343
Power Protein Mixed Green Salad, 316
Power Up Granola, 300
Power Up! Quiz, 13–14
Power yoga, 48
Prana, 48, 141
Pranayama, 149–150
Pranayama yoga, 48
Prayer, 191, 192–195
Prebiotics, 125
Pregnancy massage, 235
Pregnant women, 15
Probiotics, 85, 90, 125, 128, 129, 246–247
Processed foods, 56, 57, 105–107
Prostate cancer, 41, 104
Proteins, 63, 64, 79, 81, 96
Provigil, 5
Prozac, 30, 176
Pseudophedrine, 176
Psycho-neuro-immunology (PNI), 3, 23
Purges, 130
Push-ups, 144, 145, 158, 230
Pyruvate, 154

Qi, 46, 51, 141, 142, 217
Qi gong, 146–147, 149, 203
Qi Gong Energy Ball, 157
Quantum physics, 4, 205, 206
Quercetin, 122
Quick Italian Vegetable Soup, 304
Quinoa, 276
   with Scallions and Toasted Sesame Oil,
      328
   with Sliced Avocado, 329
   Tabouli, 330
Quiz. See Power Up! Quiz

Rapid eye movement (REM) sleep, 164,
      165, 168, 170, 178, 181, 233, 242
Reactive oxygen species. See Free radicals
Rebound sleep, 233
Recipes, 11, 298–363
   beverage, 358–363
   breakfast, 298–302
   dessert, 353–357
   fish, 337–340
   poultry, 341–343
   salad, 309–321

   side dish, 322–336
   snack, 350–352
   soup, 303–308
   vegetarian, 344–349
Recombinant bovine somatropin (rbST),
    107
Rectus abdominus, 141
Red berries, 123, 252
Red curry paste, 276
Red Curry Tofu with Basil, 345
Red Lentil Soup, 305
Red wine, 123
Reiki, 203, 204, 263
Reincarnation, 189
Relaxation, 8, 20, 21, 28, 31, 32
   botanicals (herbs) and, 53–54
   breath breaks, 36, 38–39
   guide to best exercises, 36–38
   meditation. See Meditation
   sleep and, 160, 162, 181–182
   in 21-Day Plan, 213, 231
Religion, 40, 195–197
Reproductive disorders, 93, 104, 111,
    116
Resilience, 35
Resp-e-rate, 43
Resveratrol, 85, 123
Rheumatoid arthritis, 24, 127, 129
D-Ribose, 154
Rice milk, 79
Rogan, Eleanor, 122
Rollins School of Public Health, Emory
    University, 105
Roosevelt Hospital, New York, 4
Rosemary Butternut Squash Soup,
    306
Roundup weed-killer, 105
Rozerem, 177
Runner's high, 136
Russian Arctic Root (Rhodiola rosea),
    86–87, 264

Sacks, Stefanie Bryn, 236, 273
Safecosmetics.org, 119
Safflower oil, 69
St. Luke's Hospital, Kansas City, Missouri,
    193
Salad recipes
   Antioxidant Fruit Salad, 309
   Arugula Salad with Crushed Walnuts
      and Goat Cheese, 310
   Black Bean Salad, 311

Salad recipes (*cont.*)
   Cucumber Wakame Salad, 312
   Leafy Greens and Chickpea Salad, 313
   Mediterranean Tuna Salad, 314
   Mesclun Greens with Balsamic
     Vinaigrette, 315
   Power Protein Mixed Green Salad, 316
   Savory Herb Chicken Salad, 317
   Sweet Spinach Salad, 318
   Vegetarian Cobb Salad, 319
   Warm Hijiki Salad, 320
   Watercress Arugula Salad, 321
Salk Institute, 134
Salmon, Walnut-Pesto Wild, 340
Salmonella, 102, 108
Salt, 101, 106, 241, 276
SAMe (S-adenosyl-methionine), 52–53,
   124
Saturated fats, 64, 69, 76, 81, 108, 240,
   241, 253, 258
Saunas, 121, 126
Sauteed Kale with Garlic, 331
Savory Herb Chicken Salad, 317
Savory Herb Marinated Chicken, 342
Schapiro, Mark, 118
Schizandra, 125
Schwartz, Gary, 203
Scrambled Tofu and Vegetables, 301
Screening tests, 15
Scrumptious Brussels Sprouts, 332
Seasonal affective disorder (SAD), 180
Seated Warrior (Virasana), 156
Seaweed, 85, 123, 252
Seconal, 177
Selenium, 83, 124
Self-awareness, 36, 40
Serotonin, 24, 30, 31, 41, 52, 53, 87, 133,
   137, 162
Seventh Day Adventists, 195–196
Shiatsu, 48, 235
Shitake-Miso Soup, 307
Shiva, 185–186
Shizandra (Shizandra Chinensis), 87
Shower curtains, vinyl, 222, 223
Shrimp, allergy to, 76, 77
Siberian ginseng (Eleutherococcus), 85,
   87
Side dish recipes
   Braised Chard, 322
   Cinnamon Roasted Acorn Squah, 323
   Crunchy Bok Choy with Tangy Chili
     Vinaigrette, 324
   Garlic Roasted Asparagus, 325
   Harvest Wild Rice, 326
   Juicy Sweet Roasted Broccoli, 327
   Quinoa Tabouli, 330
   Quinoa with Scallions and Toasted
     Sesame Oil, 328
   Quinoa with Sliced Avocado, 329
   Sauteed Kale with Garlic, 331
   Scrumptious Brussels Sprouts, 332
   Spiced Coconut Cauliflower, 333
   Steamed Artichokes with Lemon Aioli,
     334
   Sweet and Spicy Collard Greens, 335
   Warm French Lentils, 336
Silent Spring Institute, 93
Single-pointed meditation, 40, 42
Sinus congestion, chronic, 173–174,
   256–257
Sirtuins (SIRT 1–7), 128
Skin cancer, 83
Sleep, 8, 11, 140, 141, 159–184, 263
   acupuncture and, 182
   aging and, 169–170
   bedtime routine, 177–178, 224–225,
     238
   behavioral therapy and, 181
   case history, 159–160
   causes of bad sleep, 169–177
   dark therapy and, 180–181
   detoxification and, 62, 81, 121–130
   dreaming, 160, 163–165, 233–234
   guided imagery and, 44
   herbs and, 54
   insomnia, 159–160, 166, 170, 175–177,
     180, 181
   jet lag and, 168, 177, 183
   light therapy and, 179–180
   mattresses, 178–179, 248
   napping, 161, 162, 167, 244
   nightmares, 170, 176
   non-rapid eye movement (NREM),
     164, 165, 169, 178, 181, 242
   pillows, 178, 248
   rapid eye movement (REM), 164, 165,
     168, 170, 178, 181, 233, 242
   reasons for, 161–163
   rebound sleep, 233
   regenerative, 161–165
   relaxation and, 160, 162, 181–182
   slow-wave, 164, 165, 168, 175
   snoring, 171, 173, 256, 257
   states of, 164–165, 242

stress and, 170–171
supplements and, 182–184
in 21-Day Plan, 217, 247–248
Sleep apnea, 171–172, 174, 256–257
Sleeping pills, 5, 22, 159–160, 177
Slimfast Meal-On-the-Go, 76
Slow-wave sleep, 164, 165, 168, 175
Smoking, 21, 26, 68, 73, 96, 97, 99
Snack recipes
    Burst of Energy Trail Mix, 350
    Guacamole, 351
    Lemon Parsley Hummus, 352
Snoring, 171, 173, 256, 257
Snow World software program, 44
Soaps, 116
Social Intelligence (Goleman), 198
Sodium, 154, 155
Solvents, 115
Sominex, 177
Sonata, 177
Soup recipes
    Immune-Boost Soup, 303
    Quick Italian Vegetbale Soup, 304
    Red Lentil Soup, 305
    Rosemary Butternut Squash Soup,
        306
    Shitake-Miso Soup, 307
    White Bean Kale Soup, 308
Soy milk, 79
Spiced Apples with Pecan Crumble, 357
Spiced Coconut Cauliflower, 333
Spices, cooking with, 241
Spinach Salad, Sweet, 318
Spiritual connectedness, 4, 8, 11, 185–206,
    271
    case history, 185–186
    community and, 197–199, 265
    energy healers and, 203–204
    intimate relationships and, 199–200
    medicine and, 189–192
    music and art and, 201
    nature and, 202–203, 244
    prayer and, 191, 192–195
    religion and, 195–197
Spirulina, 85
Sports massage, 235
SSRIs (selective serotonin reuptake
    inhibitors), 30, 53, 176, 177
Staff yoga posture, 49
Statin drugs, 6, 84
Staying Well with Guided Imagery!
    (Naparstek), 37

Steamed Artichokes with Lemon Aioli,
    334
Steroids, 6, 173
Stoic acceptance, 35
Stomach cancer, 106
Strength training, 143–145
Stress, 9–10, 19–54
    acupuncture and, 45–48
    anatomy of, 26–32
    case history, 19–20, 33–34
    coping styles and, 33, 35–36, 40
    digestion and, 32
    as factor in illness, 21–22
    good vs. bad, 22, 32–35
    heart rate variability (HRV) and, 31–32
    homeopathy and, 54
    insomnia and, 160, 166, 170–171
    log, 216–217, 230, 240, 255, 261
    mind-body connection and, 22, 23–26
    sources of, 22
    supplements and, 32, 52–54
    tai chi and, 36, 51–52
    tipping point for, 34
    Type A personalities and, 33–34
    yoga and. *See* Yoga
Stress Busters, 43
Sucrose, 74
Sudafed, 176
Sugar, 63, 64, 66, 67, 73–76, 79
Sugar substitutes, 228–229
Sulfur, 61, 122
Sulfurophanes, 122
Sulfurous vegetables, 122, 251
Sun exposure, 72
Sun Salutation, 226, 227
Sunflower oil, 69
Sunscreen, 95, 101
Superoxide dismutase, 72
Supplements, 15, 82–85
    adaptogens, 86–88, 264
    antioxidants, 266
    Co-enzyme Q10 (Ubiquinone), 84
    detoxification and, 121, 124–125, 256
    exercise and, 153–155
    green drinks, 85
    Krebs Cycle Nutrient Co-Factors, 84–85
    L-theanine, 52
    SAMe (S-adenosyl-methionine), 52–53
    sleep and, 182–184
    stress and, 32, 52–54
Suspending judgment, 150
Sweet and Spicy Collard Greens, 335

Sweet Spinach Salad, 318
Swimming, 138
Sympathetic nervous system, 28, 41, 47, 52, 164, 171, 173, 175

T-cells, meditation and, 41
Tai chi, 4, 36, 51–52, 142, 146, 149
Tangerine Spritzer with Papaya Ice, 363
Tap water, 214–215
Targ, Elizabeth, 193
Teflon, 102, 222, 223
Television viewing, 254
Telomerase, 25
Telomeres, 25, 26, 93
10-Minute Evening Unwind, 261
Terman, Michael, 179
Testosterone, 11, 169
L-theanine, 52, 183, 228
Theobroma coca, 243
Theophylline, 52
Theosomatic medicine, 196
Therapeutic (healing) touch, 203–204, 263
This Is Your Brain on Music (Levitin), 201
Thistle family, 122, 251
Thyroid, 104, 165
Thyroid stimulating hormone, 30
Tibetan Buddhism, 188
Tipping point, 34
Tofu, Red Curry, with Basil, 345
Tofu Vegetable Stir-Fry, 346
Toluene, 120
Tooth or gum disease, 15
Toprol, 176
Toxic Chemistry of Everyday Products and What's at Stake for American Power, The (Schapiro), 118
Toxic intermediaries, 97
Toxins, 3, 89–130. See also Detoxification
    carpets, 89, 90, 114, 115, 222
    case history, 89–90
    cleaning products, 115–116, 223
    cosmetics, 101, 119, 120, 223
    food and nutrition and, 102–113
    heavy metals, 68, 85, 110, 115, 119, 121, 123
    household products, 114–116
    mattresses, 222
    paints, 114, 115, 222
    PCBs (polychlorinated biphenyls), 95, 99, 102, 111, 126
    plastics, 116–118

volatile organic compounds (VOCs), 90, 101, 114–116, 223
    in water, 214–215
    in workplace, 232–233
Trail Mix, Burst of Energy, 350
Trans fats, 78, 253
Transcendental meditation, 40
Transverse abdominus, 141, 142
Triclocarbon (triclosan), 116
Triclosan, 120
Tricyclics, 177
Triglycerides, 96
Triptan drugs, 30
Trout with Lemon and Herbs in Parchment, 339
True Love (Nhat Hanh), 267–268
Tryptophan, 53, 183
Tumor necrosis factor, 30, 68
Tuna Salad, Mediterranean, 314
Turkey Bolognese over Spaghetti Squash, 343
Turmeric, 71, 90, 252
21-Day Plan, 8, 11, 15, 56, 64–65, 77, 79, 81, 209–271. See also Detoxification; Exercise; Food and nutrition; Sleep; Spiritual connectedness; Stress
    menus, 277–297
    negotiating change on, 210–212
    recipes. See Recipes
    Week One, 209, 212–244
    Week Two, 209–210, 245–260
    Week Three, 210, 260–271
Twin studies, 190
Two-Minute Energy Boost, 226
Type A personalities, 33–34

Ulcerative colitis, 68
Umbilical cord, chemicals found in, 94, 118
Uncoupling protein-1 (UCP-1), 166
Universitry of Arizona, 203
University of Calgary, 41
University of California
    at Irvine, 41
    at Los Angeles, 134–135
    at Los Angeles David Geffen School of Medicine, 197–198
    at Los Angeles Neuropsychiatric Institute, 51
    at San Diego, 190
    San Francisco School of Medicine, 193

University of Chicago Department of Medicine, 167
University of Colorado Department of Medicine, 191
University of Massachusettes Department of Medicine, 41
University of Pennsylvania, 190
University of Washington Human Interface Technology Lab, 44
Urban yoga, 48
Uvulectomy, 173

Vacations, 260–261
Vacuum cleaners, 115
Vagus nerve, 28, 194
Valerian (Valeriana officinalis), 54, 183, 184
Valium, 177
Vegetable Biryani, 347
Vegetable Goat Cheese Egg-White Omelet, 302
Vegetables, 59, 65, 73–74, 79, 81, 121–122, 251
Vegetarian Chili, 348
Vegetarian Chili Burritos, 349
Vegetarian Cobb Salad, 319
Vegetarian dishes, 276
Vegetarian entrée recipes
    Lemon Parsley Hummus Wrap, 344
    Red Curry Tofu with Basil, 345
    Tofu Vegetable Stir-Fry, 346
    Vegetable Biryani, 347
    Vegetarian Chili, 348
    Vegetarian Chili Burritos, 349
Videogames, biofeedback and, 44
Vietnam Era Twin Registry, 190
Vision, poor, 15
Visualization techniques, 151, 156
Vitamin A, 263
Vitamin B1 (thiamine), 60
Vitamin B2 (riboflavin), 60
Vitamin B3 (niacin), 60
Vitamin B6 (pantothenic acid), 60, 153
Vitamin C, 60, 61, 73, 124, 263
Vitamin E, 66, 73, 82, 124, 262–263
Vitamins, 59–64, 82–83
Volatile organic compounds (VOCs), 90, 101, 114–116, 223

Walking, 138, 139, 156, 224, 229, 237, 249, 252
Walnut-Pesto Wild Salmon, 340

Walter Reed Army Hospital, 174
Warm French Lentils, 336
Warm Hijiki Salad, 320
Warm ups, 152–153
Warrior One yoga posture, 49
Washing hands, 40
Water
    consumption of, 73, 123, 153, 214
    filters, 216, 268–269
    pollution, 72
    toxins in, 214–215
    treatment plants, 101–102
    well water, 215, 268
Watercress Arugula Salad, 321
Way to Cook, The (Child), 236
Weights, 145–146
Weil, Andrew, 44
Well water, 215, 268
What to Eat (Nestle), 107
Wheat, 55, 56, 226–228
Wheat grass, 85
White Bean Kale Soup, 308
White blood cells, 30, 68, 77, 95, 174
White miso, 276
Whole grains, 56, 57, 63–64, 123
Wild Divine Project, The, 44
Wild Rice, Harvest, 326
Williams, Serena, 152
Winters, Ruth, 103

Xanthan gum, 106

Yale University, 33
Yee, Rodney, 157, 247
Yoga, 28, 31, 32, 36, 141, 142, 146–149, 156–157, 247
    benefits of, 48, 50–51
    instructors, 51
    postures, 49
    schools of, 48
Yoga: The Path to Holistic Health (Iyengar), 150
Yogurt, 123, 128, 129, 246–247

Zeaxanthin, 263
Zinc, 60, 61, 64, 66, 85, 124, 155
Zithromax, 176
Zocor, 84
Zoloft, 136

ABOUT THE AUTHORS

Woodson Merrell M.D., one of the nation's preeminent integrative medicine physicians, has been frequently featured on and quoted in the national media and was named by *New York* magazine one of ten "Leaders for the New Millennium." Dr. Merrell received his M.D. from Columbia University College of Physicians and Surgeons where he is assistant clinical professor of medicine. He is the M. Anthony Fisher Director of Integrative Medicine at the Continuum Center for Health and Healing and Chairman of the Department of Integrative Medicine at Beth Israel Medical Center, Manhattan campus of Albert Einstein College of Medicine. Since 1985 he has maintained a high-profile private practice in integrative internal medicine and acupuncture on Manhattan's Upper East Side. Dr. Merrell has chaired and been scientific director for numerous medical and consumer healthcare conferences.

Kathleen Merrell—Dr. Merrell's writing partner and spouse—is an award-winning freelance journalist specializing in holistic and preventive health whose articles have appeared in numerous national publications including *O, The Oprah Magazine, Forbes, Real Simple,* and *Allure.* The Merrells live in New York City with their two school-age daughters, Caitlin and Isabel.

Stefanie Bryn Sacks M.S., culinary nutritionist and menu and recipe developer for *Power Up,* is a professional chef with a Masters of Science in nutrition from Columbia University. She practices in the metro–New York area, counseling patients on the art, science, and simplicity of eating for well-being. Stefanie has been featured in articles in consumer magazines and on television. She lives on Eastern Long Island with her husband, Rich, and son, Jack.

To learn more about *Power Up,* visit us on the web at www.woodson merrell.com.